a LANGE medical book

UNDERSTANDING PHARMACOEPIDEMIOLOGY

Editors

Yi Yang, MD, PhD
Assistant Professor
Department of Pharmacy Administration
Research Assistant Professor
Research Institute of Pharmaceutical Sciences
School of Pharmacy
The University of Mississippi
University, Mississippi

Donna West-Strum, PhD, RPh
Chair and Associate Professor
Department of Pharmacy Administration
Research Associate Professor
Research Institute of Pharmaceutical Sciences
School of Pharmacy
The University of Mississippi
University, Mississippi

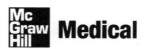
Medical

New York   Chicago   San Francisco   Lisbon   London   Madrid   Mexico City
Milan   New Delhi   San Juan   Seoul   Singapore   Sydney   Toronto

Understanding Pharmacoepidemiology

1 2 3 4 5 6 7 8 9 0 DOC/DOC 14 13 12 11 10

ISBN 978-0-07-163500-4
MHID 0-07-163500-9

> **Notice**
>
> Medicine is an ever-changing science. As new research and clinical experience broaden our knowledge, changes in treatment and drug therapy are required. The authors and the publisher of this work have checked with sources believed to be reliable in their efforts to provide information that is complete and generally in accord with the standards accepted at the time of publication. However, in view of the possibility of human error or changes in medical sciences, neither the authors nor the publisher nor any other party who has been involved in the preparation or publication of this work warrants that the information contained herein is in every respect accurate or complete, and they disclaim all responsibility for any errors or omissions or for the results obtained from use of the information contained in this work. Readers are encouraged to confirm the information contained herein with other sources. For example and in particular, readers are advised to check the product information sheet included in the package of each drug they plan to administer to be certain that the information contained in this work is accurate and that changes have not been made in the recommended dose or in the contraindications for administration. This recommendation is of particular importance in connection with new or infrequently used drugs.

This book was set in Minion by Aptara, Inc.
The editors were Michael Weitz and Robert Pancotti.
The production supervisor was Catherine H. Saggese.
Project management was provided by Samir Roy, Aptara, Inc.
The text designer was Alan Barnett; the cover designer was Anthony Landi.
RR Donnelley was printer and binder.

This book is printed on acid-free paper.

Library of Congress Cataloging-in-Publication Data

Understanding pharmacoepidemiology / editors, Yi Yang, Donna West-Strum.
    p. ; cm.
  Includes bibliographical references and index.
  ISBN-13: 978-0-07-163500-4 (pbk. : alk. paper)
  ISBN-10: 0-07-163500-9 (pbk. : alk. paper)
1. Pharmacoepidemiology. I. Yang, Yi, 1968- II. West-Strum, Donna.
  [DNLM: 1. Pharmacoepidemiology. QZ 42]
  RM302.5.U48 2010
  615′.7042–dc22
                                          2010027290

McGraw-Hill books are available at special quantity discounts to use as premiums and sales promotions, or for use in corporate training programs. To contact a representative, please e-mail us at bulksales@mcgraw-hill.com.

Contents

Authors

Benjamin F. Banahan III, PhD
Director and Research Professor, Center for
  Pharmaceutical Marketing and Management and
  Professor, Department of Pharmacy Administration,
  School of Pharmacy, The University of Mississippi,
  University, Mississippi

John P. Bentley, PhD
Associate Professor, Department of Pharmacy
  Administration, Research Associate Professor, Research
  Institute of Pharmaceutical Sciences, School of
  Pharmacy, The University of Mississippi, University,
  Mississippi

Spencer E. Harpe, PharmD, PhD, MPH
Assistant Professor, Department of Pharmacotherapy and
  Outcomes Science, Department of Epidemiology and
  Community Health, Schools of Pharmacy and
  Medicine, Virginia Commonwealth University,
  Richmond, Virginia

Heidi C. Marchand, PharmD
Office of Special Health Issues, U.S. Food and Drug
  Administration, Rockville, Maryland

David J. McCaffrey III, PhD, RPh
Professor, Department of Pharmacy Administration,
  Research Professor, Research Institute of
  Pharmaceutical Sciences, School of Pharmacy,
  The University of Mississippi, University, Mississippi

Qayyim Said, PhD
Assistant Professor, Division of Pharmaceutical Evaluation
  and Policy, College of Pharmacy, University of Arkansas
  for Medical Sciences, Little Rock, Arkansas

Douglas Steinke, MS, PhD
Assistant Professor, Pharmacy Practice and Science,
  University of Kentucky College of Pharmacy,
  Lexington, Kentucky

Donna West-Strum, PhD, RPh
Chair and Associate Professor, Department of Pharmacy
  Administration, Research Associate Professor,
  Research Institute of Pharmaceutical Sciences,
  School of Pharmacy, The University of Mississippi,
  University, Mississippi

Yi Yang, MD, PhD
Assistant Professor, Department of Pharmacy
  Administration, Research Assistant Professor,
  Research Institute of Pharmaceutical Sciences,
  School of Pharmacy, The University of Mississippi,
  University, Mississippi

Preface

Understanding Pharmacoepidemiology is an introduction to the study of medication utilization and safety in large populations of people. During the last 20 years, the discipline of pharmacoepidemiology has grown significantly. Clinicians, policy makers, researchers, academicians, marketers, and others are all interested in pharmacoepidemiology study findings. With the increasing use of medications, it is natural for there to be more interest in the use and safety of medications. The U.S. Food and Drug Administration (FDA), the pharmaceutical industry, health care professionals, and society as a whole need to understand how medications are used in the "real world" and need to ensure that medications are used appropriately and safely. We hope that this book will serve as a primer to the health care professional or student who wants to better understand pharmacoepidemiology or medication safety.

AUDIENCE

The main audience for the book is the student or health care professional who will apply information about medication safety and pharmacoepidemiology to make health care decisions at the individual or population level. The book is written primarily for health care professionals in training, specifically pharmacy and public health students. Pharmacists, public health practitioners, and other individuals who seek an introduction to the field of pharmacoepidemiology will also find the book useful. The authors of the chapters in this book are pharmacists or have faculty appointments in schools of pharmacy. Some of the authors also have training or appointments in public health. Although the book is an introduction to the topic, the reader will find it helpful if he or she already has some appreciation for research methods and statistics. The book is not intended for those who want to learn how to conduct advanced pharmacoepidemiology techniques or analyses; other books on the subject are available for the pharmacoepidemiology researcher.

PURPOSE

This book attempts to explain what pharmacoepidemiology is, how pharmacoepidemiology studies are conducted, and how to interpret pharmacoepidemiology findings. In Chapters 1 to 6, we explain the importance of pharmacoepidemiology, basic terminology used in pharmacoepidemiology research, and the data sources, study designs, and statistical analyses often employed in pharmacoepidemiology research. Chapter 7 provides examples of evaluating a pharmacoepidemiology study. Two chapters provide detailed descriptions of the use of pharmacoepidemiology to understand medication utilization (Chapter 8) and medication safety issues (Chapter 9). The final chapter discusses the perspective of the FDA on medication safety, the importance of health care professionals to the process of improving medication safety, and the ways in which pharmacoepidemiology will be a key component of future medication safety initiatives. After reading the book, the reader should have a better understanding of how to evaluate the associations between medication utilization and outcomes.

FORMAT

The heath care professional and student will find the format of the book useful in learning this material. Each chapter includes a list of learning objectives, case studies or examples, discussion questions, and tables and figures. The book also includes a glossary to help the reader to master the pharmacoepidemiology language. Moreover, faculty in schools of pharmacy or public health will find the book a useful resource when developing and teaching introductory pharmacoepidemiology courses. As mentioned in the book, the Accreditation Council for Pharmaceutical Education (ACPE) requires all pharmacy students to receive some training in pharmacoepidemiology. This requirement reinforces the importance of the topic to pharmacists and other health care professionals and the need for introductory pharmacoepidemiology textbooks.

ACKNOWLEDGMENTS

The editors want to thank all the authors for their contributions. Each chapter is written by an expert in the area and we appreciate their willingness to participate in this project. The editors also thank all the graduate students in the Department of Pharmacy Administration at The University of Mississippi, who assisted with reading various chapters and making helpful suggestions about the book.

CONCLUSION

We have enjoyed editing this book and we hope that it provides a foundation for health care professionals and students who are interested in medication use and safety in large populations of people. We also hope that this book sparks an interest for some persons to pursue advanced training in pharmacoepidemiology. The U.S. health care system needs clinicians who can interpret pharmacoepidemiology studies and apply the findings to make evidence-based decisions, as well as researchers who can employ the various pharmacoepidemiology techniques to provide insight into the relationship between medication use and outcomes.

About the Authors

Benjamin F. Banahan III, PhD, is currently the Director of the Center for Pharmaceutical Marketing and Management (CPMM) and a Professor in the Department of Pharmacy Administration at The University of Mississippi. He returned to "Ole Miss" in 2007 where he had previously served as the Coordinator of the Pharmaceutical Marketing and Management Research Program from 1984 to 2000. From 2000 to 2007, Dr. Banahan worked as a Senior Vice President at Roger Green and Associates, a pharmaceutical marketing research consulting firm. Dr. Banahan's research areas of interest include pharmaceutical marketing, medication adherence, pharmacoepidemiology, and health outcomes related to medication use. He has a BS degree in Psychology from Louisiana State University and MS and PhD degrees in Health Care Administration from The University of Mississippi.

John P. Bentley, PhD, is an Associate Professor of Pharmacy Administration and a Research Associate Professor in the Research Institute of Pharmaceutical Sciences at the University of Mississippi School of Pharmacy. He received his BS degree in pharmacy and MBA from Drake University and his MS and PhD degrees in pharmacy administration from the University of Mississippi. He recently completed an MS degree in biostatistics (2008) from the School of Public Health at the University of Alabama at Birmingham (UAB) and is currently working on a PhD in biostatistics from UAB. In the professional pharmacy curriculum, Dr. Bentley teaches elements of research design, biostatistics, epidemiology, and drug literature evaluation, and at the graduate level he teaches several applied statistics courses. He has conducted research projects in a variety of areas including quality of life, ethics, professionalism, patients' evaluation of healthcare providers, tobacco use and control, medication use and misuse, and practice management.

Spencer E. Harpe, PharmD, PhD, MPH, is an Assistant Professor in the Division of Pharmacoeconomics and Health Outcomes of the Department of Pharmacotherapy and Outcomes Science at the Virginia Commonwealth University School of Pharmacy and holds a joint appointment in the Department of Epidemiology and Community Health within the School of Medicine. He received his PharmD from the University of Mississippi. Dr. Harpe pursued graduate studies at the Ohio State University, where he earned an MS and PhD in pharmaceutical administration as well as a Master of Public Health in biostatistics. Dr. Harpe teaches research methods, statistics, and literature evaluation in the professional pharmacy program and pharmacoepidemiologic methods to graduate students. His research involves the use of secondary data sources to examine the quality, safety, and effectiveness of the use of medications, as well as refining methods for working with these data sources.

Heidi C. Marchand, PharmD, is an interdisciplinary scientist at the Office of Special Health Issues of the U.S. Food and Drug Administration (FDA). She has a PharmD degree from the Medical College of Virginia, Virginia Commonwealth University, and has held leadership positions in clinical pharmacy, pharmacy management, and the pharmaceutical industry. Dr. Marchand currently focuses upon external outreach to the health care professional organizations and has been leading the FDA's initiative to collaborate with health care professional organizations. Specifically, she has been involved with the FDA/American Association of Colleges of Pharmacy (AACP) collaboration that evaluates pharmacy curriculum dealing with the "science of safety."

David J. McCaffrey III, PhD, RPh, is a Professor of Pharmacy Administration and Research Professor in the Research Institute of Pharmaceutical Sciences at The University of Mississippi. He teaches in the professional degree program covering social and behavioral aspects of pharmacy practice and his graduate teaching responsibilities center on research methods and primary data collection techniques. His areas of interest lie within suboptimal medication utilization, pharmacists' influence on the product selection decision, the influence of direct-to-consumer advertising of medications on postexposure information search, and patient satisfaction with pharmacy services.

Qayyim Said, PhD, is an Assistant Professor at the Division of Pharmaceutical Evaluation and Policy, University of Arkansas for Medical Sciences. Dr. Said's research has focused on evaluating health and economic outcomes of pharmaceutical interventions in the areas of cardiovascular diseases, mental health, and asthma. Dr. Said has extensive experience in conducting retrospective population-based economic and epidemiologic studies using large administrative, electronic medical record, and survey databases. Dr. Said's research has been published in various medical journals. Dr. Said received his PhD in health economics from the University of Utah.

Douglas Steinke, MSc, PhD, holds a PhD in Pharmacoepidemiology from the University of Dundee, Scotland, an MS degree in Community Health and Epidemiology from Queen's University, Canada, and a BS in Pharmacy from the University of Manitoba, Canada. Dr. Steinke's research specializes in pharmacoepidemiology and health services research. Prior to becoming Assistant Professor of Pharmacy Practice at the University of Kentucky, he worked as a Research Pharmacist for the National Health Service in Scotland. He coordinates a third-year PharmD course in Pharmaceutical Policy and Public Health and participates in graduate scholarship and teaching in the Pharmaceutical Outcomes and Policy graduate program at the University of Kentucky College of Pharmacy.

Donna West-Strum, PhD, RPh, received her BS in pharmacy and her PhD from the Department of Pharmacy Administration at The University of Mississippi in 1995 and 1999, respectively. She spent 9 years at the UAMS College of Pharmacy before returning to The University of Mississippi in 2008. She is currently Chair and Associate Professor in the Department of Pharmacy Administration and a Research Associate Professor in the Research Institute of Pharmaceutical Sciences. She has taught pharmacy management, pharmaceutical policy, and pharmaceutical marketing and patient behavior. Her research interests relate to quality improvement and safety in medication use, medication adherence, and community pharmacy practice.

Yi Yang, MD, PhD, is an Assistant Professor of Pharmacy Administration and a Research Assistant Professor in the Research Institute of Pharmaceutical Sciences at The University of Mississippi School of Pharmacy. Dr. Yang received her MD degree from China Medical University, her PhD degree in Clinical Research from Chinese Academy of Medical Sciences and Peking Union Medical College, and her PhD degree in Health Science Administration with a focus on pharmacoeconomics from the University of Tennessee. In the professional pharmacy curriculum, Dr. Yang teaches pharmacoeconomics, pharmacoepidemiology, medication safety, and current issues in health care, and at the graduate level she teaches health economics and pharmacoeconomics. Dr. Yang has conducted research projects in the areas of pharmacoepidemiology, outcomes research, health literacy, and direct-to-consumer pharmaceutical marketing.

Introduction to Pharmacoepidemiology

Donna West-Strum

PHARMACOEPIDEMIOLOGY DEFINITION

Pharmacoepidemiology is the study of the use and effects of drugs in large numbers of people.[1(p3)] It is a growing discipline that applies epidemiological techniques to study drug use in a large population.[2,3] Just as the term implies, *pharmacoepidemiology* combines clinical *pharmacology* with *epidemiology*. Pharmacology is the study of the effects of medications in humans.[1(p4)] It pertains to using pharmacokinetics and pharmacodynamics of a patient to predict the drug effect on a patient. *Epidemiology* is the study of the factors that determine the occurrence and distribution of diseases in populations.[4(p3)] Epidemiologists study how much disease is in a given area, who gets it, and what specific factors put individuals at risk. Epidemiology can often be divided into infectious and chronic disease epidemiology. Chronic disease epidemiology is more dependent on complex sampling and statistical methods; which are often used in pharmacoepidemiology studies to evaluate drug exposure over time.[1(p5)] By combining the interest of pharmacology and epidemiology, a pharmacoepidemiologist applies epidemiology principles to

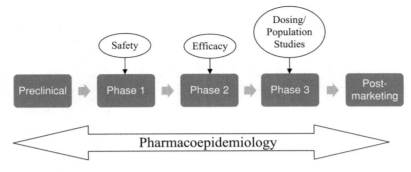

▲ **Figure 1-1.** Pharmacoepidemiology through drug development and postmarketing.

study the effects of medications in human populations.

Pharmacoepidemiology studies quantify drug use patterns and adverse drug effects.[5] For example, they are interested in understanding the patterns of drug prescribing, the appropriateness of use, medication adherence and persistence patterns, and the identification of predictors for medication use. Pharmacoepidemiologists also conduct safety studies of drug use in large populations. They are interested in common, predictable adverse drug reactions as well as the uncommon and unpredictable ones. It is important to note a few terms that are often used when discussing drug safety (see Chapter 9 for further discussion). An *adverse event* is any untoward medical occurrence that occurs while a patient is taking a drug but which does not necessarily have a causal relationship with the drug product.[6,7] An *adverse drug reaction* or *adverse drug effect* refers to an adverse outcome that is harmful or unpleasant that occurs while a patient is taking a drug product and has a causal link with the drug.[6,7] Adverse drug reactions may be dose dependent (i.e., there is a relationship between the drug dose and the outcome observed) and predictable or more idiosyncratic and unpredictable. A *side effect* is usually a dose-dependent effect of a drug that is predictable and may be desirable, undesirable, or inconsequential.[6] Another important term to consider is *medication error*, which is any preventable event that may lead to inappropriate use or patient harm.[8]

Because pharmacoepidemiology studies reveal important information about drug utilization and safety, these studies are important throughout the entire drug life cycle, beginning before receiving approval from the U.S. Food and Drug Administration (FDA) and continuing after approval (Figure 1-1). With more than $216 billion spent on prescription drug products in the U.S. in 2006 and with an average of 12.6 retail prescriptions dispensed per capita in 2007, there is a significant societal need to study the impact of drugs when used in large, diverse populations.[9]

THE U.S. DRUG APPROVAL PROCESS

In the U.S., the FDA must approve a drug product before it can be marketed to the public. The public depends on the FDA's Center for Drug Evaluation and Research (CDER) to facilitate the availability of safe and efficacious drugs, to keep unsafe or inefficacious drugs off the market, and to provide drug information for appropriate medication use. There is a great deal of pressure by the pharmaceutical industry and the public for drugs to be approved and made available for use. On the other hand, there is tremendous pressure for the FDA to keep the public safe. New drug entities and biologics are being approved each year, with 18 approved in 2007 and 24 in 2008.[10]

The FDA influences the new drug-approval process by writing and enforcing federal regulations, all of which are compiled in the U.S. Code of Federal Regulations (CFR). The FDA publishes guidelines to provide direction to pharmaceutical companies or drug sponsors who must demonstrate that the drug product is safe and efficacious. The drug approval process can take many months, even years. Through the Prescription Drug User Fee Act (PDUFA), the FDA collects fees from pharmaceutical companies to help cover the cost of new drug product reviews and expedite the drug approval process. It has had an impact on the drug approval timeline. For example, in 2008, the median number of months it took the FDA to approve a new drug application was 13 months, compared to 27 months in 1993.[10] A general overview of how a new drug entity is approved is provided; however, it is important to realize that for various conditions and patient populations there are exceptions to this general description of the FDA approval process.[11,12]

Before the FDA allows a new pharmaceutical compound to be administered to human subjects, the agency requires some evidence that the compound is reasonably safe for use in such studies. In vitro and/or animal studies are conducted to evaluate the drug's toxic and pharmacologic effects, such as absorption, distribution, metabolism and toxicity of metabolites, and excretion. When a pharmaceutical company or sponsor believes it has the data to show that a new drug is sufficiently safe to be used in initial clinical trials, the company submits an Investigational New Drug (IND) application to the FDA. This application seeks the FDA's permission to begin clinical trials in humans. The FDA will review the IND and within 30 days determine whether clinical trials should not begin.

▶ Phase 1 to Phase 3 Clinical Trials

The FDA uses clinical trial data to determine whether the drug should be approved for marketing in the U.S. Phase 1 randomized clinical trials consist of small studies of healthy volunteers. The purpose of these studies is to determine basic safety and pharmacological information in humans. They are usually short, lasting from 6 to 12 months, and they may exclude children, women of childbearing age, and other patient groups. After Phase 1 clinical trials, Phase 2 randomized clinical trials are conducted where the drug is used in a small number of subjects (e.g., 100–200 patients) who suffer from the indicated condition (i.e., indication) which the drug is intended

to treat. The drug is used cautiously in Phases 1 and 2 to ensure safety in humans before large numbers of people are exposed. Phase 2 provides safety data and begins to provide some indication of the drug's clinical efficacy. In Phase 3, the drug is used in a larger group of patients who suffer from the indicated disease or condition. These clinical trials are randomized, double blind, placebo controlled and may have several hundred to several thousand patients who actually have the disease or condition being studied. The drug sponsor can assess the safety and efficacy of the drug in a larger patient population. These studies typically take one to four years.

Upon completion of Phase 1, 2, and 3 clinical trials, the drug sponsor will seek drug approval from the FDA by submitting a New Drug Application (NDA). The NDA will consist of the results of the animal studies and clinical trials as well as relevant information such as results from foreign studies, marketing data, package insert information, and manufacturing processes. The FDA will then review the NDA to determine whether the drug is safe and efficacious as well as whether the product labeling, marketing, and manufacturing processes are adequate. The FDA may decide to approve the drug product for marketing, ask for minor revisions before it is approved, or not approve the drug. It is important to note that some products make it through Phases 1 and 2, but Phase 3 trials identify serious safety concerns or lack of efficacy, and thus, they are not approved. This entire process for drug approval can take between 10 to 15 years, and costs range from approximately $200 million to $1.3 billion per drug approved.[11,13]

▶ Clinical Trial Limitations

The FDA must make drug approval decisions on well-designed clinical trials. The drug approval process in the U.S. is rigorous and requires pharmaceutical companies to provide a tremendous amount of data about the safety and efficacy of a product. Despite the rigor associated with the approval process, there are shortcomings in it.[14,15] For example, certain patient groups like children and women of childbearing age may be excluded from clinical trials. Phase 3 clinical trials have a few thousand people enrolled, but not hundreds of thousands or millions.

By the time a drug receives FDA approval, it has only been administered to a few hundred or a few thousand people. There are some adverse events and other safety issues that only occur in one in a million, making it difficult to detect these issues in a clinical trial. As a drug product is used in unstudied patient populations or for off-label uses (i.e., used for clinical indications that are not currently approved by the FDA) in a large number of people, it is important that the use of the drug product be monitored. Another limitation is the short duration of clinical trials. The effect of taking a drug for 10, 20, or 30 years is not studied in clinical trials. Thus, in a diverse group of people who have chronic conditions and where polypharmacy (i.e., use of multiple medications by one person) is common, there is a need to monitor continually for both positive and negative effects of drug products.

POSTMARKETING SURVEILLANCE

Once a drug is approved, health care professionals begin prescribing the product in the general population. There may be millions of people who are now using the drug. Moreover, people with multiple diseases or who are taking multiple medications are using the drug, providing an opportunity for additional drug interactions, disease interactions, or other safety issues that were not seen in clinical trials to be observed. Rare adverse events may now appear. All of these possibilities lead us to our discussion of *postmarketing surveillance*. Postmarketing surveillance refers to any means of gathering information about a product after it has been approved for public use.[16] The FDA defines postmarket surveillance as the process by which a drug's safety is monitored to identify potential problems with the use of the drug after it has received FDA approval.[12]

Without postmarketing surveillance, there is limited information about the effectiveness of drugs in practice such as how a drug product is used, whether people continue to take a drug product, and what outcomes are associated with a drug product in diverse patient populations. It is important to remember that *efficacy* refers to whether the drug product can produce a specific therapeutic outcome in a controlled environment. Efficacy is measured in clinical trials. In the "real world," *effectiveness* needs to

be considered. In other words, can the drug product produce the desired therapeutic outcome in practice where the environment is not controlled?

▶ Phase 4 Clinical Trials and Postmarketing Studies

To gather information about a drug product, pharmaceutical companies and the FDA rely on the results of Phase 4 randomized clinical trials. Phase 4 trials are clinical trials conducted after the product is approved by the FDA to gather additional information about the drug, including safety information and information about its use in other indications. The FDA may require the pharmaceutical company or drug sponsor to conduct Phase 4 clinical trials after product approval.[11] In addition to Phase 4 clinical trials, other postmarketing studies like case-control or cohort studies may be used to provide information about a drug product's safety profile.[16] The FDA can use fees collected from PDUFA to increase surveillance of a new drug's safety during the first 2 years on the market. The FDA requires sponsors of approved drugs and biological products to report to the FDA annually on the progress of their postmarketing study commitments.[12]

▶ Adverse Event Reporting Systems

Because it is not feasible to learn everything about a drug product from clinical trials, the FDA, pharmaceutical companies, and other health care organizations have developed processes and systems to conduct postmarketing surveillance. Specifically, they have developed adverse event reporting systems to collect spontaneous reports of drug issues.[12] The FDA has established the *MedWatch Safety Information and Adverse Event Reporting Program* (http://www.fda. gov/MedWatch) that allows health professionals and the public to report voluntarily serious reactions and problems with medications.[12,17] The FDA uses MedWatch reports to identify and evaluate risk with a specific product, to develop interventions to modify the risk (e.g., make a product labeling change), and to communicate the risk to health care professionals and the public.[15,17] The FDA with the Centers for Disease Control and Prevention has also implemented the Vaccine Adverse Event Reporting System (VAERS) to collect information about safety issues related to vaccine use.[18]

CASE STUDY 1-1

Adverse Event Reports Lead to Further Studies

The U.S. FDA received a higher than expected number of reports through their Adverse Event Reporting System of amyotrophic lateral sclerosis (ALS i.e., Lou Gehrig's disease) in patients taking statins. Through this reporting system, the FDA decided to evaluate this signal of a possible causal association between the two. In an article published in Pharmacoepidemiology and Drug Safety *in 2008, they reported reviewing 41 controlled clinical trials. The results indicated that about 9 of 64,000 patients treated with a statin and 10 of about 56,000 patients treated with placebo were diagnosed with ALS. The FDA concluded that the use of statins does not increase the incidence of ALS. The FDA continues to evaluate the issue. Case-control studies and other epidemiologic studies evaluating the incidence of ALS and statin use are being conducted.[19]*

Pharmaceutical companies and other health care organizations worldwide are also collecting and using medication safety information. Pharmaceutical companies have toll-free numbers and websites for health care professionals and patients to report issues with medications. In turn, they report these issues to the FDA (Table 1-1). Academicians publish case reports about rare events that may be associated with drug use. Many hospitals have processes to collect the drug history of patients upon admission and then attempt to identify relationships between drug exposure and reason for hospital admission. These activities may not result in generalizable information and may be based on incomplete or inaccurate information; however, they are important for identifying unexpected adverse events for future evaluation.

All of these mechanisms for spontaneous event reports assist with *pharmacovigilance,* as discussed in Chapter 9. Pharmacovigilance relates to the identification, assessment, and prevention of adverse drug effects in medications. The adverse events reported are used as safety signals. A *safety signal* refers to reported data or information that suggest a potential link between a drug product and an adverse event.[6] When multiple reports or reports with serious outcomes are observed, this acts as a signal to investigate the possibility of a causal link between the drug product and outcome. The FDA can then use the results of these investigations to require labeling changes, issue "Dear Doctor" letters, publish journal articles, or even withdraw a product from market.

Over the past 20 years, there have been numerous drug withdrawals due to safety issues (Table 1-2).[20,21] It is important to remember that some of these withdrawals were initiated by the pharmaceutical company voluntarily and others were required by the

Table 1-1. Number of adverse events reported to FDA MedWatch over a 5-year period.[a]

Years	Reported directly to FDA	Reported to pharmaceutical company and then reported to FDA	Total reports received
2004	21,655	401,275	422,930
2005	25,312	438,507	463,819
2006	20,977	450,417	471,394
2007	23,033	459,121	482,154
2008	32,899	493,628	526,527

[a]Data from Ref. 17.

Table 1-2. Examples of U.S. drug withdrawals due to safety concerns.[a]

Brand drug name	Generic drug name	Year withdrawn	Safety concerns
Suprol	Suprofen	1987	Flank pain syndrome
Enkaid	Encainide HCl	1991	Ventricular arrhythmias
Omniflox	Temafloxacin HCl	1992	Hypoglycemia
Manoplax	Flosequinan	1993	Increased mortality
Seldane	Terfenadine	1998	Cardiac arrhythmias
Duract	Bromfenac Na	1998	Liver toxicity
Posicor	Mibefradil dihydrochloride	1998	Drug interaction
Hismanal	Astemizole	1999	Fatal arrhythmias
Raxar	Grepafloxacin HCl	1999	Torsade de pointes arrhythmias
Rezulin	Troglitazone	2000	Hepatotoxicity
Propulsid	Cisapride	2000	Cardiac arrhythmias
Baycol	Cerivastatin	2001	Rhabdomyolysis
Raplon	Rapacuronium	2001	Fatal bronchospasm
Vioxx	Rofecoxib	2004	Myocardial infarction
Bextra	Valdecoxib	2005	Myocardial infarction

[a]Adapted from Ref. 21 with permission from Elsevier.

FDA. Some of these removals received wide publicity, and many led to lawsuits. Other drug products have received publicity for safety concerns but have not been withdrawn from the market. In fact, it is estimated that at least 10% of approved drugs receive a *black box warning* after FDA approval.[22] Many of these withdrawals, black box warnings, and safety alerts have been based on the evaluation of spontaneous reports. The FDA uses the reports to determine whether further studies are needed, to change the labeling or distribution of a single product or an entire therapeutic class, and to inform health care professionals about safety issues.

Limitations of Spontaneous Event Reporting

Although spontaneous reporting contributes much to postmarketing surveillance efforts, there are several limitations. First, there is no control group. Patients exposed to a drug product cannot be compared to patients not exposed to the product. Second, it is difficult to know the frequency or the rate at which the drug effect occurs. There is not adequate information about how many patients were exposed to the drug and how many experienced the identified effect. Third, with so many factors involved with each patient, it is difficult to know whether the drug is causing the outcome or something else. Thus, causation is difficult to establish. Fourth, there may be bias from the reporter or other source, and the report may be inaccurate or incomplete.

GROWTH OF PHARMACOEPIDEMIOLOGY

In the U.S. health care system, there is evidence that the cost of medications is increasing. Polypharmacy is an issue, medications are often used to treat chronic diseases, and newer, more advanced drug therapies are approved annually.[9,11] Because of these trends, payers, policy makers, pharmaceutical companies, government agencies, clinicians, and patients all have a vested interest in the use of medications. They are interested in which drug products are cost-effective. They are interested in comparative-effectiveness research. They are encouraging evidence-based medicine to ensure patients receive quality care. They are focused on helping patients use medications appropriately. Pharmacoepidemiology provides a way to answer many questions about drug use and inform interventions or policies that may need to be developed.[23]

Given the need to study a drug's use in the "real world," the use of observational study designs and other pharmacoepidemiologic research designs to answer questions about medication use has grown. It is important that all stakeholders understand how drugs are used in the general population.[2] As previously stated, there is a need for continuous surveillance of drug use and ways to evaluate how patient characteristics influence drug utilization and clinical outcomes, both the expected and unexpected clinical outcomes.[2] This need to study drug use in large populations can be met through the use of epidemiologic research designs.

It is not realistic to believe that large, prospective clinical trials can be conducted to understand all issues of medication use in large populations. There are limited financial resources to conduct large clinical trials for every drug in various subsets of populations.[24] Payers, policy makers, and clinicians are looking for other avenues to study how medications are used. Pharmacoepidemiology research is one way for these interested parties to learn about medication use and safety without having to invest in large clinical trials.[25] A pharmacoepidemiology study is usually less expensive and can provide some evidence as to the use and safety of medications in populations.

▶ Secondary Databases in Pharmacoepidemiology

The ability to use epidemiologic study designs to investigate the effects of drugs has become more feasible with the advancement of informatics in the health care system. There are large health care databases that are being used to study drug utilization

trends, medication adherence, and medication safety issues.[25,26] Through health care databases, researchers can evaluate the use of a drug in an unstudied population or for an unlabeled use. Rare drug–drug interactions, drug–disease interactions, or other adverse drug reactions can be identified. Datasets with multiple years of patient data enable researchers to study the effect of the drug over an extended period of time.[23] The effect of a prescribing intervention or other quality-improvement initiative can be evaluated using large datasets.

A few examples of the types of databases that are used to conduct pharmacoepidemiology studies are described. These datasets provide the data for researchers to evaluate drug exposure in given populations (see Chapter 4 for more about secondary data sources and how secondary databases are used in pharmacoepidemiology).

- Administrative or transactional databases are used for billing and payment by pharmacies, third-party payers (e.g., Medicaid, Blue Cross/Blue Shield), and other health care organizations.[26] These databases may contain claims with codes for diagnoses, drug products dispensed, hospitalizations, and other medical billing events. These databases can be used to evaluate drug use patterns and to look for adverse drug reactions.

- Electronic medical records are being used by health maintenance organizations, clinics, and other health care organizations. Electronic medical records are becoming more common in the U.S., and there is much encouragement from the government and others for providers to adopt the use of electronic medical records.[27] These datasets that contain information about drug product usage and other clinical information can be used in pharmacoepidemiology research.[25]

- Researchers use data from other secondary sources such as adverse event reporting systems, patient registries, and national surveys to study medication use. Additionally, the FDA Amendments Act of 2007 called for the development of a new system for postmarketing surveillance in the U.S. This initiative is referred to as the *Sentinel Initiative*. The new system will link data from multiple sources like the Veterans Administration,

Medicare, and the private sector, which then can be used to study drug use and safety.[28] For more information about the Sentinel Initiative, refer to Chapter 10.

PHARMACOEPIDEMIOLOGY RESEARCH

With the availability of databases, epidemiological study designs, and advanced computer software and statistical techniques, researchers can study practice-relevant questions. Results of pharmacoepidemiology research can then influence current practice and policy. An example of how pharmacoepidemiology research results have had implications for practice is described.

Newer (second-generation) antipsychotics have less extrapyramidal side effects than the older, conventional antipsychotics, but they are associated with other side effects, including weight gain, alterations in glucose metabolism, and other metabolic effects. Case reports had documented the incidence of hyperglycemia or diabetes with the use of olanzapine, one of the newer antipsychotics. A group of investigators wanted to quantify the relationship between olanzapine and diabetes. They used the U.K. General Practice Research Database between 1987 and 2000. They identified 19,637 patients who had been diagnosed and treated for schizophrenia. They matched 451 incident cases of diabetes with 2,696 controls. The results indicated that patients taking olanzapine had a significantly increased risk of developing diabetes than did nonusers of antipsychotics and those taking conventional antipsychotics. The authors concluded that olanzapine is associated with a clinically important and significant increased risk of diabetes. Clinicians should consider the risk–benefit ratio of olanzapine (as well as other newer antipsychotics) for each individual patient before prescribing.[29]

▶ Association and Causation

Pharmacoepidemiology researchers are usually interested in describing drug use, identifying associations or relationships with drug use, and determining causal relationships (i.e., does an exposure to a drug/intervention cause a specific outcome?).

For example, they may want to describe the utilization of beta blockers over the past 10 years. Another option is to identify the relationship between a drug treatment (or other exposure/intervention) and an outcome. There may be no association between drug use and an observed outcome or there may be an artifactual association, which means the association or relationship between the drug and outcome was seen by chance or because of some systematic error in the study. The FDA and health care professionals are most interested in finding causal relationships.[2] Did the medication cause the outcome of interest? Did the intervention cause medication utilization to change? Study designs and statistical techniques are used to rule out artifactual associations and to find the true causal relationships, as discussed throughout this book. Guidelines for determining whether an association is causal are discussed in Chapter 6.

Experimental designs as used in clinical trials are often looking for causal effects. As previously suggested, it is not possible to always conduct an experiment. Experiments are costly, and sometimes there are ethical or practical reasons that prohibit a clinical trial from being conducted.[5,24] Thus, pharmacoepidemiology researchers are relying on nonexperimental study designs or observational study designs to evaluate causal relationships.[24] Specifically, pharmacoepidemiologists are using complex study designs and statistical analyses to address whether there is association between an exposure (e.g., drug exposure, intervention exposure) and an outcome. Chapter 3 will provide a detailed description of the various study designs used in pharmacoepidemiology research and the advantages and disadvantages of these designs. In addition, Chapters 5 and 6 discuss some of the statistical analyses and methods to handle biases used in causal research.

▶ Pharmacoepidemiology Research Questions

Regardless of whether the researcher is interested in describing medication use or identifying causal associations with medication use, pharmacoepidemiology studies can provide insight into what is occurring in practice, with the expectation that the results will inform policy- and evidence-based decision making.[23] Various stakeholders would like to know more about the benefit–risk ratio of drug products. Examples of questions that can be answered using pharmacoepidemiology research designs include the following.[16,23]

- Patterns of use
  - What are the patterns of drug utilization? How are drugs used in clinical practice?
  - How are drugs used in specific patient populations, such as women, children, the elderly, or racially diverse patients?[3]
  - How long do people take this drug? Do certain patient groups stop taking the drug? What are the medication adherence and persistence rates?
- Safety
  - What is the frequency of drug-induced outcomes? Are there rare adverse events that occur with this drug product, and if so, how often do they occur? Is this a causal relationship?
  - Are there drug–drug interactions with this drug product that have not been identified previously? How frequently do drug–drug interactions occur in the population?
  - Do certain risk factors predispose patients to adverse drug reactions?
  - Are there drug–disease interactions associated with this drug?
- Effectiveness
  - What are the clinical benefits of this drug? Is the drug effective when used in the "real world"?
  - Is drug A more effective than drug B?
  - Is a drug product effective for an off-label use?
  - What is the effect of using the drug over time?
- Economic evaluations
  - What are the economic consequences of therapy?

Table 1-3 provides examples of real-world practice questions that have been addressed through pharmacoepidemiology research. By looking at these examples, it is evident that the results of these studies have implications for clinicians, pharmaceutical companies, government agencies, and other policy makers.

Table 1-3. Examples of pharmacoepidemiology studies that address practice-based research questions.

Is there a relationship between atypical antipsychotic use and the metabolic syndrome? The investigators reviewed 70 abstracts and articles of case reports, retrospective database studies, retrospective head-to-head clinical trials, and pharmacoepidemiology studies to find the answer to this question.[a]

Is the use of antidepressants associated with the risk of hip/femur fractures? A case-control study was conducted using a Dutch database to address this question.[b]

Do medications used to treat diabetes decrease or increase the risk of cardiovascular disease? A retrospective cohort study of diabetes patients using The Health Information Network database was conducted.[c]

Have medication adherence trends for cardiovascular medications improved over time? Investigators used a retrospective cohort study of Medicare beneficiaries who were discharged from the hospital after their first myocardial infarction to address this question.[d]

How are atypical antipsychotics being used in children? A retrospective analysis of state Medicaid claims data was used.[e]

[a]Ref. 30.
[b]Ref. 31.
[c]Ref. 32.
[d]Ref. 33.
[e]Ref. 34.

▶ Users of Pharmacoepidemiology Research

Practice-based research questions are of interest to many stakeholders in the health care system.[2] Case study 1-2 provides an example of how different stakeholders are interested in medication use in the population and the results of pharmacoepidemiology studies.

Government Agencies and Health Care Plans

As previously mentioned, the FDA is certainly interested in conducting more pharmacoepidemiology studies to understand medication safety. As the agency responsible for protecting the public, they are interested in continually studying drug product safety.

Health care plans and government agencies who are informing and developing policy and managing drug therapy for large populations find pharmacoepidemiology research important. Government agencies like the Agency for Healthcare Research

Users of Pharmacoepidemiology Research

For nearly a decade, phosphodiesterase type 5 (PDE-5) inhibitors have been used worldwide and are considered safe and effective treatments of erectile dysfunction (ED). The first drug to be approved in this class by the FDA was sildenafil (Viagra) in 1998. Subsequently, vardenafil (Levitra) and tadalafil (Cialis) were approved for the treatment of ED. Drs. Egan and Pomeranz published a case report about the possible connection between the use of Viagra and blindness.[35] Additional cases were reported in the literature[36] as well as to the FDA and Pfizer, the manufacturers of Viagra. The issue appeared to be sudden vision loss when blood flow to the optic nerve was blocked. This condition is called NAION or nonarteritic anterior ischemic optic neuropathy. As of 2005, the FDA had 43 reports of this among impotence drug users: 38 for Viagra, 4 for Cialis, and 1 for Levitra. A total of 43 reports did not seem like a high number, given that more than 23 million men have taken Viagra alone

and NAION is a common cause of vision loss in older Americans. Yet blindness associated with the use of a drug product seems significant and alarming. The CBS news reported these cases of blindness and Viagra use.[37] In fact, CBS reported one patient started taking Viagra at age 57. He felt changes in his vision and eventually went blind in his right eye. He sued Pfizer. So clinicians and academicians, along with the pharmaceutical companies and the FDA, were interested in finding the answer to the question: Do drugs used to treat ED cause blindness in some patients, and if so, which patients? The FDA launched investigations into this and required the manufacturers of these drugs to update their package inserts to reflect this, in response to reports of sudden blindness in men taking the ED medications. Pharmacoepidemiology studies can be used to determine the frequency of this adverse event and whether it is a causal relationship or whether other patient pathology-specific factors are responsible for the blindness.

and Quality (AHRQ) and the Centers for Medicare and Medicaid Services (CMS) are interested in learning how drug products are used in the "real world." Results from these studies can inform policy and drive educational interventions. Health plans are responsible for providing access to medications in a quality manner, and at an affordable cost, to a variety of population groups. Pharmacoepidemiology findings may inform them when making decisions about coverage issues, educational interventions, and other policies. In addition, pharmacoepidemiology provides a means for them to evaluate interventions and policies that affect medication utilization.

Pharmaceutical Industry

Likewise, the pharmaceutical industry conducts pharmacoepidemiology research. For many reasons, they want to understand how a drug is prescribed, used, and what outcomes, both positive and negative, can be attributed to the drug product. Working with the FDA,

the company can use this information to educate the public and practitioners about the product, develop interventions to ensure safe use in practice, pursue other indications for approval, identify issues for further study, and respond to legal issues. One example of how a pharmaceutical company has utilized pharmacoepidemiology to monitor medication use is described here.

AstraZeneca developed a pharmacoepidemiology program to complement safety data obtained from randomized clinical trials and spontaneous reporting systems. This program consisted of nine studies. Four studies evaluated patient characteristics of new users of rosuvastatin compared with new users of other statins in automated databases. Four studies were safety evaluation studies that examined the rates of specific adverse events in different cohorts of statin users and determined the risk factors for these events. The other study was a prescription-event-monitoring study that monitored for significant events recorded by general practitioners after starting rosuvastatin treatment.

These studies were carried out in the United Kingdom, the U.S., Canada, and the Netherlands and collectively included more than 50,000 patients.[38]

Practitioners

Because pharmacists, physicians, nurses, public health officials, and other health care practitioners are making decisions daily about treatment for patients, they are also interested in pharmacoepidemiology research. The findings of many pharmacoepidemiology studies can help them make informed decisions at both the individual-patient level and the population level.

Academicians

Academicians, who may or may not be clinicians, are also interested in the use of drug products in large populations. They often conduct pharmacoepidemiology studies. Furthermore, they are interested in advancing the science and trying to refine techniques and methodologies to find answers to practice-related questions.

Attorneys

Given Case Study 1-2, it becomes apparent that attorneys and those in the legal system have also found pharmacoepidemiology studies useful. Findings from pharmacoepidemiology studies can be used as evidence that a drug product did or did not cause an event. Therefore, those in the legal system as well as hospital administrators, pharmaceutical companies, clinicians, and others who are aware of litigation are interested in those findings and understand the importance of monitoring medication use.

Consumers and Patients

And last but certainly not least, consumers, patients, and patient advocacy groups also rely on pharmacoepidemiology studies to learn about the safety and effectiveness of drug products. There are websites such as the Adverse Drug Reaction Electronic System (http://www.adverse-drug-reaction.net) that provides a venue for patients to look at safety information about specific drug products. Consumer groups like Public Citizens are also interested in the findings and are lobbying the FDA to act upon information

from these studies. The media also reports on medication use patterns and safety. Again referring to Case Study 1-2, *CBS* news covered the story about reports suggesting that some men who use Viagra may have suffered blindness. This prompts the question from consumers as well as the previously mentioned groups: Does Viagra cause blindness in some patients? Pharmacoepidemiology research can be conducted to answer this question.

International users

It is important to mention that there are many international efforts related to pharmacoepidemiology. It is not only those in the U.S. who are interested in understanding drug use patterns and safety in large populations but also governments, practitioners, academicians, and others from around the world are conducting pharmacoepidemiology studies. In fact, in 2008, approximately one-third of the reports made to the FDA's MedWatch were reported by someone outside the U.S.[17] The World Health Organization International Drug Monitoring Programme also collects data from 30 countries to help identify potential drug problems.[39] Moreover, many countries have national databases or national registries that provide much opportunity for pharmacoepidemiology research. For example, in the United Kingdom, there is the General Practice Research Database.[23] This database contains clinical data, including laboratory data, diagnoses, drugs prescribed, and other clinical information.

ROLE OF PHARMACISTS AND PUBLIC HEALTH PRACTITIONERS IN PHARMACOEPIDEMIOLOGY

Pharmacists have been expanding their role in the health care system and are considered drug experts. Because pharmacoepidemiology pertains to how drugs affect large populations, it is only natural that pharmacists play a role in pharmacoepidemiology. The practicing pharmacist is in a prime position to help identify issues or problems that a pharmacoepidemiologist may want to study further. For example, a pharmacist may observe that a few patients on a drug have an adverse event and report this to a hospital drug safety committee, MedWatch, or a pharmaceutical company. Although many pharmacists are providing drug therapy to individual patients, the lessons learned from individual patient encounters can be used to develop research questions. It is critical that pharmacists are identifying and reporting adverse drug events, which can then be studied using pharmacoepidemiology techniques. Currently, physicians and pharmacists have the highest rate of adverse drug event reporting among health care professionals.[17] Given that health care professionals report much of the adverse drug event data, another role for them is to provide guidance on the development of reporting forms and databases, which can provide data for pharmacoepidemiology studies.

Pharmacists and public health practitioners should be users of pharmacoepidemiology research findings. They can apply study findings at the individual patient level or at the population level. With evidence-based medicine increasingly being emphasized, practitioners should consider evidence when making drug therapy choices for an individual patient. In the alternative, study findings can be used when making formulary and payment decisions for a population. Practitioners may serve on pharmacy and therapeutics committees, patient safety committees, or other groups that require studies to be reviewed and considered when making decisions for the institution or health care plan.

Many health care organizations and hospitals have adverse drug reaction-reporting programs and drug use evaluation programs. Pharmacists often conduct drug use evaluations for drug products that are associated with risk of adverse outcomes, are of high cost,

or are of high volume. They can apply pharmacoepidemiology principles when conducting these activities. For example, a hospital pharmacist who is collecting adverse drug event reports may determine that further study is needed within the organization. The pharmacist may use a cohort study design to identify the rate of the event or risk factors. The pharmacist can then use these findings to develop guidelines or restrict use of a drug product for the institution. Pharmacists may want to determine who is getting a specific drug product, what problems are occurring, and whether there is a probable causal relationship between drug exposure and the outcomes evaluated. These findings can be used to educate prescribers about drug effectiveness and safety issues.

Pharmacists in public health roles as well as public health practitioners are often interested in what occurs in the "field" (i.e., the "real world"). For example, many pharmacists and public health practitioners are interested in medication adherence. They can monitor medication adherence rates and the outcomes associated with adherence in a large population. This type of study may inform others that an educational intervention or an adherence program is needed for a given population. Pharmacists and public health practitioners can use the findings from pharmacoepidemiology studies to develop population-based interventions.

Pharmacists and public health practitioners also have the opportunity to participate and conduct pharmacoepidemiology research. Obviously phar-

CASE STUDY 1-3
Pharmacists and Pharmacoepidemiology[40]

A pharmacist wanted to determine the frequency, severity, and preventability of adverse drug reactions (ADRs) leading to hospitalization in a medical intensive care unit (MICU). A prospective study was conducted. The pharmacist found that a total of 281 patients were admitted to the MICU over a 19-week period. Of these, 21 admissions (7.5%) were ADR related and 18 were deemed preventable. Drug interactions were the cause of 12 ADRs, which were all deemed preventable. The pharmacist suggested that physician, pharmacist, and nurse awareness of polypharmacy and continuous surveillance of medications was needed to prevent serious ADRs secondary to drug–drug interactions. Interventions and policies need to be considered at this institution.

maceutical companies, government agencies, health care plans, and others will be looking for health care professionals with training in pharmacoepidemiology. Those with advanced training will be able to design appropriate study methodologies and apply their clinical knowledge when developing study designs. They will be able to evaluate data in large databases to answer practice-related questions and then disseminate the findings.

It is apparent that the pharmacoepidemiology discipline is growing. A large number of articles relating to pharmacoepidemiology are published in *JAMA,* the *New England Journal of Medicine, Pharmacotherapy,* and other pharmacy and medical journals that relate to pharmacoepidemiology.[5,41] Academicians and researchers are identifying new methodologies and techniques that can be used when studying the effects of drugs in large populations. The International Society for Pharmacoepidemiology (ISPE), an international organization dedicated to advancing the field of pharmacoepidemiology, including pharmacovigilance, drug utilization research, comparative effectiveness research, and therapeutic risk management (http://www.pharmacoepi.org), is growing and expanding their activities.[42] Pharmacy schools, public health schools, and medical schools are including pharmacoepidemiology in the curriculum. For example, the Accreditation Council for Pharmaceutical Education (ACPE) requires all pharmacy students to receive some training in pharmacoepidemiology.[43] Health care professionals are encouraged to learn about applying epidemiology principles to the study of drug use and outcomes in large populations and how to use data repositories to identify new uses of drugs and/or identify potential drug safety issues.

SUMMARY

Pharmacoepidemiology is the study of the use and effects of drugs in populations. This field is growing because it is important for various stakeholders to understand more about drug use in practice. To provide safer and more cost-effective care, the government, pharmaceutical companies, clinicians, patients, policy makers, and others need to understand the use of drugs in large numbers of people. Pharmacoepidemiology research can contribute to postmarketing surveillance efforts, identifying new indications for drug products, evaluating interventions, describing medication use trends, and informing policy. Given the potential of pharmacoepidemiology, health care professionals need to have a better understanding of it and contribute to its advancement.

DISCUSSION QUESTIONS

1. Explain the U.S. drug development and approval process, including its strengths and limitations.

2. Do you think it is worth the cost for the U.S. to develop a nationwide database to study the effect of drugs in large populations? Why or why not?

3. What are some resources currently used to learn about the effectiveness and safety of drug use in the "real world"?

4. Write three practice-related questions that would be of interest to a pharmacoepidemiologist.

5. What type of job positions in pharmacoepidemiology may be available for pharmacists or public health practitioners in the future? What type of skills would this person likely need?

6. What do you think will be some of the strengths and limitations of pharmacoepidemiology research studies?

REFERENCES

1. Strom BL, Kimmel SE. *Textbook of Pharmacoepidemiology.* West Sussex, England: John Wiley & Sons Ltd, 2006.

2. Wertheimer AI, Andrews KB. An overview of pharmacoepidemiology. *Pharm World Sci.* 1995;17(3):61-66.

3. Luo X, Doherty J, Cappelleri JC, Frush K. Role of pharmacoepidemiology in evaluating prescription drug safety in pediatrics. *Curr Med Res Opin.* 2007;23(11):2607-2615.

4. Gordis L. *Epidemiology,* 4th ed. Philadelphia, PA: Saunders Elsevier Inc, 2009.

5. Etminan M, Samii A. Pharmacoepidemiology I: A review of pharmacoepidemiology study designs. *Pharmacotherapy.* 2004;24(8):964-969.

6. Edwards IR, Aronson JK. Adverse drug reactions: Definitions, diagnosis, and management. *Lancet.* 2000;356:1255-1259.

7. Nebeker JR, Barach P, Samore MH. Clarifying adverse drug events: A clinician's guide to terminology, documentation, and reporting. *Ann Intern Med.* 2004;140:795-801.

8. What is a medication error? National Coordinating Council for Medication Error Reporting and Prevention website. http://www.nccmerp.org/about MedErrors.html. Accessed on December 15, 2009.

9. Prescription drug trends. The Henry Kaiser Family Foundation website. http://www.kff.org. September 2008. Accessed on January 10, 2009.

10. FDA-CDER approval times for priority and standard NMEs and new BLAs. The U.S. Food and Drug Administration website. http://www.fda.gov/Drugs/DevelopmentApproval Process/HowDrugsareDevelopedandApproved/Drugand BiologicApprovalReports/default.htm. Accessed November 10, 2009.

11. Pharmaceutical research and manufacturers of America –Pharmaceutical Industry Profile 2009. PhRMA website. http://www.phrma.org. April 2009. Accessed January 8, 2010.

12. Drugs. The U.S. Food and Drug Administration website. http://www.fda.gov/Drugs/default.htm. Accessed January 13, 2010.

13. DiMasi JA, Hansen RW, Grabowski HG. The price of innovation: New estimates for drug development costs. *J Health Econ.* 2003;22:151-185.

14. Vassilev ZP, Chu AF, Ruck B, et al. Evaluation of adverse drug reactions reported to a poison control center between 2000–2007. *Am J Health-Syst Pharm.* 2009;66:481-487.

15. Wysowski DK, Swartz L. Adverse drug event surveillance and drug withdrawals in the United States, 1969-2002. *Arch Intern Med.* 2005;165:1363-1369.

16. Hennessy S. Postmarketing drug surveillance: An epidemiologic approach. *Clin Ther.* 1998;20(suppl. C):C32-C39.

17. MedWatch: The FDA Safety Information and Adverse Event Reporting Program. The U.S. Food and Drug Administration website. http://www.fda.gov/Safety/MedWatch/default.htm. Accessed January 13, 2010.

18. VAERS. The U.S. Department of Health and Human Services website. http://vaers.hhs.gov/index. Accessed January 27, 2010.

19. Colman E, Szarfman A, Wyeth J, et al. An evaluation of a data mining signal for amyotrophic lateral sclerosis and statins detected in FDA's spontaneous event reporting system. *Pharmacoepidemiol Drug Saf.* 2008;17(11):1068-1076.

20. Tufts Center for the Study of Drug Development. Drug safety withdrawals in the U.S. not linked to speed of FDA Approval. *Tufts Impact Rep.* 2005;7(5):1-4.

21. Bunniran S, McCaffrey DJ, Bentley JP, Bouldin AS. Pharmaceutical product withdrawal: Attributions of blame and its impact on trust. *Res Social Adm Pharm.* 2009;5:262-273.

22. Nardinelli C, Lanthier M, Temple R. Drug-review deadlines and safety problems. *N Engl J Med.* 2008;359(1):95-96.

23. Garcia Rodriquez LA, Gutthann SP. Use of UK general practice research database for pharmacoepidemiology. *Br J Clin Pharmacol.* 1998;45:419-425.

24. McMahon AD, MacDonald TM. Design issues for drug epidemiology. *Br J Clin Pharmacol.* 2000;50(5):419-425.

25. Etminan M, Gill S, FitzGerald M, Samii A. Challenges and opportunities for pharmacoepidemiology in drug-therapy decision making. *J Clin Pharmacol.* 2006;46(1):6-9.

26. Hennessy S. Use of health care databases in pharmacoepidemiology. *Basic Clin Pharmacol Toxicol.* 2006;98(3):311-313.

27. Jha AK, DesRoches CM, Campbell EG, et al. Use of electronic health records in U.S. hospitals. *N Engl J Med.* 2009;360(16):1628-1638.

28. FDA's Sentinel initiative. The U.S. Food and Drug Administration website. http://www.fda.gov/Safety/FDAsSentinelInitiative/default.htm. Accessed January 13, 2010.

29. Koro CE, Fedder DO, L'Italien GJ, et al. Assessment of independent effect of olanzapine and risperidone on risk of diabetes among patients with schizophrenia: Population-based nested case-control study. *BMJ.* 2002;325:243-245.

30. Kabinoff GS, Toalson PA, Healy KM, McGuire HC, Hay DP. Metabolic issues with atypical antipsychotics in primary care: Dispelling the myths. *J Clin Psychiatry.* 2003;5:6-14.

31. van den Brand MWM, Samson MM, Pouwels S, et al. Use of anti-depressants and the risk of facture of the hip or femur. *Osteoporos Int.* 2009;20:1705-1713.

32. Margolis DJ, Hofstad MA, Strom BL. Association between serious ischemic cardiac outcomes and medications used to treat diabetes. *Pharmacoepidemiol Drug Saf.* 2008;17(8):753-759.

33. Choudhry NK, Setoguchi S, Levin R, Winkelmayer WC, Shrank WH. Trends in adherence to secondary prevention medications in elderly post-myocardial infarction patients. *Pharmacoepidemiol Drug Saf.* 2008;17(12):1189-1196.

34. Pathak P, West DS, Martin BC, Helms M, Henderson C. Evidence-based use of second-generation antipsychotics in a state Medicaid pediatric population, 2001-2005. *Psychiatr Serv.* 2010;61(2):123-129.

35. Egan R, Pomeranz H. Sildenafil (Viagra) associated anterior ischemic optic neuropathy. *Arch Ophthalmol.* 2000;118:291-292.

36. Pomeranz HD, Bhavsar AR. Nonarteritic ischemic optic neuropathy developing soon after use of sildenafil (Viagra): A report of seven new cases. *J Neurovirol.* 2005;25:9-13.

37. Cosgrove-Mather B. Feds eye Viagra-blindness reports: Drug alters blood flow in body, may alter circulation to optic nerve. CBS Broadcasting Inc website. http://www.cbsnews.com/stories/2005/05/26/eveningnews/main698124.shtml. May 2006. Accessed January 13, 2010.

38. Johansson S, Ming EE, Wallander M, et al. Rosuvastatin safety: A comprehensive, international pharmacoepidemiology program. *Pharmacoepidemiol Drug Saf.* 2006;15(7): 454-461.

39. Medicines: Safety, efficacy, and utilization. World Health Organization website. http://www.who.int/medicines/areas/quality_safety/safety_efficacy/en/index.html. Accessed December 5, 2009.

40. Rivkin A. Admissions to a medical intensive care unit related to adverse drug reactions. *Am J Health-Syst Pharm.* 2007;64:1840-1843.

41. Draugalis JR, Plaza CM. Emerging role of epidemiologic literacy. *Ann Pharmacother.* 2006;40(2):229-233.

42. International Society for Pharmacoepidemiology website. http://www.pharmacoepi.org.

43. Accreditation standards and guidelines for the professional program in pharmacy leading to the doctor of pharmacy degree. Accreditation Council for Pharmacy Education website. http://www.acpe-accredit.org/pdf/ACPE_Revised_PharmD_Standards_Adopted_Jan152006.pdf. January 2006. Accessed January 13, 2010.

Principles of Epidemiology Applied to the Study of Medication Use

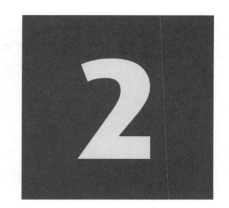

Yi Yang

OVERVIEW OF EPIDEMIOLOGY

As discussed in Chapter 1, pharmacoepidemiology is the study of the use and the effects of drugs in large numbers of people.[1] It is a relatively new discipline employing the methods of epidemiology in the study of drug use and drug effects in populations.

Epidemiology is the study of the factors that determine the occurrence and distribution of diseases in populations.[2] Specifically, epidemiology focuses on who is likely to develop a disease under what circumstances. This reflects the basic principle in epidemiology that disease does not occur randomly in a population; rather, certain people are at higher risks to develop certain conditions compared to others.

Individual genetic characteristics, behaviors, socioeconomic status, environmental milieu, and probably the interaction among these factors have an impact on the development of disease. Epidemiologic studies are conducted to examine the frequency or distribution of disease in groups of people, to determine the cause of or risk factors for a disease, and to evaluate the effectiveness of preventive and therapeutic measures to control the disease.

▶ Infectious Disease Epidemiology

In history, mankind had long been plagued by infectious diseases. For example, in 1900, the leading causes of death in the U.S. were pneumonia and

Table 2-1. Leading causes of death in the U.S., 1900.[a]

Rank[b]	Cause	Number	Rate[c]
1	Pneumonia (all forms and influenza)	40,362	202.2
2	Tuberculosis (all forms)	38,820	194.1
3	Diarrhea, enteritis, and ulceration of the intestines	28,491	142.7
4	Diseases of the heart	27,427	137.4
5	Intracranial lesions of vascular origin	21,353	106.9
6	Nephritis (all forms)	17,699	88.6
7	All accidents	14,429	72.3
8	Cancer and other malignant tumors	12,769	64.0
9	Senility	10,015	50.2
10	Diphtheria	8,056	40.3

[a]Data from the Centers for Disease Control and Prevention. http://www.cdc.gov/nchs/data/dvs/lead1900_98.pdf.
[b]Rank based on number of deaths.
[c]Crude mortality rate, per 100,000 population.

influenza; tuberculosis; and diarrhea, enteritis, and ulceration of the intestines (Table 2-1). As a fundamental medical science to study the frequency and occurrence of disease, historically, epidemiology has been considered the study of infectious diseases in large populations.[3] From this perspective, epidemiology has focused on how infectious disease is distributed in populations and the factors that determine this distribution. Infectious diseases have some special features:[3]

- There is usually the presence of a single, known, identifiable cause. Infectious disease can be caused by bacteria, viruses, fungi, or parasites. For example, cholera, an acute diarrheal infection, is caused by ingestion of the bacterium *Vibrio cholera*. The 2009 H1N1 flu is caused by the swine-origin influenza A (H1N1) virus.
- Infectious disease has the potential of transmission from one person or species to another. Some infectious diseases may be spread from person to person by means of direct or indirect contact or airborne small particles, some may be transmitted via animal or insect bites, and some may be transmitted through contaminated food or water.

- Individuals with infectious disease, sometimes even without being recognized as a case, may become a risk factor for other people. For example, a person infected with influenza virus can be infectious to another person 1 day before illness onset.
- People may be immune from getting the disease in the first place, for example, people who have had measles will not get it again.
- Vaccines can prevent the debilitating, and sometimes fatal, consequences of many infectious diseases, such as measles and chickenpox. Vaccines not only protect the vaccinated individual but also protect the community as a whole. When the majority of people in the community are vaccinated, the few who cannot be vaccinated for various reasons, such as those with a life-threatening allergic reaction to any component of a vaccine, often are indirectly protected because of group immunity.

▶ **Chronic Disease Epidemiology**

The leading causes of death have changed from infectious diseases to chronic diseases over the course of the past century.[4] Today, the leading causes of deaths

Table 2-2. Leading causes of death in the U.S., 2006.[a]

Rank[b]	Cause	Number	Rate[d]
1	Diseases of heart	631,636	211.0
2	Malignant neoplasms	559,888	187.0
3	Cerebrovascular diseases	137,119	45.8
4	Chronic lower respiratory diseases	124,583	41.6
5	Accidents (unintentional injuries)	121,599	40.6
6	Diabetes mellitus	72,449	24.2
7	Alzheimer's disease	72,432	24.2
8	Influenza and pneumonia	56,326	18.8
9	Nephritis, nephrotic syndrome and nephrosis	45,344	15.1
10	Septicemia	34,234	11.4

[a]Data from the Centers for Disease Control and Prevention. http://www.cdc.gov/NCHS/data/nvsr/nvsr57/nvsr57_14.pdf.
[b]Rank based on number of deaths.
[c]Crude mortality rate, per 100,000 population.

are heart disease, cancer, and stroke, which are all chronic in nature (Table 2-2). As the impact of chronic diseases on society has become increasingly prominent, the discipline of epidemiology has also evolved and incorporated the study of chronic diseases.

Specific Features of Chronic Disease Epidemiology

- Unlike infectious diseases, the causes of chronic diseases are usually complex, and sometimes no single cause can be identified; instead, a large number of risk factors contribute to the occurrence of disease. For example, blood pressure, total and high-density lipoprotein cholesterol, cigarette smoking, and diabetes are established risk factors of coronary artery disease.[5,6] Each of these factors is an independent predictor of major coronary disease events, but none of them is the single cause of coronary heart disease.

- Chronic disease is usually not contagious in nature; that is, it does not spread from person to person in the community. Some chronic diseases have strong genetic basis, yet they also interact with environmental factors. For example, family history of type 2 diabetes is one of the strongest risk factors for getting the disease, but other factors such as food intake and sedentary lifestyle also play an important role in determining the risk of developing type 2 diabetes.

- In chronic diseases, the disease process is usually lengthy and involves a preclinical or asymptomatic phase. Therefore, early detection and early treatment become crucial in chronic disease management.[4] Also because of the long-lasting or recurrent nature of chronic diseases, interventions to manage chronic diseases must be carried out persistently and on a long-term basis.

- Chronic diseases are usually incurable and potentially detrimental to the individual's life expectancy and quality of life.[4] Successful management of chronic disease involves slowing down the disease progression and preventing or delaying the occurrence of complications. For example, in rheumatic arthritis the individual's physical function will decline over time. The goals of treatment, therefore, become relief of symptoms, reduction of joint deformity and preservation of functions, and maintenance or improvement of quality of life.

Over time, the discipline of epidemiology has grown from systematic observation of natural occurrence of diseases, to the investigation of causes and risk factors of diseases, and now to the evaluation of measures to prevent and control diseases in populations. Pharmacoepidemiology applies the concepts and methodologies of chronic disease epidemiology to the study of drugs in populations. The remainder of this chapter will lay out the basic definitions and concepts of chronic disease epidemiology that can be adapted to the study of drug utilization patterns and drug effects. The applications of these concepts in pharmacoepidemiology will also be described.

TYPES OF CALCULATIONS: RATES, RATIOS, AND PROPORTIONS

In epidemiology, the presence and absence of disease and other dichotomous outcomes are often measured using rates, ratios, and proportions.[7] *Rate* is an expression of the frequency with which an event occurs in the population at risk during a specified time period, such as a day, 6 months, or a year. A rate is a comparison of two numbers, and it has four components: a numerator, which is the frequency of event; a denominator, which is the population at risk for the event; a specified time period; and a multiplier.[8] Rates are often used in epidemiology to make comparisons between subgroups of the population over time. For instance, the infant mortality rate measures the annual rate of deaths in children less than 1 year of age per 1,000 live births in a specific year.[8] Infant mortality rate is often used as an indicator of the level of health in a community. The infant mortality rate in the United States has shown a consistent downward trend over time, from 47.02 per 1,000 live births in 1940 to 6.69 in 2006.[9]

A *ratio* is the value obtained by dividing one number by another. It describes the relationship between the numerator and the denominator, which are two separate and unconnected quantities. Thus, an important feature of ratios is that the numerator and the denominator are not necessarily related. The numerator is not included in the denominator, and

vice versa. A ratio can range from zero to infinity. For example, what is the ratio of women to men in the U.S. population? This is expressed as a fraction, with the numerator equal to the number of women in the population and the denominator equal to the number of men in the population. According to Census 2000, there were 143.4 million women and 138.1 million men in the U.S..[10] The female to male ratio was 1.04 in 2000.

A *proportion* is also obtained by dividing one number by another. However, unlike a ratio, the numerator and the denominator are always related in a proportion. The numerator is always a subset of the denominator. Proportion is often expressed as a percentage ranging from 0% to 100%. For example, the proportion of acute myocardial infarction (AMI) patients without beta-blocker contraindications who are prescribed a beta-blocker at hospital discharge is used by the Centers for Medicare and Medicaid Services (CMS) as a national hospital inpatient-quality indicator.[11] In this example, AMI patients without contradictions to beta-blockers who are discharged with a beta-blocker are a subset of all AMI patients without contraindications to beta-blockers who are discharged from hospitals. The proportion of AMI patients who are discharged with a beta-blocker and the proportion of AMI patients who are discharged without a beta-blocker should add up to 100% because these two proportions are collectively exhaustive.

MEASURING MORBIDITY

Morbidity is defined as "any departure, subjective or objective, from a state of physiological or psychological well-being."[8] The synonyms of morbidity include sickness, illness, and morbid condition. The first step in understanding morbidity is to be able to measure it appropriately.

There are two types of basic measures of the frequency of disease occurrence in a population—*incidence* and *prevalence*. Whereas incidence measures the occurrence of new cases of a disease or the onset of disease, prevalence measures the number of cases of a disease already present in a population. The following section will define the measures of disease incidence and prevalence, present ways to quantify them, and discuss the relationship between incidence and prevalence measures. The applications of incidence and prevalence measures in pharmacoepidemiology will also be illustrated.

▶ Incidence

Incidence of a disease is defined as the number of new cases that occurs in a population at risk for developing the disease during a specified time period (usually a year). The individuals at risk are initially disease free. For common diseases, incidence may be expressed as a percentage or number of new cases per 1,000 population, whereas for rare conditions incidence is usually expressed with a larger denominator, for example, per 100,000 population.

There are two critical elements in the definition of incidence. First, incidence measures the occurrence of new cases of disease. It measures disease occurrence in persons who did not have the condition before. For diseases that can occur more than once during the specified period of time, incidence only measures the first occurrence of the disease. Second, the denominator of incidence calculation should include all persons who are at risk for developing the disease of interest, who are often referred to as the "population at risk" or the "candidate population." Any person who is included in the denominator must have the possibility to become a member in the numerator. For example, suppose that we wish to calculate the incidence of prostate cancer in the U.S. in 2009, we could find the number of new prostate cancer cases registered during 2009 and divide that number by the total number of men in the U.S. population in 2009, because women are not at risk for developing prostate cancer.

There are two types of incidence measures: *cumulative incidence*, when the denominator is people in the candidate population who are observed throughout the entire period of time, and, *incidence rate*, when the denominator takes the form of person-time when all people are not followed for the entire period of time. Although they both measure the occurrence of new cases, or the transition from no disease to disease, cumulative incidence and incidence rate have different characteristics.

Cumulative Incidence

Cumulative incidence measures the proportion of the population at risk that develops the disease of interest over a specified period of time. All persons in the denominator must be observed for the entire duration of follow-up. The choice of time period is arbitrary, though a period of 1 year is often used in reporting cumulative incidence. Cumulative incidence is a measure of risk in a group of people. When risk is measured for a single person, it is simply referred to as risk.[12] Cumulative incidence is sometimes referred to as the incidence proportion. The cumulative incidence is calculated as follows:

$$\text{Cumulative incidence} = \frac{\text{Number of new cases of a disease during a specified period}}{\text{Number of persons at risk for developing the disease during that period}}$$

Note that in the foregoing equation, number of new cases and number of persons at risk must be measured for the same defined period of time. Cumulative incidence can be expressed as a percentage or the number of new cases per 1,000 or per 100,000 populations.

Cumulative incidence is primarily used in fixed populations when in-migration equals out-migration and there are no losses to follow-up. Now let us consider a hypothetical example: There were 80 obese (BMI ≥ 30) people attending a 1-year educational program, and among them, 60 did not have type 2 diabetes mellitus at the start of the program in January 2009. All 80 people were followed throughout 2009. At the end of the program in December 2009, 6 of the 60 participants had been diagnosed with type 2 diabetes. This results in a cumulative incidence of type 2 diabetes among those without diabetes at the start of the program of 10% or 100 per 1,000 participants during the 1-year period.

Figure 2-1 presents an example of using cumulative incidence in measuring disease occurrence in large populations, the cumulative incidence of diagnosed diabetes per 1,000 population among those aged 18 to 79 years from 1980 to 2007. We notice

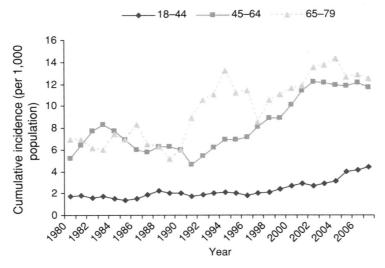

▲ **Figure 2-1.** Cumulative incidence of diagnosed diabetes per 1,000 population aged 18 to 79, by age, in the U.S., 1980 to 2007. Data from the Centers for Disease Control and Prevention. http://www.cdc.gov/diabetes/statistics/incidence/fig3.htm.

from Figure 2-1 that across all age groups, the cumulative incidence of diagnosed diabetes changed slightly during the 1980s. However, cumulative incidence of diagnosed diabetes started to increase in all age groups in the 1990s. During the 2000s, cumulative incidence of diagnosed diabetes continued to increase among those aged 18 to 44 years. There were some encouraging signs in those in the age group of 45 to 64 years and 65 to 79 years; that is, the rate of increase in cumulative incidence appeared to have slowed down in these two older age groups.

Incidence Rate

In epidemiologic studies, sometimes, not every individual in the population at risk has been observed during the entire period of time for a variety of reasons. Some individuals enter the observation period after it has started, whereas others may be lost to follow-up. The length of follow-up time will therefore not be the same for each individual. When the study population is dynamic, that is, when different individuals are followed for different lengths of time, incidence rate will be used to measure how fast new

cases of a disease occur, accounting for the varying observation time for different individuals. Incidence rate is also referred to as incidence density. Incidence rate is calculated as follows:

$$\text{Incidence rate} = \frac{\text{Number of new cases of a disease during a specified period}}{\text{Total person-time of observation in population at risk during that period}}$$

The numerator for incidence rate is the same as that of cumulative incidence; the difference between the two measures lies in the denominator. The denominator of incidence rate is the sum of the time periods that each person in the population at risk for developing disease has contributed. Incidence rate, therefore, measures the number of people who become new cases of a disease during a specified period of time as a proportion of the total time at which individuals in a population at risk are observed.

Now let us assume that there is a 5-year study (Figure 2-2). Participant A entered the study at Year 0

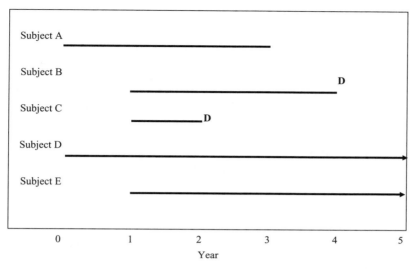

▲ **Figure 2-2.** Hypothetical study of five participants. The solid horizontal line indicates time followed while the participants are at risk for developing the disease; D indicates a case.

and was followed until the end of Year 3; Participant B entered the study at the beginning of Year 1 and became a case at the end of Year 4; Participant C entered the study at the beginning of Year 1 and developed the disease at the end of Year 1; Participant D entered the study at the beginning of the study and was followed for the entire period of the study without developing the disease of interest; Participant E entered at the beginning of Year 1 and was also observed till the end of the study. One person at risk who is monitored for 1 year equals one person-year. In this hypothetical example, Participants A and B each contribute 3 person-years, Participant C contributes 1 person-year, Participants D and E contribute 5 and 4 person-years, respectively, yielding a total of 16 person-years. Notice that the total number of person-years of follow-up is obtained by simply summing all of the years contributed by each participant. Also, we know that in this hypothetical example two new cases developed during the observation, the calculated incidence rate is 0.125/person-year, or 12.5/100 person-years. This means that one would expect, on average, about 12.5% of patients per year would develop the disease of interest among patients similar to those in

the example. The choice of person-time units in the denominator is arbitrary. The time unit used in calculating incidence rate can be year, month, and even day, depending on the nature of the disease under study. For diseases that take a long time to develop, such as diabetes mellitus, person-year is commonly used, whereas for diseases that develop rapidly, such as influenza, person-month or person-day are usually used.

In many instances, computing person-times for a large population, for example, for the entire population in New York City, by separately counting the person-years at risk for each individual using the method described in Figure 2-2 would be impractical. In epidemiology, person-time for a large population can often be calculated by multiplying the average size of the population at risk by the average length of time the population is under observation. In many situations, relatively few people in the population develop the disease of interest, and the population under observation remains relatively stable during the period of observation. In such instances, the average size of the population at risk can be estimated using the size of the entire population, which can be obtained from the U.S. Census Bureau. Suppose that we wish to calculate the incidence rate of breast cancer in women in the U.S. in 2006, we would use the total number of new breast cancer cases in 2006 divided by the total number of women in 2006, assuming that each woman was observed for the entire year of 2006. On the basis of Surveillance and Epidemiology End Results data maintained by the U.S. National Cancer Institute, the author found that the age-adjusted (see age-adjusted mortality rate later in this chapter) incidence rate of breast cancer was 123.8 per 100,000 women per year,[13] or 123.8 per 100,000 woman-years.

▶ Prevalence

The prevalence of disease is defined as the number of existing cases (old and new) in the population (sick, healthy, at risk, and not at risk). It focuses on disease status and measures the proportion of the population who has the disease of interest. Some individuals may have developed the disease of interest a long time ago, and some may have developed the disease more recently. However, all of them must have the disease of interest at the time of assessment. There are two types of prevalence measures: *point prevalence* and *period prevalence.*

Point Prevalence

Point prevalence is the number of people who have the disease of interest at a single point in time, divided by the number of people in the population at that specific time, for example, on a given day. Point prevalence is calculated as follows:

$$\text{Point prevalence} = \frac{\text{Number of persons who have the disease at a specified time}}{\text{Number of persons in the population at that specified time}}$$

Point prevalence can be thought of as a single snapshot of the population; that is, the calculation of point prevalence is based on a single examination at one point in time, such as a calendar date, or the day of hospital admission. Suppose that we are interested in knowing the point prevalence of methicillin-resistant *Staphylococcus aureus* (MRSA) nasal colonization in all hospitalized patients in intensive care units (ICU) in a state, we would obtain MRSA nasal cultures on all ICU patients, including patients known to be MRSA positive on a chosen day, to determine the number of patients with positive MRSA culture on that day. We will then divide this number by the total number of ICU patients in the state on that day. The resulting proportion is the point prevalence of MRSA nasal carriage in ICU in the state on that particular day. Point prevalence can be expressed as a percentage or number of cases per 1,000 or per 100,000 persons in the population, depending on the frequency of the disease of interest. Notice that in some situations the survey for point prevalence would actually take longer than a single day.

Period Prevalence

The second type of prevalence measure is period prevalence. Period prevalence refers to the number of persons who have the disease at any point during a period of time, divided by the number of persons in the population during that period of time. Period prevalence is calculated as follows:

$$\text{Period prevalence} = \frac{\text{Number of persons who have the disease at any time during a specified period}}{\text{Number of persons in the population during that specified period}}$$

Period prevalence is calculated in the same way as point prevalence, except the numerator is the number of people who have the disease at any time during a specified time period. The numerator includes cases that were present at the beginning of the period as well as cases developed during the specified period. Period prevalence can be thought of as a series of snapshots of a population during a specified period of time; it tells us how much of a particular disease is present in a population over a time period. Period prevalence can be calculated for a week, month, year, decade, or any other specified length of time.

Period prevalence is a less commonly used term. In the literature, the term *prevalence* is often used without

Table 2-3. Characteristics of incidence and prevalence measures.

Characteristics	Cumulative incidence	Incidence rate	Point prevalence	Period prevalence
Type of cases	New	New	Existing	Existing
Type of measure	Proportion	Rate	Proportion	Proportion
Unit of measure	None	Cases/person-time	None	None
Range	0 to 1	0 to ∞	0 to 1	0 to 1
Synonyms	Risk, incidence proportion	Incidence density	None	None

a modifier, and it usually refers to the disease status at a specified point in time, that is, *point prevalence.*[14]

Relationship between Incidence and Prevalence

As summarized in Table 2-3, cumulative incidence, incidence rate, point prevalence, and period prevalence have the following major differences. First, these measures reflect different phases of a disease. Cumulative incidence and incidence rate measure the occurrence of new disease, or a change from health to disease, whereas prevalence reflects existing cases, or the burden of disease in a population. Second, the measures differ in what is actually measured. Cumulative incidence measures the probability that an individual will become ill over a specified period of time, and incidence rate measures the rapidity with which new cases occur, whereas the two prevalence measures determine the proportion of population with the disease of interest at a specific point in time or during a given period of time. Lastly, these measures have different units. Incidence rate has units of new cases per unit of person-time, whereas cumulative incidence and prevalence measures have no units.

Disease incidence and prevalence are also closely related in that disease incidence affects prevalence. The greater the incidence, the more people will have the disease of interest. Clearly, prevalence is also influenced by the duration of the disease. Let us consider the following scenarios: first, the longer the duration of the disease, the greater the prevalence. For example, in essential hypertension the incidence rate is high, the duration of the disease is long, and

the prevalence is high. Second, diseases with a shorter duration may have a low prevalence even if the incidence rate is high; this is especially true for benign diseases. For example, the incidence rate of roseola infantum, a viral illness commonly affecting young children between the ages of 6 months and 2 years, is high. But the prevalence of roseola infantum may be low because, after a brief period (roseola infantum is typically marked by 3 to 7 days of high fever, followed by a distinctive rash just as the fever breaks lasting from hours to a few days), most young children recover from the infection and are no longer in the disease state. Third, prevalence may also be low for a severe disease that leads to rapid death because the duration is short. For instance, the prevalence of sudden cardiac arrest is low even though it has a high incidence, because it usually causes death if not treated within minutes. In this case, the low prevalence means that at any given time, there will only be a small proportion of people suffering from a sudden cardiac arrest. And lastly, some diseases have a long duration, so even if the incidence rate is low, the prevalence is still high. Alzheimer's disease and Parkinson's disease are examples.

A person who becomes ill adds one to the incidence of the disease. He also adds one to the prevalence of the disease for the duration of his illness, until he recovers or dies. If the prevalence of a disease is low in a relatively stable population, the relationship between prevalence and incidence rate can be roughly expressed as:

$$P \approx I \times D$$

where P is prevalence, I is the incidence rate, and D is the average duration of disease. This means that in a relatively stationary population where an equal number of people entering and exiting during any point in time, prevalence of a disease equals the product of incidence rate and the average duration of the disease.[15] For example, if the incidence rate of a disease is 2% and the incidence has been relatively steady over the years, and if the approximate duration of the disease is 15 years, the prevalence of the disease would be approximately 30%.

To further illustrate the relationship between incidence and prevalence, let us look at a hypothetical cohort study (see Chapter 3 for a description of cohort study). The use of a new drug, Drug A, was studied for prevention of seasonal allergies in patients who have already had seasonal allergies in the past. All 50 patients who received Drug A developed seasonal allergies during follow-up. The 50 patients were observed for a total of 700 person-days before first developing allergy symptoms; at the end of the study, about 20% of the patients reported having allergy symptoms. Thus, the cumulative incidence of developing seasonal allergy was 50/50 = 1 in this group of patients, the incidence rate was 50/700 = 0.071 cases/person-day = 7.1 cases/100 person-days, and the prevalence was 20%. Now let us look at the data of the untreated group: All 50 patients developed seasonal allergies, and assume that the incidence rate was 0.12 cases/person-day. About 30% of the patients in the untreated group reported having allergy symptoms. The cumulative incidence of one in both the treated and untreated groups suggests that treatment with Drug A does not ultimately prevent seasonal allergies or reduce risk of developing seasonal allergies. However, the incidence rate was lower in the treated group, indicating that Drug A may have slowed or delayed the onset of seasonal allergies. In addition, the prevalence was lower in the treated group, suggesting that treated patients are less likely to have allergy symptoms on an average day.[16]

Uses of Incidence and Prevalence in Pharmacoepidemiology

Incidence and prevalence are measures used to describe disease occurrence. Prevalence is most useful for determining the burden of disease in a community; for example, the prevalence of cancer in a community is useful in predicting the need for cancer diagnostic and treatment facilities in that community. On the other hand, incidence is most useful for studying the cause of the disease and evaluating the effectiveness of programs in preventing disease from developing in the first place. For instance, the incidence of diabetes in a population is useful information in designing educational programs to increase patient adherence with medical recommendations intended to prevent diabetes complications from occurring. In pharmacoepidemiology, in addition to their standard epidemiologic uses, the concepts of incidence and prevalence can be applied to study the uses and effects of drugs. They can be used to measure drug events, such as identifying new users of drugs, measuring existing drug uses, and so on. A pharmacoepidemiologic analysis of drug utilization is, by nature, population based. For example, to increase the use of statin medications among members with diabetes or coronary artery disease who had not filled a prescription for statins in the previous 6 months, a pharmacy benefit management company delivered educational interventions to prescribers. The study shows that 12.1% of members whose prescribers received the intervention and 7.3% of the control group started statin therapy during a 4-month follow-up period.[17] This is an example of applying the concept of cumulative incidence in pharmacoepidemiology. New users of drugs are also referred to as *incident users* in pharmacoepidemiology.

Because prevalence is a measure of status, it is also used to describe the frequency of characteristics other than disease in a population.[15] For example, the proportion of a population that receives a certain drug therapy would be described as the prevalence of drug therapy. In another study of statin users, existing statin uses were identified prior to hospital admissions for pneumonia. This study reported that among 29,900 eligible patients hospitalized due to pneumonia, 1,372 patients were current statin users (or prevalent users), which was defined as at least one filled prescription within 125 days before the hospitalization with pneumonia.[18]

CASE STUDY 2-1

A Study of Antidepressant Prescribing and Changes in Antidepressant Mortality and Suicide

In a study of primary care prescription records in England from 1993 to 2004, Morgan et al.[19] examined the prevalence of antidepressant treatment and association between antidepressant use and adverse health outcomes, including suicide and poisoning mortality. Antidepressant prescription data were obtained from the

Department of Health. Suicide and poisoning mortality data were obtained from the Office for National Statistics. Age-and sex-specific antidepressant prescribing data were obtained from the Health Improvement Network primary care data. Figure 2-3 shows the prevalence of antidepressant treatment per 1,000 patients

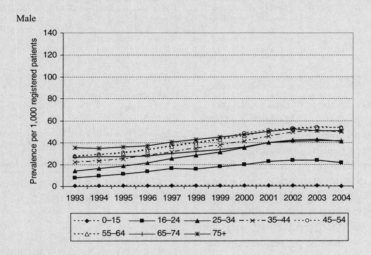

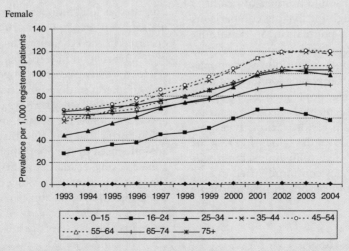

▲ **Figure 2-3.** Prevalence of antidepressant treatment per 1,000 patients registered with a general practitioner by age group and sex, in England, 1993 to 2004. (Reprinted from Ref. 19 by permission of Oxford University Press.)

registered with a general practitioner by age group and sex in England, 1993 to 2004. We can see from this figure that there is a general trend of increased prevalence of antidepressant treatment from 1993 to 2004 for both sexes and all age groups, except for men aged between 15 and 24 years and women aged between 15 and 24 years, and 25 and 34 years, where there was a decline in treatment prevalence.

The increase in antidepressant prevalence was mainly explained by the rapid increase in selective serotonin reuptake inhibitor prescribing, with a gradual increase of other antidepressants. Age-standardized suicide rate and antidepressant mortality rate were reported as per million population. General suicide rates declined steadily from 1993 to 2004, so did non-drug poisoning rate. Antidepressant poisoning mortality rates had a slight increase from 1996 to 1997, followed by a decline up to the end of the study. Multivariate regression results suggest that after controlling for age and sex, increased treatment with antidepressants was not associated with antidepressant poisoning mortality or suicide in England, at a population level.[19]

MEASURING MORTALITY

Mortality refers to the occurrence of death, and mortality data are of great interest in epidemiology. Mortality data can be used in evaluating the health of a population or comparing health across different segments of a population. Mortality is also an index of the severity of disease; thus, mortality data can be used by health care practitioners and public health professionals in identifying the diseases and conditions frequently associated with death and evaluating the effectiveness of health services in preventing premature death. However, absolute number of deaths is rarely informative enough for making comparisons between segments of a population or examining changes over time because it is influenced heavily by population size and the age composition of the population. For example, a larger population tends to have more deaths than a smaller population, or a population with a large elderly segment also tends to generate more death events.[20] As a result, various measures of mortality are used to describe the risk of dying in a population. The following section will present the mortality rates commonly used in epidemiology and their applications in pharmacoepidemiology.

Crude Mortality Rate

Crude mortality (or death) rate is the total number of deaths from all causes per 1,000 persons in a population during a specified period of time divided by the total number of persons in the population during that period of time.

$$\text{Crude mortality rate} = \frac{\text{Number of deaths for all causes during a specified period}}{\text{Number of persons in the population during that period}} \times 1{,}000$$

Crude mortality rate is usually reported for a 1-year period. Crude mortality rate can also be expressed as total number of deaths per 100,000 population. For example, in 2006, 2,426,264 deaths occurred in the U.S. among an estimated population of 299,398,484 on July 1, 2006,[9,21] yielding an annual crude mortality rate of 810.4 per 100,000 population in 2006. Because the population changes over time, the population size at midyear is often used as an approximation of the number of persons in the population during that year. Note that crude mortality rates are influenced by the population's age composition.[20] Hence, using crude mortality rates in examining changes over time or making comparisons between subgroups in a population can often be misleading. As such, *age-specific mortality rate* is used to compare mortality risks between age groups.

Age-Specific Mortality Rate

Age-specific mortality rate measures the total number of deaths from all causes among individuals in a specific age category. Age-specific mortality is usually expressed as per 1,000 or per 100,000 population for a 1-year period. For example, we might be interested in the mortality rate in children younger than 10 years of age. Age-specific mortality rate can be computed using the following equation:

$$\text{Age-specific mortality rate} = \frac{\substack{\text{Number of deaths for}\\\text{all causes during a}\\\text{specified period in a}\\\text{specified age category}}}{\substack{\text{Number of persons}\\\text{in that age category}\\\text{in the population}\\\text{during that period}}} \times 1{,}000$$

Age-specific mortality rates allow one to compare mortality risks for a particular age group across different subpopulations. For example, in 2006, the age-specific mortality rate for children between ages 1 and 4 was 28.4 per 100,000 population for both sexes in the U.S., whereas the age-specific mortality rates for men and women were 30.5 and 26.3 per 100,000 population, respectively.[9]

▶ Age-Adjusted Mortality Rate

To account for variation in age distributions on comparisons of crude mortality rates over time or across segments in population, it might be desirable to have a summary measure of mortality risk. Thus *age-adjusted mortality rate* was developed.[20] Age-adjusted mortality rate is defined as "the death rate that would occur if the observed age-specific death rates were present in a population with an age distribution equal to that of a standard population."[20] Computing age-adjusted mortality rate requires the choice of a standard population, that is, a population with "standard" age distribution. This selection is arbitrary to some extent because there is no such standard population in existence. Prior to 1999, the 1940 standard population was used in computing age-adjusted mortality rate in the U.S.; beginning with 1999, age-adjusted mortality rate is calculated on the basis of the 2000 standard population.[20]

The commonly used method to compute age-adjusted mortality rate is the method of direct stan-

dardization, although indirect standardization may also be used. For technical details on how to compute age-adjusted mortality rate, please refer to other sources.[20,22] Figure 2-4 shows the trends of annual crude and age-adjusted mortality rates, per 100,000 population in the U.S. from 1940 to 2006.[9]

Age-adjusted mortality rates afford one the ability to compare mortality risks between population groups and across geographic locations; they also allow one to compare mortality trends over time. However, age-adjusted mortality rate cannot replace crude mortality rate or age-specific mortality rate because the calculated age-adjusted mortality rate is based on a "standard" population and does not reflect the mortality risk of any "real" population.[20,22]

▶ Cause-Specific Mortality Rate

Cause-specific mortality rate measures the total number of deaths from a specific cause. Cause-specific mortality rate restricts the mortality to a specific cause or a specific diagnosis. It is usually expressed as per 1,000 or per 100,000 population for a 1-year period.

$$\text{Cause-specific mortality rate} = \frac{\substack{\text{Number of deaths for}\\\text{a specific cause during}\\\text{a specified period}}}{\substack{\text{Number of persons}\\\text{in the population}\\\text{during that period}}} \times 1{,}000$$

For example, coronary heart diseases caused 425,425 deaths in 2006 and is the single leading cause of death in the U.S..[23] With an estimated population of 299,398,484 on July 1, 2006,[21] the resulting annual mortality rate for coronary artery disease is 142.1 per 100,000 population in 2006.

Immediate and underlying causes of death and other significant conditions contributing to death are reported on death certificates and are determined using the applicable revision of the International Classification of Diseases (ICD) codes.[22] The underlying cause of death refers to the single selected cause of death, which is the disease or injury that initiates the series of events leading to the death. All other reported causes are the nonunderlying causes of death. A death event may have

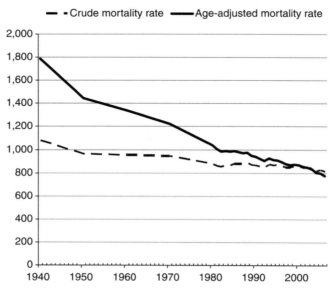

— - Crude mortality rate　——Age-adjusted mortality rate

▲ **Figure 2-4.** Annual crude and age-adjusted mortality rates, per 100,000 population in the U.S., 1940–2006. Data from the Centers for Disease Control and Prevention. http://www.cdc.gov/NCHS/data/nvsr/ nvsr57/nvsr57_14.pdf.

multiple causes, including both the underlying and nonunderlying causes.[22,24] The underlying cause of death is used in computing cause-specific mortality rate. Note that misclassification and miscoding can affect the accuracy of reported cause-specific mortality rate.

Similarly, one can put a restriction on other demographic characteristics, such as sex, race, and geographic areas to compute characteristic-specific mortality rate, such as race-specific mortality rates. In addition, one can place restrictions on more than one characteristic simultaneously, for example, to compute age-adjusted mortality rate for women for a certain race. Such restrictions must be placed on both the numerator and the denominator simultaneously so that everyone in the denominator will be at risk for becoming a part of the numerator. Figure 2-5 shows the age-adjusted mortality rate by sex and race in U.S. populations, 1960 to 2006.

▶ **Case Fatality**

Case fatality measures the propensity of a disease to cause the death of affected persons. Although often referred to as case fatality *rate,* it is not a true rate, but a proportion. Case fatality is usually expressed as a percentage. Case fatality is calculated as follows:

$$\text{Case fatality} = \frac{\begin{array}{c}\text{Number of deaths from a disease}\\\text{during a specified period}\end{array}}{\begin{array}{c}\text{Number of persons with the specified}\\\text{disease during that period}\end{array}} \times 100$$

In other words, case fatality represents the proportion of individuals affected with a disease who die from it. For example, between August 30 and October 31, 2009 (the beginning of the 2009–2010 influenza season), there were 672 deaths associated with the laboratory-confirmed influenza viruses reported to the Centers for Disease Control and Prevention (CDC). During that period, there were 45,585 cases with positive influenza viruses in the U.S..[25] The case fatality for influenza was calculated to be 1.47% for the 2-month period.

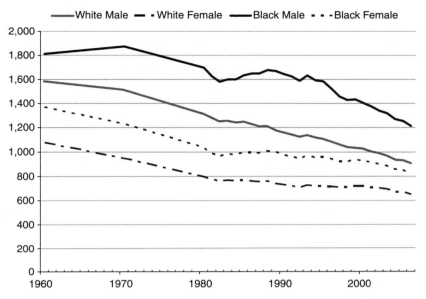

▲ **Figure 2-5.** Age-adjusted mortality rate, by race and sex, in the U.S., 1960 to 2006.
Data from the Centers for Disease Control and Prevention. http://www.cdc.gov/nchs/data/nvsr/nvsr57/nvsr57_14.pdf.

Notice that in computing crude mortality rate for a disease the denominator includes all persons in a population who are at risk for getting the disease; however, in calculating case fatality, the denominator only includes those who have the disease of interest. Some diseases, such as pancreatic cancer, may have a low crude mortality rate, as the disease is rare. However, the case fatality is high, as once a person is affected with the disease, the likelihood of the disease to cause death is high.

Proportionate Mortality

Proportionate mortality is the proportion of deaths that are attributable to a specific cause. For example, one can ask, "Of all the deaths that have occurred in the U.S. in 2006, what proportion is attributable to heart diseases?" Although sometimes called proportionate mortality ratio, proportionate mortality is not a ratio or a rate; it is a proportion because the numerator is always a part of the denominator. Proportionate mortality is usually expressed as a percentage. Proportionate mortality can be computed as follows:

$$\text{Proportionate mortality} = \frac{\substack{\text{Number of deaths from a disease} \\ \text{during a specified period}}}{\substack{\text{Total number of deaths during} \\ \text{that period}}} \times 100$$

To find out the proportion of deaths that are caused by heart diseases in the U.S. in 2006, we use the number of deaths caused by heart disease divided by the total number of deaths in 2006; the proportionate mortality from heart diseases in the U.S. in 2006 is 631,636/ 2,426,264 × 100 = 26%. The 15 leading causes of death in 2006 accounted for 85.1% of all deaths occurred in the U.S.. Table 2-4 summarizes the 15 leading causes of death in 2006 and the crude mortality rate, age-adjusted mortality rate, and proportionate mortality for each cause.[9]

▶ Uses of Mortality Measures in Pharmacoepidemiology

Mortality has been recognized as a benchmark measure of health outcomes as we evaluate the risks and benefits of treatments or preventive measures. Drug

Table 2-4. Crude mortality rate, proportionate mortality, and age-adjusted mortality rates, for the 15 leading causes of death for the total population in 2006, in the U.S..

Rank	Cause of death	Number	Crude mortality rate	Age-adjusted mortality rate	Proportionate mortality
	All causes	2,426,264	810.4	776.5	100
1	Diseases of heart	631,636	211.0	200.2	26.0
2	Malignant neoplasms	559,888	187.0	180.7	23.1
3	Cerebrovascular diseases	137,119	45.8	43.6	5.7
4	Chronic lower respiratory diseases	124,583	41.6	40.5	5.1
5	Accidents (unintentional injuries)	121,599	40.6	39.8	5.0
6	Diabetes mellitus	72,449	24.2	23.3	3.0
7	Alzheimer's disease	72,432	24.2	22.6	3.0
8	Influenza and pneumonia	56,326	18.8	17.8	2.3
9	Nephritis, nephrotic syndrome, and nephrosis	45,344	15.1	14.5	1.9
10	Septicemia	34,234	11.4	11.0	1.4
11	Intentional self-harm (suicide)	33,300	11.1	10.9	1.4
12	Chronic liver disease and cirrhosis	27,555	9.2	8.8	1.1
13	Essential hypertension and hypertensive renal disease	23,855	8.0	7.5	1.0
14	Parkinson's disease	19,566	6.5	6.3	0.8
15	Assault (homicide)	18,573	6.2	6.2	0.8
	All other causes (residual)	447,805	149.6	NA	18.5

Crude mortality rates on an annual basis per 100,000 population; age-adjusted rates per 100,000 U.S. standard population. Data from Heron M, Hoyert D L, Murphy SL et al. Final data for 2006. *National Vital Stat Report.* 57(14). http://www.cdc.gov/nchs/data/nvsr/nvsr57/nvsr57_14.pdf.

therapy, like many other treatments in health care, may have intended (beneficial) and/or unintended (beneficial or adverse) effects on patients. Death may occur as a failure of having fully realized the intended beneficial effects of treatments; an unintended, adverse effect of treatments; or a result of nontreatment. Adverse effects can range in severity from trivial to life threatening. In pharmacoepidemiology, mortality measures have been used to examine the association between drug exposure and patient outcome. Both all-cause mortality and cause-specific mortality are commonly used in the pharmacoepidemiology literature, sometimes with restrictions on other individual characteristics, such as all-cause mortality for a certain age group, or cause-specific mortality for men versus women. Mortality measures are either used alone or in combination with other outcome measures. Cause-specific mortality has great specificity, but there are uncertainties inherent in the ascertainment of cause of death.[26] Misclassification biases may be a threat to its validity. These all-cause mortality measure avoids the bias in the determination of causes of death, but it lacks the specificity that cause-specific mortality measures provide.[26,27] Preferably, cause-specific mortality should be reported alongside crude (all-cause) mortality.

CASE STUDY 2-2[28]

A Study of a Prevalent Adverse Effect of Warfarin that Leads to Regulatory Action by the Food and Drug Administration (FDA)

The clinical effectiveness of oral anticoagulant warfarin sodium in prevention and treatment of thromboembolic disorders has been established in a number of well-designed clinical trials and for a number of conditions, including venous thrombolism, pulmonary thrombolism, atrial fibrillation, artificial heart valve replacement, and stroke. The most common complication with warfarin therapy is bleeding. In a study of several national databases, Wysowski et al.[29] reviewed warfarin prescription data from the National Prescription Audit plus database of IMS Health from 1998 to 2004, and the prevalence of serious bleeding complications associated with warfarin use, using the FDA's Adverse Event Reporting System from 1993 to 2006. They also obtained the annual number of U.S. death events in which anticoagulants were listed as the underlying cause of death or as total mentions (the sum of mentions of anticoagulants as the immediate, contributing, or underlying cause or as a significant condition leading to death) from the National Center for Health Statistics Web site for the period between 1998 and 2004. The National Hospital Ambulatory Care Survey data from 1999 to 2003 were used to determine the number of emergency department visits associated with warfarin and warfarin-related bleeding. They reported that warfarin use increased by 45%, from 21.1 million in 1998 to 30.6 million in 2004. During that period, the number of deaths attributed to anticoagulants as the underlying cause of death has increased, from 0.45 per

100,000 to 0.52 per 100,000 U.S. resident population. The results of this study show the urgency for placement of a boxed warning in the product's labeling about warfarin's bleeding risk. As a result, the FDA requested that the makers of both brand name and generic warfarins include a "black box" on their product labeling warning of the bleeding complication. For example, Bristol-Myers Squibb, the maker of warfarin, Coumadin®, has placed a "black box" warning on the product labeling, including medication guide, which reads:

WARNING: BLEEDING RISK

Warfarin sodium can cause major or fatal bleeding. Bleeding is more likely to occur during the starting period and with a higher dose (resulting in a higher INR). Risk factors for bleeding include high intensity of anticoagulation (INR >4.0), age ≥65, highly variable INRs, history of gastrointestinal bleeding, hypertension, cerebrovascular disease, serious heart disease, anemia, malignancy, trauma, renal insufficiency, concomitant drugs, and long duration of warfarin therapy. Regular monitoring of INR should be performed on all treated patients. Those at high risk of bleeding may benefit from more frequent INR monitoring, careful dose adjustment to desired INR, and a shorter duration of therapy. Patients should be instructed about prevention measures to minimize risk of bleeding and to report immediately to physicians signs and symptoms of bleeding.[30]

Now let us look at an example of using mortality measures in the study of drug effects: a retrospective cohort study of medication nonadherence (see Chapter 8 for a detailed discussion of adherence) and adverse health outcomes among patients with diabetes. The extent of nonadherence was assessed for three classes of medications that are important for managing patients with diabetes, including oral hypoglycemics, antihypertensives,

and statin medications.[28] Results of this study suggest that nonadherence to prescribed medications is prevalent among patients with diabetes and nonadherence is associated with increased all-cause mortality and hospitalization.[28] In this study, all-cause mortality was used as one of the adverse health-outcome measures. Case 2-2 illustrates the use of cause-specific mortality in pharmacoepidemiology.

MEASURING ASSOCIATIONS BETWEEN EXPOSURES AND OUTCOMES

In epidemiology, *association* refers to a statistical relationship between two or more variables. *Exposure* refers to having any *potential* causal characteristics, such as a behavior (e.g., smoking) or a treatment (e.g., a drug therapy). Epidemiologists are often interested in assessing the associations between exposures and outcomes; for example, "Is there an excess risk of developing disease X given exposure to Y?" The *risk ratio* (RR) and the *odds ratio* (OR) are the two most commonly used measures of association in epidemiology. They measure the strength of association between an exposure and the outcome of interest. The magnitude indicates how more or less likely the exposed is to have the outcome as compared to the unexposed group. The remainder of this chapter will describe measures of associations in epidemiology and their applications in pharmacoepidemiology.

▶ Risk Ratio

When faced with an array of risk factors for disease or mortality, we need to assess how strongly exposure and outcomes are associated. Risk ratio is the ratio of the risk of developing the event (disease or death) in exposed individuals (R_e) to that in unexposed individuals (R_u).

$$RR = \frac{R_e}{R_u}$$

In the above equation, R_e is the risk (cumulative incidence) in the exposed group and R_u is the risk (cumulative incidence) in the unexposed group. In the epidemiology literature, RR is also referred to as *relative risk*. The term *relative risk* is sometimes used to describe both RR and rate ratios (i.e., the comparison of the exposed and unexposed groups in terms of incidence rates or mortality rates).[15]

Let us consider a hypothetical cohort study (see Chapter 3 for a description of cohort study) in which 500 current smokers (the exposed group) and 500 individuals who never smoked (the unexposed group) were followed for 5 years. Assume that after 5 years, researchers released data that 25 individuals in the exposed group and 5 individuals in the unexposed group developed lung cancer. What is the RR of developing lung cancer in the exposed group as compared to those in the unexposed group? Based on definition, the RR of developing lung cancer in the exposed group (smokers) to that of the unexposed group (nonsmokers) can be calculated as:

$$RR = \frac{25/500}{5/500} = 5.0$$

The risk of developing lung cancer in the smoker group is 5 times the risk in the nonsmoker group; in other words, there is a 400% increase in risk of developing lung cancer in the smoker group. An RR of 1 or close to 1 indicates that the risk of event (disease or death) is equal in the exposed and unexposed groups and that exposure is unlikely to cause the event of interest; an RR greater than 1 means that exposure is associated with the event, and the greater the RR, the stronger the association; an RR of 0 or close to 0 suggests that the exposure has protective effects against the event in some way; that is, the risk of event is much lower in exposed individuals.

▶ Odds Ratio

Odds is the ratio of the probability of the event of interest (e.g., disease of interest or death) to that of the nonevent. The ratio of two odds, that is, the odds ratio (OR), is an extremely popular measure of association in case-control studies (see Chapter 3 for a description of case-control study). The OR of disease development or death is the ratio of the number of events and nonevents in cases to the number of events and nonevents in the control group.

In epidemiology, it has been demonstrated that the OR of disease (OR_{dis}) is mathematically equivalent with the OR of exposure (OR_{exp}).[31] Table 2-5 presents the cross-tabulated data of a typical case-control study.

OR can be calculated as follows:

$$OR_{exp} = \frac{a/c}{b/d} = \frac{ad}{bc} = \frac{a/b}{c/d} = OR_{dis}$$

Table 2-5. Cross-tabulation of a case-control study.

Exposure	Outcome		
	Present	Absent	Total
Yes	a	b	a+b
No	c	d	c+d
Total	a+c	b+d	a+b+c+d

The OR can be any nonnegative numbers. An OR of 1 is a baseline for comparison. An OR greater than 1 indicates that the odds for event is higher in the exposed (or disease) group than in the unexposed (or nondisease) group; OR of less than 1 suggests that an event is less likely in the exposed group than in the unexposed group.[32]

As seen in a hypothetical case-control study of hypertension and stroke in Table 2-6, stroke "present" is the case and stroke "absent" is the control group; stage 2 hypertension and normal blood pressure are the exposures. In this example, the OR is

$$OR = \frac{417/83}{744/752} = \frac{417 \times 752}{83 \times 744} = 5.08$$

An OR of 5.08 suggests that stroke is 5.08 times as frequent in stage 2 hypertension group as compared to the normal blood pressure group.

Estimates of RR and OR are both used to measure the strength of association between exposure and outcome. In summary, both measures can range from 0 to infinity with the same general interpretation. An RR or OR equal to 1 indicates there is no association between exposure and outcome; an RR or OR value greater than 1 means a positive association; that is, the risk of outcome is greater when exposed to the specific risk factor. A value of less than 1 indicates that exposure reduces the risk or odds of outcome, a negative association between exposure and outcome.[32] Note that the OR can be used to estimate RR when the probability of event is small (i.e., <10%); this is referred to as "rare disease assumption."[32] A further discussion of the relationship between OR and RR is available in Chapter 5.

▶ Measuring Therapeutic Effects

Epidemiologists are often interested in measuring the effects of interventions in increasing the likelihood of positive health outcomes or reducing the risk of developing negative outcomes, such as disease or death. There are four measures of therapeutic effects that are commonly used: *relative risk reduction* (RRR), *absolute risk reduction* (ARR), *number needed to treat* (NNT), and *number needed to harm* (NNH). These measures are also measures of association. They are presented separately for the reason that these measures are often used to assess the effects of a treatment or therapy, such as a new drug or a new surgical procedure.

Relative Risk Reduction

Sometimes we need to consider the consequences of exposure versus nonexposure or treating versus not treating. RRR measures the extent to which an

Table 2-6. Hypothetical case-control study of stroke in relation to systolic hypertension.

Systolic blood pressure status[a]	Stroke		
	Present	Absent	Total
Stage 2 systolic hypertension	417 (a)	744 (b)	1,161 (a+b)
Normal blood pressure	83 (c)	752 (d)	835 (c+d)
Total	500 (a+c)	1,496 (b+d)	1,996 (a+b+c+d)

[a]Stage 2 systolic hypertension is defined as systolic blood pressure ≥160 mm Hg; normal blood pressure is defined as systolic blood pressure <120 mm Hg.

exposure (therapy) reduces a risk, in comparison with individuals in the unexposed group (not receiving therapy). It is usually expressed as a proportion of risk in the untreated group. In other words, RRR is the difference in the event rates expressed as a proportion of the event rate in the unexposed group. RRR can be calculated as follows:

$$RRR = \frac{R_u - R_e}{R_u}$$

As discussed in the Risk Ratio section, RR is the ratio of the risk of event (developing the disease or death) in exposed individuals to that in unexposed individuals. Then the RRR equation can be rewritten as:

$$RR = 1 - \frac{R_e}{R_u} = 1 - RR$$

To illustrate the calculation of RRR, let us turn to Table 2-7. Table 2-7 shows the results of a retrospective cohort study of a new drug in the primary prevention of heart attack in high-risk individuals. In this cohort study, individuals in the treated group received this new drug for 3 years; individuals in the untreated group did not receive the new drug. The primary endpoint was the occurrence of heart attack.

From Table 2-7, the proportion (risk) of the untreated group who experienced at least one heart attack was 9.5%; the proportion of the treated group who experienced at least one heart attack was 7.5%.

$$RRR = \frac{9.5\% - 7.5\%}{9.5\%} = 21.0\%$$

Therefore, we conclude that the RRR with the new drug is 21%. Note that this example is oversimplified.

Table 2-7. Results of a hypothetical cohort study to evaluate the therapeutic effect of a new drug to prevent heart attack in high-risk population.

Drug treatment	Heart attack		
	Present	Absent	Total
Yes	75	925	1,000
No	95	905	1,000
Total	170	1,830	2,000

Please refer to Chapter 3 for a detailed explanation of cohort study and Chapter 6 for bias and confounding in epidemiologic studies.

Absolute Risk Reduction

ARR is the simplest measure of therapeutic effect. ARR is defined as the absolute value of the arithmetic difference in the event rates of the exposed (or treated) and unexposed (or untreated) groups; it is also called risk difference. ARR can be calculated as follows:

$$ARR = |\, R_e - R_u \,|$$

In the example in Table 2-7, ARR was calculated as $|7.5\% - 9.5\%| = 2.0\%$; that is, the difference between the heart attack rates in the treated and the untreated groups is 2.0%. Note that unlike RRR, ARR does not give any idea of the proportional reduction between the treated and untreated groups. ARR becomes small when the event rates are low in both the treated and the untreated groups, whereas the estimation of RRR often is not influenced by the magnitude of the event rates. When the event rate in the treated group is greater than that of the untreated group, this absolute measure of risk difference is also referred to as absolute risk increase. Note that ARR is sometimes referred to as attributable risk in the epidemiology literature. However, the term *attributable risk* has also been used to describe several other different concepts. To avoid confusion, it is recommended that the term *attributable risk* be avoided completely.[15]

Number Needed to Treat

NNT is a measure related to ARR. It is defined as the number of individuals who would have to receive the treatment for one of them to benefit from the treatment over a specified period of time.[33,34] It is usually expressed as the reciprocal of the ARR. For example, how many people with diabetes would have to be treated with oral hypoglycemic agents for

5 years to avoid one death due to diabetes complications? NNT is useful both on a large scale when treatments are compared and on the individual level when treatment decisions are made. When a particular individual is given a treatment, NNT also reflects the likelihood this individual will benefit from the treatment. A calculated NNT of 10 indicates that for a given treatment to be beneficial to one person, 10 persons would have to be treated with the particular therapy. When treatment is administered to an individual, a NNT of 10 also indicates that for each person who received the treatment, he or she would have a 1 in 10 chance of benefiting from the treatment.[33]

If ARR is large, the calculated NNT would be small, which means that only a small number of persons need to be treated for one of them to benefit. However, it should be noted that NNTs can only be directly compared when the same outcome of treatments are evaluated.[33] For example, a NNT of 5 for a minor benefit, such as preventing people from getting common cold, may be less important than a NNT of 10 for preventing people from having a heart attack.

Number Needed to Harm

In medicine, treatments, including drugs and other therapeutic interventions, may harm patients in many different ways; some are mild, and some may be severe, resulting in disability or death. The relative significance of harms caused by drugs and other therapies depends on the condition being treated and the nature and severity of the harm. For example, in a minor illness such as common cold, a potentially life-threatening adverse event would not be acceptable even if the chance of experiencing the adverse event is small. If a condition is fatal in itself, the risk of death or disability from the treatment is likely to be acceptable.[35] NNH is a measure of the number of persons who would have to be treated for one person to experience an adverse event. It is calculated as 1 divided by the absolute risk increase. A large NNH indicates that adverse events are rare, whereas a small NNH suggests adverse events are common.

Uses of Association Measures in Pharmacoepidemiology

With the help of tools in epidemiology, pharmacoepidemiology studies are able to generate knowledge on who uses a drug, for what reasons (diagnoses), and when patients use the drug. Pharmacoepidemiology is also able to generate knowledge on the associations between drug uses and health outcomes, such as cases cured or improved, negative outcomes prevented, adverse drug events, and mortality.

For example, in a prospective cohort study of patients aged 18 years or older, who stayed in a large academic medical center for 3 or more days during 2004 to 2007, Herzig et al.[36] examined the association between acid-suppressive medication use and hospital-acquired pneumonia. Among a total of 63,878 eligible hospital admissions, they found that acid-suppressive medication was used in 52% of them and hospital-acquired pneumonia occurred in 3.5% of admissions. After controlling for confounders (see Chapters 5 and 6 for a detailed explanation of confounding and confounders) using multivariable logistic regression and matched propensity-score analysis (see Chapters 5 and 6 for more on multivariable logistic regression and matched propensity-score analysis), they reported that the adjusted OR of hospital-acquired pneumonia was 1.3 [95% confidence interval (95% CI), 1.1–1.4] in the group exposed to acid-suppressive medication, which means that use of acid-suppressive medication was associated with a 30% increase in the odds of hospital-acquired pneumonia. In subset analyses, the association was only significant for proton-pump inhibitors (OR, 1.3; 95% CI, 1.1–1.4) but not for histamine$_2$-receptor antagonists (OR, 1.2; 95% CI, 0.98–1.4). In this pharmacoepidemiologic cohort study, the association between exposure (acid-suppressive medication use) and outcome (incidence of hospital-acquired pneumonia) was measured using the OR, which is a good approximation of the RR, because the incidence of event was low (3.5%).

SUMMARY

In this chapter, we first discussed different approaches to measuring disease morbidity and mortality. Incidence and prevalence are two basic measures of morbidity. Incidence measures the occurrence of new cases, and prevalence measures existing cases of a disease. Many mortality measures that are commonly used in public health have also been discussed and differentiated. We have also reviewed ways of measuring associations of exposures and outcomes in epidemiology. All these commonly used measures in epidemiology can be applied to study drug uses and drug effects in populations.

DISCUSSION QUESTIONS

1. What is the relationship between disease incidence and prevalence? Give two examples of uses of incidence and prevalence measures in pharmacoepidemiology.

2. What is the best measure to estimate the rapidity with which new cases of H1N1 influenza occur among students on a college campus?

3. Suppose that in a population of 1,000 people, 20 people die. Can you calculate a crude mortality rate based on the data? Explain.

4. What is the best mortality measure to estimate the likelihood of death for patients diagnosed with breast cancer?

5. Briefly describe the main similarities and differences between each of the following:

    a. Incidence and prevalence

    b. Cumulative incidence and incidence rate

    c. Crude mortality rate and age-adjusted mortality rate

    d. Relative risk reduction and absolute risk reduction

6. Suppose that a city has a population of 13,000 on July 1, 2009. About 150 new cases of diabetes occurred between January 1 and December 31, 2009. The total number of individuals with diabetes was 1,430 in 2009, and 26 individuals died from diabetes in 2009. What is the incident rate of diabetes in 2009? What is the prevalence of diabetes in 2009? What is the case fatality of diabetes?

7. Explain how to interpret risk ratio and odds ratio estimates.

REFERENCES

1. Strom BL, Kimmel SE. *Textbook of Pharmacoepidemiology.* West Sussex, England: John Wiley & Sons Ltd, 2006.
2. Gordis L. Introduction. *Epidemiology,* 4th ed. Philadelphia, PA: Elsevier Saunders, 2009:3-17.
3. Giesecke J. What is special about infectious epidemiology? *Modern Infectious Disease Epidemiology,* 2nd ed. London, UK: Arnold, 2002:3-7.
4. McKenna MT, Taylor WR, Marks JS, Koplan JP. Current issues and challenges in chronic disease control. In: Brownson RC, Remington P, Davis JR, eds. *Chronic Disease Epidemiology and Control,* 2nd ed. Washington, DC: American Public Health Association, 1998:1-26.
5. Wilson PW. Established risk factors and coronary artery disease: The Framingham Study. *Am J Hypertens.* 1994;7(7 Pt 2):7S-12S.
6. Wilson PW, D'Agostino RB, Levy D, Belanger AM, Silbershatz H, Kannel WB. Prediction of coronary heart disease using risk factor categories. *Circulation.* 1998;97(18): 1837-1847.
7. Aschengrau A, Seage GR III. Measures of Disease Frequency. In: *Essentials of Epidemiology in Public Health.* SudBury, MA: Jones and Bartlett Publishers, 2003:33-57.
8. Last JM. *Dictionary of Epidemiology,* 2nd ed. New York: Oxford University Press, 1988.
9. Heron M, Hoyert DL, Murphy SL, Xu J, Kochanek KD, Tejada-Vera B. Deaths: Final data for 2006. *Natl Vital Stat Rep.* 2009;57(14):1-134.
10. U.S. Census Bureau. Profiles of general demographic characteristics. *2000 Census of Population and Housing.* U.S. Census Bureau Web site. http://www.census.gov/prod/cen2000/dp1/2kh00.pdf. Accessed January 26, 2010.
11. National Quality Measures Clearinghouse Web site. http://www.qualitymeasures.ahrq.gov/summary/summary.aspx?doc_id=13201. Accessed January 26, 2010.
12. Rothman KJ, Greenland S. Measures of occurrence. In: Rothman KJ, Greenland S, Lash TL, eds. *Modern Epidemiology,* 3rd ed. Philadelphia, PA: Lippincott Williams & Wilkins, 2010: 32-50.
13. National Cancer Institute Web site. http://seer.cancer.gov/statfacts/html/breast.html. Accessed January 26, 2010
14. Gordis L. Measuring the occurrence of disease: I. Morbidity. In: *Epidemiology,* 4th ed. Philadelphia, PA: Elsevier Saunders, 2009:37-58.
15. Greenland S, Rothman KJ, Lash TL. Measures of effect and measures of association. In: Rothman KJ, Greenland S, Lash TL, eds. *Modern Epidemiology,* 3nd ed. Philadelphia, PA: Lippincott Williams &Wilkins, 2008:51-70.
16. Greenberg RS, Daniels SR, Flanders WD, Eley JW, Boring JR. Epidemiologic measures. In: *Medical Epidemiology,* 2nd ed. Stamford, CT: Appleton & Lange, 1996:15-26.
17. Stockl KM, Tjioe D, Gong S, Stroup J, Harada AS, Lew HC. Effect of an intervention to increase statin use in Medicare

members who qualified for a medication therapy management program. *J Manag Care Pharm.* 2008;14(6):532-540.

18. Thomsen RW, Riis A, Kornum JB, Christensen S, Johnsen SP, Sorensen HT. Preadmission use of statins and outcomes after hospitalization with pneumonia: Population-based cohort study of 29,900 patients. *Arch Intern Med.* 2008;168(19): 2081-2087.

19. Morgan O, Griffiths C, Majeed A. Antidepressant prescribing and changes in antidepressant poisoning mortality and suicide in England, 1993–2004. *J Public Health (Oxf).* 2008;30(1): 60-68.

20. Anderson RN, Rosenberg HM. Age standardization of death rates: Implementation of the year 2000 standard. *Natl Vital Stat Rep.* 1998;47(3):1-16, 20.

21. U.S. Census Bureau Web site. http://www.census.gov/popest/states/NST-ann-est2006.html. Accessed January 26, 2010.

22. Gordis L. Measuring the occurrence of disease: II. Mortality. In: *Epidemiology,* 4th ed. Philadelphia, PA: Elsevier Saunders, 2009:59-84.

23. American Heart Association Web site. http://www.american heart.org/presenter.jhtml?identifier=4478. Accessed January 26, 2010.

24. Centers for Disease Control and Prevention Web site. http://www.cdc.gov/nchs/icd/icd10.htm. Accessed January 26, 2010.

25. Centers for Disease Control and Prevention. Update: Influenza activity—United States, August 30–October 31, 2009. Available at CDC Web site. http://www.cdc.gov/mmwr/preview/mmwrhtml/mm5902a3.htm. Accessed January 26, 2010.

26. Black WC, Haggstrom DA, Welch HG. All-cause mortality in randomized trials of cancer screening. *J Natl Cancer Inst.* 2002;94(3):167-173.

27. Kopans DB, Halpern E. Re: All-cause mortality in randomized trials of cancer screening. *J Natl Cancer Inst.* 2002;94(11): 863-866.

28. Ho PM, Rumsfeld JS, Masoudi FA, et al. Effect of medication nonadherence on hospitalization and mortality among patients with diabetes mellitus. *Arch Intern Med.* 2006;166(17): 1836-1841.

29. Wysowski DK, Nourjah P, Swartz L. Bleeding complications with warfarin use: A prevalent adverse effect resulting in regulatory action. *Arch Intern Med.* 2007;167(13):1414-1419.

30. Bristol-Myers Squibb Company Web site. http://www.access data.fda.gov/drugsatfda_docs/label/2006/009218s102lbl.pdf. Accessed January 26, 2010.

31. Szklo M, Nieto FJ. Measuring associations between exposures and outcomes. In: *Epidemiology: Beyond the Basics.* Gaithersburg, MD: Aspen Publishers, Inc., 2000:91-121.

32. Agresti A. Contingency tables. In: *An Introduction to Categorical Data Analysis,* 2nd ed. New York: John Wiley & Sons, Inc., 2007:21-64.

33. Barratt A, Wyer PC, Hatala R, et al. Tips for learners of evidence-based medicine: 1. Relative risk reduction, absolute risk reduction and number needed to treat. *CMAJ.* 2004;171(4): 353-358.

34. Schechtman E. Odds ratio, relative risk, absolute risk reduction, and the number needed to treat—which of these should we use? *Value Health.* 2002;5(5):431-436.

35. Zermansky A. Number needed to harm should be measured for treatments. *BMJ.* 1998;317(7164):1014.

36. Herzig SJ, Howell MD, Ngo LH, Marcantonio ER. Acid-suppressive medication use and the risk for hospital-acquired pneumonia. *JAMA.* 2009;301(20):2120-2128.

Study Designs for Pharmacoepidemiology

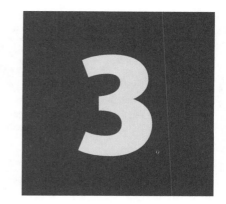

Spencer E. Harpe

▼ OBJECTIVES

At the end of the chapter, the reader will be able to:

1. Identify the general purposes of research
2. Discuss the important principles of study design
3. Distinguish between experimental, quasi-experimental, and observational approaches to pharmacoepidemiologic research
4. Describe various quasi-experimental study designs used in pharmacoepidemiology
5. Describe various observational study designs used in pharmacoepidemiology
6. Discuss the relative advantages and disadvantages of the various study designs
7. Describe the role of meta-analysis in pharmacoepidemiology

OVERVIEW OF STUDY DESIGN

▶ Purposes of Research

Before selecting a particular study design, it is important to consider the general goal of performing a given research study. It can be useful to categorize a study as serving one of three general purposes: description, identification/exploration of associations, or determination of causal relationships (Table 3-1). Because certain study designs may be better suited than others for a given research purpose, identifying what is expected from the standpoint of the research objective can help in guiding the selection of an appropriate study design. For example, if the goal is to identify potential risk factors for a given outcome, selecting a study design that merely describes the occurrence of the outcome will be of little value.

Another way of conceptualizing the purpose of research is to determine whether one wants to develop potential hypotheses (i.e., hypothesis generation) or to formally test hypotheses that were previously developed (i.e., hypothesis testing). The traditional epidemiologic designs (e.g., cohort and case-control) are useful in allowing a researcher to develop hypotheses. The process of formally testing a

Table 3-1. General purposes of research and examples.

Purpose	Potential study designs	Example research questions
Description	Case studies, case series, prevalence studies, cross-sectional studies	• How many patients are adherent to the drug regimen? • How many physicians switch drug therapy because of adverse effects?
Identification/exploration of associations	Quasi-experiments, cohort studies, case-control studies, cross-sectional studies	• What factors are associated with patient adherence to drug therapy? • Are physicians who switch drug therapy more likely to have patients reporting adverse effects than those who do not switch therapy?
Determination of causal relationships	Randomized controlled trials, quasi-experiments	• Does a new patient adherence program result in increased adherence? • Does the introduction of a new electronic alert reduce the rate of the prescribing of inappropriate medications?

hypothesis is aimed at making some causal statement (e.g., taking drug X will cause a reduction in blood pressure) and is frequently the underlying purpose of conducting research.[1] Some sort of interventional study, such as a randomized controlled trial or a quasi-experiment, is usually considered necessary to test a hypothesis formally and arrive at a causal conclusion; however, advances in statistical techniques have increased the strength of causal statements from some observational study designs.[2] A more formal discussion about principles of causality is provided in Chapter 6.

▶ Principles of Study Design

When designing research studies, certain concepts are important to consider regardless of the particular approach being used. The ability to make accurate statements or conclusions is arguably one of the most important considerations. This idea of accuracy is at the core of the concept of *validity*. The concept of validity can be separated into two complementary parts: *internal validity* and *external validity*.[3] One common way of conceptualizing internal validity is the degree to which any statements of effects are actually the result of the exposure of interest (e.g., some drug or program) and not from some other interfering variable. External validity can be thought of as the extent to which the conclusions from a given study

can be extended, or generalized, beyond the current sample and target population to the general population or to another setting. Randomized controlled trials (RCTs) are typically designed to maximize internal validity, which is necessary to make firm causal statements. Unfortunately, this can be at the expense of external validity. One of the strengths of the epidemiological approach to research is that it uses data outside of experimental settings, which can increase the potential external validity. This is one reason why RCTs are useful in assessing drug efficacy, whereas other epidemiologic study designs are useful in examining drug effectiveness.[4] Validity is most often affected by the introduction of some sort of *systematic error*, or *bias*, through inappropriate study design, improper subject sampling, or inappropriate data analysis. Common threats to internal validity in the epidemiologic context include confounding bias, selection bias, and information bias.[3] These are discussed in greater detail in Chapter 6.

In addition to validity, *reliability* is another important concept when designing studies. Reliability is often described as the precision of an estimate, its consistency over time or across study subjects, or the extent to which the estimate is reproducible. Within the context of the measurement process, reliability can be thought of as being affected by *random error*. Any measurement theoretically includes both systematic and random errors, but the measurement process should be developed such that both of these sources of error are minimized.[5] When considering exposure to a drug, self-reported drug use, for example, may be a less reliable measurement method than using data from prescription claims.

The process of study design involves both selecting the appropriate design for the research question at hand and the development and implementation of procedures to ensure that valid conclusions can be made. In order to arrive at these valid conclusions, care must be taken to minimize bias and to ensure appropriate measurement and analysis methods. There are various methods available to reduce bias, but they can generally be classified based on whether they are implemented when designing the study or when performing the statistical analyses.[6,7] These methods are discussed in Chapters 5 and 6.

▶ Reporting Guidelines

There are various guidelines that provide guidance to researchers in reporting the results of research studies. Although these are commonly used when preparing the results of a study for publication, they can be useful even when designing pharmacoepidemiologic studies since the concepts important in the accurate and transparent reporting of study results can be helpful when considering the design of a study. The Consolidated Standards of Reporting Trials (CONSORT) guidelines[8] for RCTs are probably the most familiar of the reporting statements; however, they are focused on RCTs. The same principles motivating CONSORT's development have resulted in a variety of other guidelines that may be of use in conducting pharmacoepidemiologic research. Table 3-2 provides some common reporting guidelines that may be of particular interest.

EXPERIMENTAL AND QUASI-EXPERIMENTAL DESIGNS

Collectively, *experimental* and *quasi-experimental* study designs can be conceptualized as interventional studies since the researcher is, to varying degrees, actively implementing some intervention or treatment. Although there are other differences, the primary characteristic that distinguishes an experimental design from a quasi-experimental design is that randomization of subjects to treatment groups is not performed in quasi-experiments.[9] *Randomization* or *random assignment* is the process of assigning individuals to one or more groups based on an accepted method that gives each subject the same probability of being in any given group (e.g., treatment or placebo group). The RCT is routinely viewed as the strongest design in biomedical research from the standpoint of testing hypotheses and making firm causal conclusions.[2,10] RCTs are probably familiar to most readers given their routine use in the biomedical literature. Quasi-experiments on the other hand may be less familiar and are discussed in slightly more detail.

In the more traditional sense, epidemiologic studies do not involve active manipulation of some variable of interest (i.e., an intervention). Instead, epidemiologists use observational methods that seek to determine a subject's exposure status as accurately as possible. There are, however, some situations where an interventional approach may be useful in studying drug usage, such as when some program has been developed to improve the use of drugs (e.g., appropriate prescribing). For example, Saltvedt et al.[11] used a randomized trial to examine prescribing patterns among frail older adult patients admitted to the hospital. Upon admission, each patient was randomized to either the geriatric evaluation and management unit or the general medical ward. Appropriate prescribing, as defined by the Beers' criteria,[12] was compared between the two groups. At the end of the study, the authors found prescribing patterns that were significantly better among those patients randomized to the geriatric unit instead of the general medical ward.

As mentioned previously, the absence of random assignment to treatment groups is an important characteristic of quasi-experiments. One general quasi-experimental approach that is particularly useful in pharmacoepidemiologic research is the *interrupted time series design*. This design involves repeated measurements taken before and after an intervention or distinct change occurs. This design is often used to evaluate the effects associated with the implementation of a new program or policy. For example, this design may be used when a formulary change is made to determine the impact of the formulary change on

Table 3-2. Reporting statements or guidelines that can be useful when conducting pharmacoepidemiologic research.

Guideline/statement	Comments
Strengthening the Reporting of Observational Trials in Epidemiology (STROBE)	Includes information unique to various epidemiologic study designs; does not necessarily address issues unique to the use of secondary databases; published in *Ann Intern Med.* 2007;147(8):573-577 or available online at www.strobe-statement.org
Transparent Reporting of Evaluations with Nonrandomized Designs (TREND)	Originally developed for behavioral and public health interventions; particularly useful with quasi-experiments; published in *Am J Public Health.* 2004;94(3):361-366 or available online at www.trend-statement.org
ISPE Guidelines for Good Pharmacoepidemiology Practices	Provides guidelines to assist researchers with issues surrounding the planning, conduct, and evaluation of pharmacoepidemiologic research; separate sections are included for adverse event reporting and communicating results; published in *Pharmacoepidemiol Drug Saf.* 2008;17(2):200-208
ISPOR Checklist for Retrospective Database Studies	Addresses issues unique to the use of retrospective databases for research purposes; may be used with other reporting guidelines; published in *Value Health.* 2003;6(2):90-97 or available online at www.ispor.org/ workpaper/healthscience/ret_dbTFR0203.asp
ISPOR Checklist for Medication Compliance and Adherence Studies Using Retrospective Data	Addresses issues unique to the use of retrospective databases in studies looking at drug compliance and persistence; may be used with other reporting guidelines; published in *Value Health.* 2007;10(1):3-12 or available online at www.ispor.org/workpaper/MedComplianceChecklist.asp
Standards for Quality Improvement Reporting Excellence (SQUIRE)	Developed to help authors to improve the reporting of quality improvement efforts; focuses on accurately and consistently reporting local efforts to improve care so that they might be applied at other sites; published in *Qual Saf Health Care.* 2008;17(suppl. 1):i13-i32 or available online at www.squire-statement.org
Preferred Reporting Items for Systematic Reviews and Meta-Analyses (PRISMA)	Developed to guide authors in conducting and reporting systematic reviews and meta-analyses of randomized controlled trials; formerly known as the QUOROM statement; published in *Ann Intern Med.* 2009;151(4):264-269 or available online at www.prisma-statement.org
Meta-analysis of Observational Studies in Epidemiology (MOOSE)	Similar to the PRISMA statement except that it is aimed at meta-analyses of observational studies; published in *J Am Med Assoc.* 2000;283(15):2008-2012

ISPOR, International Society for Pharmacoeconomics and Outcomes Research; ISPE, International Society for Pharmacoepidemiology. Modified, with permission, from Ref. 57.

physician prescribing behavior. Some variations of this general design involve the addition of a control group that did not experience the intervention or event of interest or the subsequent removal (or revocation) of the intervention of interest (Figure 3-1). These designs are particularly useful in situations where randomization is not possible (e.g., a policy is applied to everyone in the population), but data are available to allow repeated measurements before and after the change. By examining the trend in the observations before the intervention or change in policy, the researcher can establish a pattern of the outcome of interest that can be compared with the pattern after the intervention or change. For example, Chen et al.[13] examined the monthly usage of antidepressants and antipsychotics for the 12-month period before and the 12-month period after Medicare Part D was implemented. The authors noted a steady increase in antidepressant usage before the implementation of Medicare Part D. After Medicare Part D was implemented, the upward trend in monthly antidepressant use increased significantly. With

Nonequivalent control group design

```
    O   X   O
    -------
    O       O
```

Interrupted time series designs

(a) O O O O O O O O X O O O O O O O O

(b) O O O O O O O O X O O O O O O O O

     O O O O O O O O   O O O O O O O O

(c) O O O O O O O O ✗ O O O O O O O O

▲ **Figure 3-1.** Selected quasi-experimental designs that may be useful in pharmacoepidemiologic research. O represent time points where an observation or measurement took place (e.g., the use of a given drug during a month), X represents the initiation of some intervention, program, or policy (e.g., implementation of pharmacists consultation for drug selection among frail older adults), and ✗ represents the removal (or elimination) of the program, policy, or intervention. Keep in mind that an X may be something that is under the control of the researcher or something of interest that happened during the time period that was not under the direct control of the researcher (e.g., a change in institutional policy).

antipsychotics there was a trend of decreased use of antipsychotic agents before Medicare Part D. That trend actually reversed and antipsychotic use increased in the months after Part D coverage began. Time series designs are quite useful in examining how events that affect entire groups of people simultaneously, such as the introduction of Medicare Part D[14,15] or the introduction of various quality improvement activities[16,17] or direct-to-consumer advertising,[18] may influence drug use.

Another quasi-experimental design that may be of use in pharmacoepidemiologic research is the *nonequivalent control group design* (Figure 3-1). This design can be thought of as similar to the traditional RCT except that group membership is determined through some nonrandom process. Given that the allocation of subjects to treatment groups is no

longer a random process, the groups cannot be considered "equivalent" in the statistical sense, hence the term "nonequivalent" in the name of the design. The nonequivalent control group design is quite strong from an internal validity standpoint.

Two common situations give rise to nonrandom group membership. One is *self-selection* whereby some intervention is offered to an individual subject who determines whether or not to participate (e.g., an automatic refill program offered by a community pharmacy to improve medication adherence). The fact that the treatment groups were not formed by random assignment leaves the potential for *selection bias*, which is probably the most important threat to internal validity for this design. The extent of selection bias can vary depending on how the groups were formed, with self-selection offering a greater chance for bias than other methods.[19]

The other common situation is where the researcher is working with subjects that are in preformed groups (e.g., patients using a particular physician's practice, health care providers within a particular hospital or in a particular geographic area). Although this situation may seem like self-selection, the difference is that the intervention is applied categorically to one or more groups rather than being offered to one subject at a time. Quality improvement initiatives that are applied to groups of health care providers within a geographic region are one example of the idea of applying an intervention to an intact group. For example, Martens et al.[20] examined the effects of disseminating cooperatively developed multidisciplinary guidelines on prescribing behavior in the Netherlands. A random selection of providers in the Maastricht region served as the intervention group, while a random selection of providers outside the region was used as the control group. A similar study was carried out in Wisconsin by sending letters about the appropriate use of dipyridamole to providers in three sections of the state with a fourth section serving as the control group.[21]

There are a number of other experimental and quasi-experimental studies that are less commonly used in pharmacoepidemiologic research. These studies have been used to varying degrees in other areas of health care research, such as medical informatics[22] and quality improvement.[23] Given the relative low frequency of their use in pharmacoepidemiology, a detailed discussion is not provided here.[a]

OBSERVATIONAL DESIGNS

In the absence of experimentation, observational studies have a long, albeit somewhat controversial, history of use in biomedical research.[10,24–27] In many situations, however, intervening in a population is not possible from either an experimental or a quasi-experimental standpoint. Moreover, in some situations, experimentation may be unnecessary, inappropriate, or even unethical.[7] It is becoming increasingly recognized that RCTs are probably not the best research approach to use when examining patterns of drug use or the outcomes of drug use, especially in safety-related outcomes where premarketing studies frequently lack sufficient sample sizes to detect anything but relatively common adverse effects.[28,29] Still, observational study designs are extremely useful in the study of the use of drugs and their associated outcomes, including unintended beneficial effects of drugs.[30]

▶ Case Reports and Case Series

The role of the *case report* and the *case series* cannot be ignored from a study design perspective. A case report is a study design that describes the clinical experience of one patient with a particular drug, whereas a case series is similar to a case report except that it describes the experience of multiple patients. Although these are only descriptive studies, they can provide useful information that serves as the basis for generating hypotheses for further refinement or formal testing. These types of studies are commonly seen as published adverse drug event reports. It is important to remember that these studies need not be limited only to unintended adverse drug effects, as they can be useful to identify novel uses of drugs or unintended beneficial effects that deserve future investigation.[31–33] Given the design of these studies, there is typically no manner of control or randomization. As such, these reports do not offer sufficient evidence to make any causal determinations. They can, however, be useful in further clarifying previously determined causal relationships.[34]

▶ Ecologic Studies

In some situations, data are not available at the individual *patient level*, but *group*, or *aggregate*, *level data* may be available. One may ask why group-level data may be available instead of at the patient level. There can be situations where obtaining patient-level data is either cost-prohibitive or almost infeasible given the regulations surrounding health care data. One way to work around this is to gather information in the aggregate so that individuals are not identified (or even approached). For example, it might be quite difficult (from a logistical and/or regulatory standpoint) for a researcher to gather patient-level data from a local chain of community pharmacies or from a group of health plans. On the other hand, it may be easier to obtain the number of prescriptions dispensed or the number of claims approved for a certain drug. Using these aggregate-level data result in *ecologic studies*. Some group-level data commonly used in pharmacoepidemiology involve drug usage at the national or state level. Similar situations can arise when entire physician practices, health plans, or hospitals are examined. It is not uncommon to see ecological studies conducted over multiple time points to examine trends. Case Study 3-1 describes an example of an ecological study using hospital-level data over multiple years to examine the relationship between antibiotic use and bacterial resistance.[35]

Although ecological studies can be useful, it is important to understand their limitations. The major drawback of an ecological study is that *confounding* can be a particularly important source of bias since information is not collected at the individual patient level. In patient-level studies, this extra information could be controlled for through statistical analysis. Ecological studies must be interpreted carefully to avoid the *ecological fallacy*, or the fallacy of making conclusions at the individual patient level when only aggregate data are used. This is the complement to the *atomistic fallacy* where conclusions for the aggregate level are made when the data are collected on individual patients.[36] Typically, the same *unit of analysis* is

---

[a]See Ref. 19 for more information on causal inference from quasi-experimentation.

An Ecological Study of the Relationship Between Fluoroquinolone Use and Bacterial Resistance

Bacterial resistance to antibiotic agents is an important concern within health care. One of the commonly cited causes of resistance is the increased, and often inappropriate, use of antibiotics, especially broad-spectrum agents. MacDougall et al.[35] used an ecological approach to examine the relationship between fluoroquinolone use and resistance in Pseudomonas aeruginosa and Staphylococcus aureus in a group of hospitals. Information on the use of levofloxacin, moxifloxacin, gatifloxacin, and ciprofloxacin by each hospital was collected as the number of defined daily doses (DDD; see Chapter 4) and normalized to 1,000 patient days (i.e., DDD/1,000 patient days). Similarly, hospital-level bacterial resistance was measured as the percentage of isolates of P. aeruginosa resistant to fluo-roquinolones and the percentage of isolates of S. aureus labeled as methicillin-resistant S. aureus (MRSA). These data were collected annually for each participating hospital over the period from 1999 to 2003. Using linear regression analysis, the level of fluoroquinolone usage was associated with P. aeruginosa and S. aureus resistance in the same year for 3 of the 5 years examined. Similar results were found when the analysis was repeated separately for levofloxacin and ciprofloxacin. When the method of generalized estimating equations was used to take into account previous levels of resistance (i.e., the relationship between fluoroquinolone usage and resistance in 2001 taking into account the level of resistance in 2000), the only significant relationship was between levofloxacin use and MRSA.

used for both the exposure and the outcome variables. For example if drug use is measured at the state level, then state-level outcome data (e.g., mortality rates and disease incidence rates specific to the states under study) are considered. With the increased availability and use of multilevel modeling techniques,[36,37] more studies are incorporating both aggregate and patient-level data into the same study.[38,39]

▶ Cross-Sectional Studies

As the name implies, a *cross-sectional study* involves looking at a sample of a population of interest at a given point in time (i.e., a cross-section), typically the present. Unlike the other epidemiologic study designs, the outcome of interest and the exposure of interest are determined simultaneously (Figure 3-2). This requires only one, single data collection point, which provides certain efficiencies from logistical and financial perspectives since the researcher does not have to wait for an outcome to occur. Although cross-sectional studies cannot provide estimates of incidence, they are well suited to provide estimates of the prevalence of a condition or exposure. In fact, cross-sectional studies may sometimes be referred to as prevalence studies. As an example, Stang et al.[40] conducted a study with a primary objective of describing the prevalence of the coprescription of contraindicated drugs with statins [i.e., 3-hydroxy-3-methylglutaryl (HMG) coenzyme A reductase inhibitors] despite warnings about the dangers of certain drug combinations. By describing the prevalence of the outcome in the exposed group and the prevalence of the outcome in the unexposed group, potential relationships between exposures and outcomes can be identified. These relationships should not, however, be interpreted as causal relationships due in large part to the inability to determine whether the exposure occurred before the outcome. Instead, they are best viewed as hypotheses for future examination and testing.

Although cross-sectional studies typically involve only one point in time, they can be conducted over multiple time points, or serial cross-sections. Liberman et al.[41] examined the use of antihypertensive, antidiabetic, and dyslipidemic medications in children and adolescents. The authors used data from a large pharmacy benefits management firm to examine

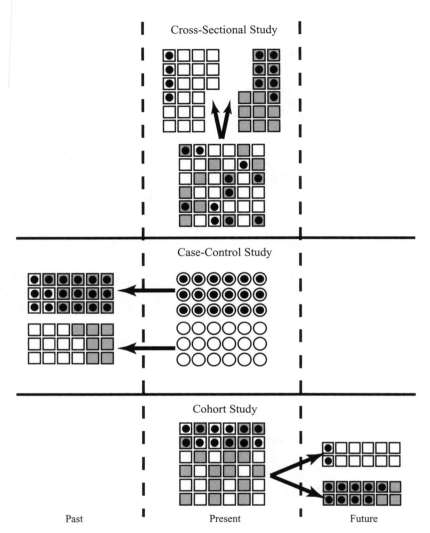

▲ **Figure 3-2.** Observational study designs that may be used in pharmacoepidemiologic research. A shaded square represents an exposed subject while unexposed subjects are not shaded. A solid circle within the square represents an outcome of interest is present. Those squares without the circle are outcome free.

the monthly prevalence of each of these drug classes from September 2004 to June 2007. Studies with multiple cross-sections are useful to examine changes in prevalence across time and may be used to approximate data from a similarly conducted longitudinal study; however, this is contingent on accurate data collection within the data source.[42]

True longitudinal studies, such as cohort studies, are stronger than multiple cross-sections since there are multiple measurements for each subject over time allowing each subject to serve as its own control and because the exposure is known to have occurred before the outcome. Longitudinal studies offer the ability to look at changes both within the study unit and across units. Unlike cross-sectional studies, changes within individuals can be separated from individual baseline differences in true longitudinal studies.[43]

▶ Case-Control Studies

Case-control studies are a widely used study design within epidemiology.[44] These studies can be particularly useful when the outcome being examined is relatively rare. This is one reason that case-control studies have been frequently used to study the adverse effects of drugs, such as in cancer[45,46] or renal failure,[47] or the occurrence of prescribing errors.[48] Case-control studies begin by identifying a sample of individuals with the outcome of interest (e.g., cancer or death) to serve as the cases and another sample without the outcome of interest to serve as the controls (Figure 3-2). Within both of these samples, the researcher then determines the exposure status of each individual. The relative proportions of those exposed within the cases are compared with those in the controls giving rise to the *odds ratio* (odds of exposure in cases vs. odds of exposure in controls).[49] Case-control studies offer a certain amount of efficiency over prospective approaches since the study begins with the outcome of interest rather than waiting for the outcome to occur. Like cross-sectional studies, the case-control approach is particularly useful for developing hypotheses. Case-control studies are also useful in that they allow the examination of multiple exposures or risk factors of interest for a given outcome. As long as sufficient data are available, the relationships between any number of different exposures and the outcome could be examined, but it is important to ensure that the exposure occurred prior to the outcome. To do this, each case can be assigned an index date based on the date the outcome was noted. Exposure status is then determined in the period before the index date. Although controls would not have an actual index date since the outcome did not occur, an index date may be assigned to them that is the same as their matched control (if cases and controls are matched) or randomly selected based on the study period or from the available index dates of the cases.

Although the incidence of an outcome cannot be estimated from a case-control study because the entire population at risk is not identified at the start of the study, the odds ratio calculated from a case-control study should be a valid estimate of the rate ratio or risk ratio in certain circumstances. First, the cases are representative of the identified source population. Depending on the size of the population, all cases may be used or a random sample can be drawn. Both of these should result in cases that are representative. Second, controls should be selected from the same population that gave rise to the cases. Given the relatively larger size of the pool of potential controls, it is not uncommon to see random sampling performed for control selection. Finally, the controls should be sampled without respect to exposure status.[44,49] One way to ensure this is to develop and apply the same eligibility criteria to both cases and controls.[34]

There are, however, a number of important drawbacks to consider. First, case-control studies can be particularly susceptible to certain biases as further described in Chapter 6. From a *selection bias* standpoint, cases and/or controls who are included in a study may be systematically different than those who are not included. When the process of study inclusion or participation is also related to exposure or outcome, then the exposure–outcome relationship estimated from study could be biased. *Information bias* can be another important consideration. Within case-control studies, information bias could be the result of measurement error or misclassification. This latter concept is particularly worrisome when it occurs in a differential manner. For example, in studies examining the adverse effects of drugs, it is possible that cases (i.e., those with the adverse outcome of interest) have more data collected and possibly collected in greater detail than controls who came from the general population. This differential misclassification is problematic as it may result in an unpredictable overestimation or underestimation of potential relationships between the exposure and outcome.[3] *Recall bias* is also an important source of bias that can be conceptualized as a type of information bias. Whenever exposure, or outcome, information is gathered by self-report or interview, the potential for error is larger. For example, those individuals experiencing an adverse event, or even the health care providers of those individuals, may be more likely to remember detailed information about their drug use than those without an adverse event. The use of data from automated collection sources or from information recorded before outcome occurrence can help reduce the potential for information bias.[50] Another potential drawback of case-control studies is that they are ill-suited to study drugs that are rarely used.[34]

One common variation of the case-control study is to match cases and controls on one or more extraneous variables thought to be confounders (see Chapter 6). Matching may be a useful tool to increase the accuracy and statistical power of a case-control study, but it also has some limitations, notably the introduction of bias in the estimation of the odds ratio. This limitation can be avoided by using an analytical strategy that takes the matching factor into account.[51] For example, in a matched case-control study one case might be matched to one control resulting in a series of matched pairs. The odds ratio should be calculated taking the matching into account in order to avoid biased estimates of the odds ratio or an underestimation of the standard error associated with the odds ratio as a result of the matching process.[52] This would be calculated as the ratio of the number of pairs where the controls were unexposed and the cases were exposed to the number of pairs where the controls were exposed and the cases were unexposed.[b] This is an example of how the chosen analytical strategy must be appropriate for the study design being used (see Chapter 5). Depending on the nature of the study, there may be more than one control matched with each case. A method to determine the appropriate number of matched controls has been suggested by Hennessy et al.[53]

---

[b]In a matched pair analysis (or individual matching), typically only those pairs where the exposure status of the case and control within the pair do not match are used (i.e., discordant pairs) in the analysis. This is because pairs where both cases and controls are exposed or both are unexposed (i.e., concordant pairs) do not contribute to the calculation of the odds ratio. For more information, see Ref. 52.

▶ Cohort Studies

The other commonly used study design in epidemiology is the *cohort study*. The cohort study approach may be desirable when the intentional exposure of a subject to some drug or intervention, as in an experimental manner, is either impossible or unethical.[54] The general purpose of these studies is to estimate the risk or rate of some outcome among a cohort of individuals.[55] In order to estimate these values, all subjects in the study (i.e., the cohort) must be free from the outcome of interest when the study begins (Figure 3-2). The identification of an initial outcome-free cohort can be seen in contrast to the case-control study where a group of individuals with the outcome of interest and a group without the outcome are identified first. Once the initial study cohort is identified, each subject is classified based on exposure status. This allows the calculation of a risk or rate for each exposure status and the subsequent comparison through a risk ratio or rate ratio. Generally speaking, the cohort study can be viewed as a modified approach to an RCT where assignment to treatment group is not random and is not under the control of the researcher. For this reason, the cohort study is often seen as a strong method, more so than the case-control approach. The main reason for this methodological strength is that all subjects included in the study are known to be at risk for the outcome since they are outcome free at study initiation, just as in RCTs. The availability of outcome-free subjects and accurate exposure information allows temporal relationships between exposure and outcome to be identified, which is an important consideration in causal inference.[34,56]

Cohort studies may be conducted in a wholly prospective fashion where identification of the outcome-free cohort begins in the present and the subjects are followed into the future. Alternatively, *retrospective cohort* studies involve looking into the past to identify a point in time where the subjects were outcome free and then following them through to the present or into the future to determine whether an outcome occurs. The ability to conduct a retrospective cohort study depends on having sufficient information to facilitate the accurate determination of outcome status, as well as the

CASE STUDY 3-2

Retrospective Cohort Study of Thromboembolic Outcomes

The retrospective cohort study is a way to maintain methodological strength while gaining some efficiencies associated with using existing data. Doepker et al.[58] used a retrospective cohort approach to examine the relationship between incidence of venous thromboembolism (VTE) and the use of vasopressin in patients with shock. The authors examined the medical record to identify all patients aged 18 and older who were admitted to the surgical or medical intensive care unit from September 2001 to June 2004 with a diagnosis code for shock. To ensure that the selected subjects were free of the outcome at the beginning of the study, the authors excluded any patients admitted to the critical care units with active treatment for VTE. The authors also excluded subjects with a past history of VTE prior to vasopressin therapy, as well as those receiving vasopressin for any reason other than the treatment of shock (e.g., variceal hemorrhage). Using the above criteria, the authors
selected a random sample of 350 subjects for the study. With this designated study cohort, subjects were separated into two groups based on exposure status: vasopressin plus catecholamine therapy (e.g., epinephrine and dopamine) or catecholamine therapy alone. Each subject could have a different index (start) date based on admission to the critical care unit since this was an open cohort. Subjects' medical records were examined for the occurrence of VTE after initiation of vasopressin or catecholamine therapy. To reduce the potential for bias in identifying the outcome, the authors required positive evidence of a VTE from either a Doppler ultrasound or a spiral computer tomography scan or a documented diagnosis for VTE on the official hospital discharge summary. The incidence of VTE in the vasopressin group was 7.4% compared with 8% in the catecholamine therapy group. This was not significantly different and remained so after adjusting for potential confounders.

sequencing of exposure information. The use of secondary databases (see Chapter 4) may allow retrospective cohort studies to be conducted more easily.[57] Chart reviews within hospitals is one method of conducting a retrospective cohort study, such as the study by Doepker et al.[58] (see Case Study 3-2).

In addition to the prospective and retrospective options, cohort studies may also examine open or closed cohorts. An open cohort, or dynamic cohort, is one in which the size of the cohort is not fixed and can vary over time as individuals join and leave the cohort. Some sources recommend describing such studies as using an open, or dynamic, population rather than an open cohort.[56] Cohort studies using prescription-event monitoring data often involve open cohorts since individuals may enter or leave the cohort based on varying dates of drug initiation or stopping the drug before having an outcome under study. Open cohorts often include an "enrollment" period where outcome-free subjects can enter the study cohort. When referring to the exposed group, each subject's particular

index date, or start date, is defined as the initiation of exposure, such as the first filled prescription of a particular drug.[50] For unexposed individuals, the index date would be the beginning of follow-up or enrollment in the study. The idea of an open cohort can be contrasted with a fixed cohort where all individuals are defined with respect to exposure at the beginning of the study and no one enters the study or switches from the exposed to unexposed group, or vice versa. Although no additional subjects can be added to this fixed cohort, it is possible that some individuals may be lost to follow-up over time. Special care must be taken to ensure that loss to follow-up is minimized since significant losses can introduce bias into the study. A closed cohort is similar to a fixed cohort in that exposure is defined at the beginning of the study and no additional subjects can be added after the initiation of follow-up; however, there are no losses to follow-up in a closed cohort resulting in the time under observation, or follow-up time, being equal for all members of the cohort allowing the direct examination of risk (or cumulative incidence).[55] In the situation of open cohorts or fixed cohorts, the time under observation is slightly different for each member of the cohort because of differences in entry into the cohort or loss to follow-up. Studies using with these types of cohorts typically focus on the measurement of person-time and the calculation of an incidence rate (or incidence density) rather than risks as in closed cohorts.[43]

Despite their inherent strengths, cohort studies do have certain limitations. When compared with some other epidemiologic approaches, cohort studies can be relatively expensive and time-consuming to conduct. This is especially true of prospective cohort studies where the researcher must wait for time to pass for outcomes to develop. For this reason, cohort studies may not be well suited to examine relatively rare outcomes. How much time is required to pass before outcomes are theoretically possible depends in part on the required induction period.[56] The induction period is the period of time between exposure and the occurrence of an outcome. When examining the effects of drug use, the induction period may be dictated by various biological mechanisms. The induction period concept can also apply to programs or policies designed to influence drug usage (e.g., an educational program to improve the quality of prescribing in older adults). Although a study 2 years in duration may be appropriate to examine the effects of a program on improved prescribing practices, it will probably not be sufficient to examine the effects of a drug on either causing or preventing cancer because of differences in induction periods. Although retrospective cohort studies can draw on the availability of existing exposure and/or outcome data, the potential need to collect additional data cannot be dismissed, which could increase both the costs and time associated with conducting the study. As with case-control studies, accurate information is an important consideration in cohort studies. With prospective studies, the researcher may have a greater amount of control over what is collected, as well as how it is collected. Still, the information source has important implications. Recall bias can be an important limitation when asking subjects to remember distant exposure information. In a study using data from the Nurses' Health Study, Curhan et al.[59] used self-reported lifetime analgesic use to examine the risk of decline in renal function. The potential for recall bias should be obvious in this situation, as it can be difficult for an individual to recall accurate estimates of their life-time use of non-narcotic analgesics, even if those subjects are themselves health care professionals.

▶ Other Observational Designs

In addition to the more traditional epidemiologic studies discussed up to this point, there are a handful of other potentially useful designs that deserve a brief discussion. These designs often provide a sort of hybridization of other study designs to maintain methodological rigor associated with cohort studies while increasing efficiency, as seen with case-control studies. Two designs are discussed in this section.

Nested Case-Control Studies

Nested case-control studies represent a case-control study conducted within a well-defined cohort. Since the full cohort is defined, it is possible to sample cases and controls randomly from within that cohort. The nested case-control approach is stronger than the traditional case-control approach because the researcher is guaranteed that only incident cases are used since the original study cohort was outcome-free by definition. Also, with *risk-set* (or *density*) *sampling*, the odds ratio more closely approximates the rate ratio that would be calculated from a similar cohort study.[60] In this sampling approach, a random sample of controls is selected from among those who were at risk for the outcome when a case is identified. This results in a control series that has approximately the same person-time contribution as the cases.[44] From an efficiency standpoint, the nested case-control approach allows the use of a smaller sample of subjects, which can be helpful when some of the information requires expensive tests or measures to determine exposure status (e.g., laboratory assays).[61]

Case-Crossover Studies

The *case-crossover design* can be thought of as the epidemiologic analog of the randomized crossover design in experimental clinical research. As in the experimental version, each subject experiences a period of exposure and a period of nonexposure and some outcome of interest is measured following each period. In this manner, each subject serves as his or her own control thus eliminating potential confounding related to differences in subjects that might normally be seen in other study designs. As in most epidemiological designs, the subject rather than the researcher determines their sequence and frequency of exposure. In the simplest form, a case-crossover study would compare the exposure status during the time period immediately before an outcome with the exposure status in a time period where an outcome did not occur. Since these time periods come from the same individual, each subject serves as its own self-matched control.[62] Some have suggested that case-control studies provide an answer to the question "Why me?," whereas case-crossover studies answer the question "Why now?" by considering the differences in exposure status in the outcome and outcome-free periods within the same subject.[63] The case-crossover design is particularly useful for examining intermittent or transient exposures, as well as outcomes that may be transient in nature,[62,64,65] but it has been shown to be useful in studying exposures that occur in longer time frames.[66] Some examples of outcomes and exposures that have been studied using the case-crossover design include the use of benzodiazepines and motor vehicle crashes,[67] medication use and the risk of falls in the elderly,[68] and adherence to statin medications and provider follow-up.[69]

META-ANALYSIS

As published research in the area of pharmacoepidemiology continues to grow, some method to combine the results of various studies in a given area would be useful. *Meta-analysis* is a statistical technique that allows the combination of studies to produce overall estimates of effect.[70] This formal quantitative combination of results from numerous studies is what separates meta-analyses from the more traditional *systematic review*.[71] Meta-analyses have four general purposes: (1) to increase the power to examine primary end points or perform subgroup analyses, (2) to resolve discrepancies between the results of different studies, (3) to improve estimates of effect size or estimate the overall effect size, and (4) to examine issues not originally included as objectives in the initial studies.[72] The steps in conducting a meta-analysis include formulating an appropriate research question, defining the data necessary to answer the question, identifying and collecting the appropriate studies, extracting data from the identified studies, and analyzing the data.[73] The

process of data analysis when conducting a meta-analysis may be as simple as calculating the weighted effect estimate (e.g., odds ratio or risk ratio) or using more complicated techniques, such as *meta-regression*.[74]

As with other studies, there are certain important biases when conducting a meta-analysis. Publication bias can result from the failure to include unpublished studies. This is important since there is the tendency for studies with nonsignificant or unfavorable results not to be published. Aggregation bias is the same fundamental concept as the ecological bias and can be important when interpreting meta-analyses. Transparency in the selection and recording of studies to be included in a meta-analysis are also very important. Guidelines exist to help researchers in describing the methods used in and reporting the results of their meta-analyses. The Preferred Reporting Items for Systematic Reviews and Meta-Analyses (PRISMA) statement[75] has been developed for systematic reviews and meta-analyses of RCTs, and the Meta-analysis of Observational Studies in Epidemiology (MOOSE) statement[76] is available for meta-analyses of epidemiologic studies.

▼ SUMMARY

Selecting an appropriate study design is an important step in conducting any type of research. A variety of study designs are useful in pharmacoepidemiology. These range from the traditional observational study designs, such as the cohort study or case-control study, to various interventional designs, such as the RCT or quasi-experiments. Each particular study design has certain strengths and weaknesses that should be taken into consideration. The chosen study design should reflect the desired research objective and appropriate steps should be taken to ensure that the study is developed in such a way to allow valid conclusions.

DISCUSSION QUESTIONS

1. What is the primary difference between the experimental approach to research and the quasi-experimental approach?

2. Briefly describe what self-selection is and why it can introduce bias into a research study.

3. Briefly define the ecological fallacy and explain how it differs from the atomistic fallacy.

4. Why are cross-sectional studies sometimes referred to as prevalence studies?

5. You are interested in examining the relationship between the use of adherence aids (e.g., a daily pill box) and medication adherence. In designing the study, you look through pharmacy records over the past year to identify 100 patients who are adherent. You do the same to identify 100 patients who are not adherent. Within each group, you ask each patient whether or not they use any sort of adherence aid. On the basis of this description, explain which type of study design was used.

6. In a cohort study of the relationship between type of hospital room (private vs. shared) and developing a hospital acquired infection (HAI), the researchers used the electronic medical record to identify all patients admitted to the hospital over the past 6 months. The type of room was determined for each patient. If a patient switched from a shared room to a private room, or vice versa, during their stay they were excluded. The incidence of HAIs was noted among patients of each room type.

   a. Explain whether this is a prospective cohort or retrospective cohort study.

   b. Is the cohort described above an open or closed cohort?

7. Compare the advantages and disadvantages for a case-control study and a cohort study.

8. How does a nested case-control study differ from a "traditional" case-control study?

9. In what situations are case-crossover studies particularly useful?

10. What are two reasons that one might want to conduct a meta-analysis?

REFERENCES

1. Newman TB, Browner WS, Hulley SB. Enhancing causal inference in observational studies. In: Hulley SB, Cummings SR, Browner WS, Grady DG, Newman TB, eds. *Designing Clinical Research*, 3rd ed. Philadelphia, PA: Lippincott Williams & Wilkins, 2007:127-146.

2. Rubin DB. The design versus the analysis of observational studies for causal effects: Parallels with the design of randomized trials. *Stat Med.* 2007;26(1):20-36.

3. Rothman KJ, Greenland S, Lash TL. Validity in epidemiologic studies. In: Rothman KJ, Greenland S, Last TL, eds. *Modern Epidemiology*, 3rd ed. Philadelphia, PA: Lippincott Williams & Wilkins, 2008:128-147.

4. Gandhi SK, Salmon JW, Kong SX, Zhao SZ. Administrative databases and outcomes assessment: An overview of issues and potential utility. *J Manag Care Pharm.* 1999;5(3):215-222.

5. Hulley SB, Martin JN, Cummings SR. Planning the measurements: Accuracy and precision. In: Hulley SB, Cummings SR, Browner WS, Grady DG, Newman TB, eds. *Designing Clinical Research*, 3rd ed. Philadelphia, PA: Lippincott Williams & Wilkins, 2007:37-49.

6. Rothman KJ, Greenland S, Lash TL. Design strategies to improve study accuracy. In: Rothman KJ, Greenland S, Last TL, eds. *Modern Epidemiology*, 3rd ed. Philadelphia, PA: Lippincott Williams & Wilkins, 2008:168-182.

7. Black N. Why we need observational studies to evaluate the effectiveness of health care. *BMJ.* 1996;312(7040):1215-1218.

8. Moher D, Schulz KF, Altman DG. The CONSORT statement: revised recommendations for improving the quality of reports of parallel-group randomized trials. *Ann Intern Med.* 2001; 134(8):657-662.

9. Friis RH, Sellers TA. *Epidemiology for Public Health Practice*, 2nd ed. Gaithersburg, MD: Aspen Publishers, 1999:190-191.

10. Concato J, Shah N, Horwitz RI. Randomized, controlled trials, observational studies, and the hierarchy of research designs. *New Engl J Med.* 2000;342(25):1887-1892.

11. Saltvedt I, Spigset O, Ruths S, Fayers P, Kasa S, Sletvold O. Patterns of drug prescription in a geriatric evaluation and management unit as compared with the general medical wards: A randomised study. *Eur J Clin Pharmacol.* 2005;61(12):921-928.

12. Beers MH. Explicit criteria for determining potentially inappropriate medication use by the elderly. An update. *Arch Intern Med.* 1997;157(14):1531-1536.

13. Chen H, Nwangwu A, Aparasu R, Essien E, Sun S, Lee K. The impact of Medicare Part D on psychotropic utilization and financial burden for community-based seniors. *Psychiatr Serv.* 2008;59(10):1191-1197.

14. Yin W, Basu A, Zhang JX, Rabbani A, Meltzer DO, Alexander GC. The effect of Medicare Part D prescription drug benefit on drug utilization and expenditures. *Ann Intern Med.* 2008; 148(3):169-177.

15. Schneeweiss S, Patrick AR, Pedan A, et al. The effect of Medicare Part D coverage on drug use and cost sharing among seniors without prior drug benefits. *Health Aff (Millwood).* 2009;28(2):w305-w316.

16. Grégoire JP, Moisan J, Potvin L, Chabot I, Verreault R, Milot A. Effect of drug utilization reviews on the quality of in-hospital prescribing: A quasi-experimental study. *BMC Health Serv Res.* 2006;6:33.

17. MacBride-Stewart SP, Elton R, Walley T. Do quality incentives change prescribing patterns in primary care? An observational study in Scotland. *Fam Pract.* 2008;25(1):27-32.

18. Law MR, Majumdar SR, Soumerai SB. Effect of illicit direct to consumer advertising on use of etanercept, mometasone, and

tegaserod in Canada: Controlled longitudinal study. *BMJ.* 2008;337:a1055.

19. Shadish WR, Cook TD, Campbell DT. *Experimental and Quasi-Experimental Designs for Generalized Causal Inference.* Boston, MA: Houghton Mifflin, 2002:156-158.

20. Martens JD, Winkens RAG, van der Weijden T, de Bruyn D, Severens JL. Does a joint development and dissemination of multidisciplinary guidelines improve prescribing behaviour: A pre/post study with concurrent control group and a randomised trial. *BMC Health Serv Res.* 2006;6:145.

21. Collins TM, Mott DA, Bigelow WE, Zimmerman DR. A controlled letter intervention to change prescribing behavior: results of a dual-targeted approach. *Health Serv Res.* 1997; 32(4):471-489.

22. Harris AD, McGregor JC, Perencevich EN, et al. The use and interpretation of quasi-experimental studies in medical informatics. *J Am Med Inform Assoc.* 2006;13(1):16-23.

23. Eccles M, Grimshaw J, Campbell M, Ramsay C. Research designs for studies evaluating the effectiveness of change and improvement strategies. *Qual Saf Health Care.* 2003;12(1): 47-52.

24. Pocock SJ, Elbourne DR. Randomized trials or observational tribulations? *New Engl J Med.* 2000;342(25):1907-1909.

25. Benson K, Hartz AJ. A comparison of observational studies and randomized, controlled trials. *New Engl J Med.* 2000;342 (25):1878-1886.

26. Liu PY, Anderson G, Crowley JJ. Observational studies and randomized trials. *New Engl J Med.* 2000;343(16):1195–1197.

27. Kunz R. Randomized trials and observational studies: Still mostly similar, still crucial differences. *J Clin Epidemiol.* 2008; 61(3):207-208.

28. Schneeweiss S. Developments in post-marketing comparative effectiveness research. *Clin Pharmacol Ther.* 2007;82(2):143-156.

29. Perfetto EM, Epstein RS, Morris LS. Assessing patient outcomes of drug therapy: The role of pharmacoepidemiology. In: Hartzema AG, Porta MS, Tilson HH, eds. *Pharmacoepidemiology: An Introduction*, 3rd ed. Cincinnati, OH: Harvey Whitney Books, 1998:182-212.

30. Strom BL, Melmon KL. The use of pharmacoepidemiology to study beneficial drug effects. In: Strom BL, ed. *Pharmacoepidemiology*, 4th ed. New York: Wiley, 2005:611-628.

31. Rubeiz BJ, Marrone CM, Leclerc JR. Treatment of heparin-induced thrombocytopenia with drotrecogin alfa (activated). *Pharmacotherapy.* 2006;26(3):428-434.

32. Darrouj J, Puri N, Prince E, Lomonaco A, Spevetz A, Gerber DR. Dexmedetomidine infusion as adjunctive therapy to benzodiazepines for acute alcohol withdrawal. *Ann Pharmacother.* 2008;42(11):1703-1705.

33. Brahm NC, Fast GA, Brown RC. Buspirone for autistic disorder in a woman with an intellectual disability. *Ann Pharmacother.* 2008;42(1):131-137.

34. Edlavitch S. Pharmacoepidemiology study methodologies. In: Hartzema AG, Porta MS, Tilson HH, eds. *Pharmacoepidemiology: An Introduction*, 3rd ed. Cincinnati, OH: Harvey Whitney Books, 1998:69-114.

35. MacDougall C, Harpe SE, Powell JP, Johnson CK, Edmond MB, Polk RE. Pseudomonas aeruginosa, Staphylococcus aureus,

and fluoroquinolone use. *Emerg Infect Dis.* 2005;11(8):1197-1204.

36. Diez-Roux AV. Bringing context back into epidemiology: Variables and fallacies in multilevel analysis. *Am J Public Health.* 1998;88(2):216-222.

37. Greenland S. Principles of multilevel modelling. *Int J Epidemiol.* 2000;29(1):158-167.

38. Ohlsson H, Lindblad U, Lithman T, et al. Understanding adherence to official guidelines on statin prescribing in primary health care—a multi-level methodological approach. *Eur J Clin Pharmacol.* 2005;61(9):657-665.

39. Johnell K, Råstam L, Lithman T, Sundquist J, Merlo J. Low adherence with antihypertensives in actual practice: The association with social participation—a multilevel analysis. *BMC Public Health.* 2005;5:17.

40. Stang P, Morris L, Kempf J, Henderson S, Yood MU, Oliveria S. The coprescription of contraindicated drugs with statins: Continuing potential for increased risk of adverse events. *Am J Ther.* 2007;14(1):30-40.

41. Liberman JN, Berger JE, Lewis M. Prevalence of antihypertensive, antidiabetic, and dyslipidemic prescription medication use among children and adolescents. *Arch Pediatr Adolesc Med.* 2009;163(4):357-364.

42. Rothman KJ. *Epidemiology: An Introduction.* New York: Oxford University Press, 2002:89-91.

43. Diggle PJ, Heagerty P, Liang KY, Zeger SL. *Analysis of Longitudinal Data*, 2nd ed. New York: Oxford University Press, 2002:1–14.

44. Rothman KJ, Greenland S, Lash TL. Case-control studies. In: Rothman KJ, Greenland S, Last TL, eds. *Modern Epidemiology*, 3rd ed. Philadelphia, PA: Lippincott Williams & Wilkins, 2008:111-127.

45. Coogan PF, Rosenberg L, Palmer JR, Strom BL, Zauber AG, Shapiro S. Statin use and the risk of breast and prostate cancer. *Epidemiology.* 2002;13(3):262-267.

46. Velicer CM, Heckbert SR, Lampe JW, Potter JD, Robertson CA, Taplin SH. Antibiotic use in relation to the risk of breast cancer. *JAMA.* 2004;291(7):827-835.

47. Fored CM, Ejerblad E, Lindblad P, et al. Acetaminophen, aspirin, and chronic renal failure. *New Engl J Med.* 2001;345 (25):1801-1808.

48. Fijn R, Van den Bemt PMLA, Chow M, De Blaey CJ, De Jong-Van den Berg LTW, Brouwers JRBJ. Hospital prescribing errors: Epidemiological assessment of predictors. *Br J Clin Pharmacol.* 2002;53(3):326-331.

49. Etminan M, Samii A. Pharmacoepidemiology I: A review of pharmacoepidemiologic study designs. *Pharmacotherapy.* 2004;24(8):964-969.

50. Newman TB, Browner WS, Cummings SR, Hulley SB. Designing cross-section and case-control studies. In: Hulley SB, Cummings SR, Browner WS, Grady DG, Newman TB, eds. *Designing Clinical Research*, 3rd ed. Philadelphia, PA: Lippincott Williams & Wilkins, 2007:109-126.

51. Rothman KJ, Greenland S, Lash TL. Design strategies to improve study accuracy. In: Rothman KJ, Greenland S, Lash TL, eds. *Modern Epidemiology*, 3rd ed. Philadelphia, PA: Lippincott Williams & Wilkins, 2008:168-182.

52. Greenland S. Application of stratified analysis methods. In: Rothman KJ, Greenland S, Lash TL, eds. *Modern Epidemiology*,

3rd ed. Philadelphia, PA: Lippincott Williams & Wilkins, 2008:283-302.

53. Hennessy S, Bilker WB, Berlin JA, Strom BL. Factors influencing the optimal control-to-case ratio in matched case-control studies. *Am J Epidemiol.* 1999;149(2):195-197.

54. Waning B, Montagne M. *Pharmacoepidemiology: Principles and Practice.* New York: McGraw-Hill, 2000:56-58.

55. Rothman KJ, Greenland S. Cohort studies. In: Rothman KJ, Greenland S, Lash TL, eds. *Modern Epidemiology*, 3rd ed. Philadelphia, PA: Lippincott Williams & Wilkins, 2008: 100-110.

56. Rothman KJ, Greenland S, Poole C, Lash TL. Causation and causal inference. In: Rothman KJ, Greenland S, Lash TL, eds. *Modern Epidemiology*, 3rd ed. Philadelphia, PA: Lippincott Williams & Wilkins, 2008:5-31.

57. Harpe SE. Using secondary data sources for pharmacoepidemiology and outcomes research. *Pharmacotherapy.* 2009;29 (2):138-153.

58. Doepker BA, Lucarelli MR, Lehman A, Shirk MB. Thromboembolic events during continuous vasopressin infusions: A retrospective evaluation. *Ann Pharmacother.* 2007;41(9): 1383-1389.

59. Curhan GC, Knight EL, Rosner B, Hankinson SE, Stampfer MJ. Lifetime nonnarcotic analgesic use and decline in renal function in women. *Arch Intern Med.* 2004;164(14):1519-1524.

60. Etminan M. Pharmacoepidemiology II: The nested case-control study—a novel approach in pharmacoepidemiologic research. *Pharmacotherapy.* 2004;24(9):1105-1109.

61. Cummings SR, Newman TB, Hulley SB. Designing a cohort study. In: Hulley SB, Cummings SR, Browner WS, Grady DG, Newman TB, eds. *Designing Clinical Research*, 3rd ed. Philadelphia, PA: Lippincott Williams & Wilkins, 2007:97-107.

62. Maclure M, Mittleman MA. Should we use a case-crossover design? *Annu Rev Public Health.* 2000;21:193-221.

63. Maclure M. 'Why me?' versus 'why now?'—Differences between operational hypotheses in case-control versus case-crossover studies. *Pharmacoepidemiol Drug Saf.* 2007;16(8): 850-853.

64. Schneeweiss S, Stürmer T, Maclure M. Case-crossover and case-time-control designs as alternatives in pharmacoepi-

demiologic research. *Pharmacoepidemiol Drug Saf.* 1997;6 (suppl. 3):S51-S59.

65. Delaney JAC, Suissa S. The case-crossover study design in pharmacoepidemiology. *Stat Methods Med Res.* 2009;18(1): 53-65.

66. Wang PS, Schneeweiss S, Glynn RJ, Mogun H, Avorn J. Use of the case-crossover design to study prolonged drug exposures and insidious outcomes. *Ann Epidemiol.* 2004;14(4):296-303.

67. Hebert C, Delaney JAC, Hemmelgarn B, Lévesque LE, Suissa S. Benzodiazepines and elderly drivers: A comparison of pharmacoepidemiological study designs. *Pharmacoepidemiol Drug Saf.* 2007;16(8):845-849.

68. Neutel CI, Perry S, Maxwell C. Medication use and risk of falls. *Pharmacoepidemiol Drug Saf.* 2002;11(2):97-104.

69. Brookhart MA, Patrick AR, Schneeweiss S, et al. Physician follow-up and provider continuity are associated with long-term medication adherence. *Arch Intern Med.* 2007;167(8): 847-852.

70. Petitti DB. *Meta-Analysis, Decision Analysis, and Cost-Effectiveness Analysis.* New York: Oxford University Press, 2000:13-15.

71. Berlin JA, Kim CJ. The use of meta-analysis in pharmacoepidemiology. In: Strom BL, ed. *Pharmacoepidemiology*, 4th ed. New York: Wiley, 2005:681-708.

72. Sacks HS, Berrier J, Reitman D, Ancona-Berk VA, Chalmers TC. Meta-analyses of randomized controlled trials. *New Engl J Med.* 1987;316(8):450-455.

73. Einarson TR. Meta-analysis of the pharmacotherapy literature. In: Hartzema AG, Porta MS, Tilson HH, eds. *Pharmacoepidemiology: An Introduction*, 3rd ed. Cincinnati, OH: Harvey Whitney Books, 1998:310-346.

74. Greenland S, O'Rourke K. Meta-analysis. In: Rothman KJ, Greenland S, Lash TL, eds. *Modern Epidemiology*, 3rd ed. Philadelphia, PA: Lippincott Williams & Wilkins, 2008:652-682.

75. Moher D, Liberati A, Tetzlaff J, Altman DG. Preferred reporting items for systematic reviews and meta-analyses: The PRISMA statement. *Ann Intern Med.* 2009;151(4):264-269.

76. Stroup DF, Berlin JA, Morton SC, et al. Meta-analysis of observational studies in epidemiology: A proposal for reporting. *JAMA.* 2000;283(15):2008-2012.

Using Secondary Data in Pharmacoepidemiology

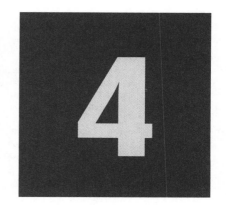

Spencer E. Harpe

▼ OBJECTIVES

At the end of the chapter, the reader will be able to:

1. Identify the two major types of data for pharmacoepidemiologic studies
2. Discuss the relative advantages and disadvantages of secondary data
3. Describe the various sources of data for pharmacoepidemiologic studies
4. Describe various coding schemes for drugs, procedures, and diagnoses
5. Describe methods for measuring exposure and outcomes
6. Discuss some special considerations when using secondary data

---

COLLECTING DATA FOR PHARMACOEPIDEMIOLOGY STUDIES

After the research question and study design are identified, an appropriate source of data must be identified. Pharmacoepidemiology studies may involve either data collected prospectively (i.e., *primary data*) for the purpose of the study or data that were already collected for some other purpose (i.e., *secondary data*). Primary data are collected for a specific purpose and represent data not previously available in a consolidated manner. This type of data may be collected through a variety of means, including questionnaires, interviews, or chart reviews. Primary data generally offer increased control over the type and amount of information that is available when compared to secondary data. If you need information about some specific medication-taking behavior, for example, how frequently a dose of med-

ication is taken with a meal, you can ask this of a participant in a study that uses primary data collection. This information would most likely not be available in secondary data that comes from prescription dispensing data provided by a pharmacy. Although manual chart reviews can provide an increased level of detail in the collected data, it can be extremely time consuming and can quickly become cost prohibitive from a time and/or financial standpoint, as the sample size increases and additional chart reviewers are required. In a similar fashion, conducting interviews can be extremely time consuming despite the rich data that can be generated. This relatively high cost from a time and financial standpoint is often considered one of the limitations of using primary data.[1,2]

Secondary data are comprised of preexisting data that were collected for some other purpose, such as

Table 4-1. Advantages and disadvantages of primary and secondary data sources.

	Primary data	Secondary data
Advantages	• High level of control of type and amount of data obtained for study subjects • Data can usually be validated by the investigator (e.g., examining the medical record or interviewing the patient) • Patient samples are often relatively homogeneous given inclusion and exclusion criteria in randomized trials • Groups are usually comparable (if primary data come from randomized trials)	• Typically less expensive than collecting new data • Large samples and long follow-up times may be readily available • May allow the study of rare conditions or drugs • Time required to obtain data can be relatively short • Representative of "real-world" practice settings • Available patient samples can be heterogeneous in terms of demographics and disease states
Disadvantages	• Can be very expensive, especially if sample is large and detailed data collection is required • Often requires long time periods to account for subject responses or follow-up periods • Possible susceptibility to biases associated with data collection procedures (e.g., recall bias) • Not necessarily representative of patients or drug usage under actual practice conditions	• Lack of control over data included from study participants • Validation may be difficult or impossible, although certain quality checks can be performed (e.g., no males were admitted for childbirth) • May not have been originally collected for research purposes • Potential problems associated with upcoding • Depending on the source, certain information may not be available (e.g., lab data from a claims database) • Groups may be difficult to compare due to certain biases

for a previous research question (e.g., a randomized controlled trial [RCT]) or to facilitate some process (e.g., hospital discharge records). These secondary data may offer a distinct advantage in terms of efficiency, when compared to primary data, because extended time need not be devoted to data collection. Depending on the particular data source, secondary data may also offer advantages in terms of sample size and generalizability.[3] These strengths have resulted in the use of secondary data to study a wide variety of topics, including physician prescribing, drug utilization, and medication adherence; unintended drug effects (both adverse and beneficial); and health policy issues.[4] There are some potential limitations to using secondary data for research purposes. Although some secondary data may have been originally collected for research purposes or with research in mind (e.g., RCT datasets or patient registries), the most frequently acknowledged limitation of secondary data is that secondary data are typically not collected for the specific purpose of answering the research question at hand; thus, there may be certain validity threats that must be considered when these sources are used for research purposes. By relying on secondary data, the researcher does not have the same level of control over the amount and accuracy of information as with primary data collection.[4] This is why pharmacoepidemiology studies may use sophisticated statistical methods or study designs to maximize internal validity. Table 4-1 compares the relative advantages and disadvantage of primary and secondary data. The focus of this chapter will be on using secondary data sources, given their unique considerations and important place in pharmacoepidemiologic research.

TYPES OF SECONDARY DATA SOURCES

Secondary data may be available in a variety of different sources, ranging from billing databases to electronic medical records and spontaneous reporting systems. The number and types of data sources available are increasing as information technology is implemented to a greater extent in the U.S. health care system. Individual sources vary with respect to type of information included, the level of detail of the information, and the number of individuals included. With the increasing scope and complexity of some available data sources, it is relatively common to find multiple types of data within one data source (e.g., both financial and utilization data at both the facility and provider level).

This may actually be advantageous, as it can simplify the process of obtaining the data for a project.

Regardless of the specific data source that is being used, it is important to understand the general structure of any given data source. Data sources typically have various amounts of documentation associated with them. One very important piece of documentation is the *data dictionary*. This is basically an explanation of all of the variables in the data source, as well as the contents of those variables, and what valid entries are for the variables. The meanings of coded variables are also provided in the documentation (e.g., Gender: 1 = Female, 2 = Male, 3 = Other, 8 = Unknown, 9 = Missing). The data dictionary, or some reduced version, may be available when preparing a request for data from a given data source. Once the data are actually obtained, a version of the data dictionary that contains the variables for your dataset should be provided.

Automated Health Care Databases

As technology has been implemented in various parts of the U.S. health care system, a large amounts of data are collected automatically whenever a patient encounters the health care system and some type of event occurs, such as a hospital admission or a filled prescription. Data on these encounters are captured in an automated fashion, often electronically. These *automated health care databases*, or transactional databases, are a source of secondary data that have become quite common over the past few decades.[5] Generally speaking, these databases are created to facilitate the reimbursement of health care practitioners whenever services are provided to a patient. Automated databases offer a number of advantages, including minimizing the cost of the study, access to rare conditions or understudied/underrepresented populations, and the potential for large sample sizes.[6] These large sample sizes are important to provide sufficient power to study rare outcomes, such as some adverse events.[7] Since automated health care databases represent the use of drugs in actual clinical practice, studies using these sources are typically viewed as having increased generalizability and allow the study of effectiveness rather than efficacy, as studied in randomized controlled trials.[3,8] Another potential advantage of these

automated health care databases is that they offer protection against some biases introduced by direct observation of research participants or self-reporting of information (e.g., recall bias).[8,9,10]

One of the most important limitations of automated health care databases is whether they accurately reflect what actually happened from an exposure and/or outcome standpoint. For example, identifying a valid prescription claim for a person does not necessarily mean that individual actually took the medication. Similarly, over-the-counter drugs or dietary supplements usually are not reported in pharmacy claims data. Either of these situations can result in misclassification of exposure or outcome status. Although some validation studies have suggested that automated data for prescription drugs have a fairly high degree of accuracy, especially when compared to self-reporting of drug use,[11,12] other research suggests that the potential inaccuracies of medication data is still an important limitation to consider when using automated health care databases.[13] Information about medical conditions and procedures may be less accurate than drug data due to coding errors.[14,15] Although mistakes in coding diagnoses and procedures may be the result of human error, there may be direct or indirect incentives to selectively code those conditions that result in higher levels of reimbursement.[8,16,17] Although there is relatively little that can be done to combat these miscoding practices, the potential bias they introduce should be taken into consideration.

Another important consideration is that information in automated databases is only captured when an individual has an encounter with the health care system (e.g., a filled prescription or a hospital admission).[4] Those individuals who are frequently ill or who are in poorer health generally have more health care encounters than those who are less ill. The result is that those individuals with greater amounts of information are typically "sicker" than those without much information.[18]

Administrative Claims Data

When an individual covered by some form of health insurance receives health care services, a claim is submitted to the insurer for payment or reimbursement. This may be submitted electronically or in paper format by the individual patient or filed by the provider on the patient's behalf. Regardless of the submission process, these claims are required by health plans for payment or reimbursement for covered services.[8] In processing these claims, health plans generate and store large amounts of data detailing services provided and the level of payment for those services. To support the processing of these claims, additional information such as medical diagnoses may also be submitted on claim forms. In addition, health plans also maintain basic demographic information about covered individuals, such as age, gender, and race. Taken together, this information can serve as a useful tool for research purposes.

Some examples of administrative claims data include inpatient or outpatient medical claims from a private insurance plan (e.g., Anthem or Humana) or pharmacy claims data maintained by a pharmacy-benefits manager (e.g., Express Scripts or Medco Health). Claims submitted for services reimbursed under Medicaid or Medicare are examples of data from the public sector. Administrative claims data can include a variety of different health care services, including outpatient medical office visits, inpatient hospitalizations, prescription drug events, and durable medical equipment. One important consideration when using administrative claims data is that different types of claims may not reside in the same database depending on the particular plan's design. For example, pharmacy claims may be processed separately from the rest of the medical claims by a pharmacy benefits manager.[8] Although some questions can be answered by using any one source in isolation, bringing the various sources together can greatly improve the utility of the data. The process of *data linkage* allows separate data sources to be combined into one cohesive database.[19] This is discussed in more detail later in the chapter.

There are certain challenges associated with using administrative claims data. One common challenge is the turnover rate of individuals in health plans. Whenever a covered individual changes jobs, or if the employer changes health plans in the case of employer-sponsored insurance, claims for that individual (and any others associated with the covered individual) will no longer be captured. To overcome this challenge, eligibility data are typically used to identify people in the administrative data who are continuously eligible for benefits during the course of the study. If this eligibility information is not taken into consideration, an abrupt stop in claims data may appear as the discontinuation of drugs or the resolution or "cure" of a medical condition when in reality the person is no longer covered by the same health plan. Changes in coding practices are another potential challenge with administrative claims data that are particularly important when considering studies that cover many years. These coding changes may be the result of changes in reimbursement policies, changes in documentation practices, or even changes in the codes themselves. An awareness of major changes in coding practices is useful. For example, the International Classification of Diseases, Ninth Revision, Clinical Modification (ICD-9-CM) is currently used to code diseases and conditions. At some point in the future, the next version (ICD-10-CM) will be introduced, marking a significant change in medical coding.[8] This will be particularly important if a study is examining a period of time that overlaps the switch from ICD-9-CM to ICD-10-CM. Even minor modifications or updates within the ICD-9-CM system are important to consider. Another challenge when using administrative claims data that are particularly important for pharmacoepidemiologic studies is that certain drug-related information may not be captured. This is most notable with hospital admissions. Because reimbursement for hospital stays is typically based on diagnosis-related groups (DRGs), a hospital receives a prespecified amount for a given diagnosis.[20] Although the amounts are adjusted for geographic variations, the institution's case mix, and the patient's severity of illness,[21] the drugs do not factor into the reimbursement so they are typically not reported. This may be an issue for other types of data that are not required for reimbursement purposes (e.g., laboratory results).[8] Fortunately, this information is usually captured in other data sources.

Other Transactional and Operational Data

Data that are collected as the result of activities that support the provision of a service, such as medical care, can be generally referred to as transactional or operational data. The administrative claims data previously discussed actually represent a specific subset of transactional data that arise from the submission of health care claims for reimbursement. As mentioned previously, a large amount of information is collected about various "transactions" that take place during health care encounters. Some of this information, like drug dispensing and sales or laboratory results, may not be required for reimbursement but could still be useful for research purposes.[20] To continue with a previous example, inpatient-drug data are one situation where information may not be available in administrative claims data, but it is most likely available in other transactional data. The pharmacy information system at hospitals may be a stand-alone computer system or one module of an integrated suite of other clinical programs. In either case, the pharmacy system plays a vital role in the ordering, dispensing, and management of drug therapy within the hospital. Information about actual medication administration may also be available from the pharmacy information system.[22] From a research standpoint, medication dispensing and administration data can be used to examine drug use at the individual patient, nursing unit, or hospital level. In addition to pharmacy, other inpatient information systems, such as laboratory or microbiology, may be important sources of data. Gathering and combining data from these separate sources can be tedious but is possible and often necessary to conduct meaningful research. Despite this effort, data from these transactional systems are often available in near real-time fashion because they come from systems used to support the operations of the health care organization. Many health systems have made efforts to consolidate information from various sources, such as pharmacy, laboratory, diagnosis, and patient demographic data, into one data warehouse that can be used to support a variety of functions, including clinical decision support, utilization review, or clinical research.[23–25]

Transactional data can also be found outside of health systems. Whereas prescription drugs are typically captured in administrative claims data, uninsured patients or those paying with cash are not represented in pharmacy claims data. Information about the dispensing of prescription drugs could be obtained for a given pharmacy or a group of pharmacies in a certain area (e.g., the local community pharmacy or all pharmacies from the same supermarket chain in a given region). In a similar fashion, information about the sales of drug products could be obtained from pharmacies, which may be particularly useful if over-the-counter or alternative medicine products are being studied. At the national and international level large research firms, such as IMS Health, can provide drug dispensing and sales data. Although it may be difficult to link sales data to individual patients for research purposes, sales data can be useful at the aggregate level to describe overall drug utilization.[26] Sales data have also been used as a method of syndromic surveillance to predict disease outbreaks.[27,28]

▶ Electronic Medical Records

Despite the expanding role of information technology in health care, the implementation of *electronic medical records* (EMRs) is relatively low among hospitals and outpatient medical practices, but it is growing.[29,30] Although there is no standard definition of an EMR, these systems generally involve immediate, electronic access to information about care provided to an individual over time.[31] A wide array of functions, ranging from electronic clinical notes and reporting of laboratory results to advanced clinical decision support and viewing diagnostic imaging, may be included in various EMR implementations.[30]

The information contained in EMRs can provide a wealth of information for research purposes. One obvious advantage of using an EMR for research is the efficiencies offered over manual chart review. EMRs typically offer a greater level of detail than is available in data from administrative claims or patient or provider questionnaires. As the EMR is based on real-time data, the latency period between the generation of the data and its availability for research can be minimal or nonexistent, especially if an EMR at a local institution is being used.[31,32] This can be compared to the 3- to 6-month lag time for some administrative claims-based research data sources or national surveys, which may take more than a year before being made available for public use.

There are some important considerations when using EMRs for research purposes. The data contained in EMRs are typically quite complex, given the longitudinal nature and volume of information included. Such data can require extra effort to prepare for any statistical analysis. The use of information from one institution (i.e., a single-site study) can be a limitation. Some EMR vendors have worked with their clients to create warehouses containing data from multiple institutions. These multisite sources can offer advantages in terms of sample size, but there may be issues with data consistency because documentation practices and implemented functions may vary across the participating sites. Another consideration is the lack of standardization of the actual data structure across EMR vendors. Although this may not be important when working with data from one institution, it can be problematic when gathering data from multiple institutions that use different EMR vendors.[31] The actual coding habits of the providers can still be an important consideration. From a practical standpoint, the manner in which information is captured is an important consideration. Textual data, such as clinical notes or laboratory reports, can be coded or captured as structured text or unstructured (free form) text. Analysis of coded data (e.g., antibiotic susceptibility reported as 1 = Susceptible, 2 = Intermediate, 3 = Resistant) is fairly straightforward. Analysis of structured text or unstructured text may require the use of complicated text-mining techniques.[33,34] In some situations, the complete EMR may not be made available for research purposes. For example, unstructured text entries like clinical notes, problem lists, and some pathology reports may not be provided when EMR-based data are made available for research.[35]

National Surveys or Datasets

Some governments make selected data available for research purposes. These sources can provide a great deal of information and frequently have extensive documentation and user communities that can be very helpful by providing a great deal of informal support through direct contact and previous publications. Table 4-2 provides a brief description of some data sources maintained by national or regional governments that are frequently used to study drug-related questions.

In the United States, Medicare and Medicaid claims data, including Part D data, are available for a fee to researchers for projects approved by the Centers for Medicare and Medicaid Services (CMS). In addition to these administrative claims data, CMS conducts periodic surveys of Medicare beneficiaries through the Medicare Current Beneficiary Survey (MCBS). This survey examines health status and functioning, sources of health care costs and payments, and insurance coverage among Medicare beneficiaries. Long-Term Care Minimum Data Set (MDS) data are also available for research. These data represent a broad assessment of all residents in long-term care facilities that receive Medicare and Medicaid reimbursements. The Research Data Assistance Center (ResDAC) is a government contractor that serves to facilitate access to data resources generated by and housed within CMS.[36]

In addition to CMS data, various federal government agencies maintain data sources. The Agency for Healthcare Research and Quality (AHRQ) maintains two useful sources: the Healthcare Cost and Utilization Project (HCUP) and the Medical Expenditure Panel Survey (MEPS). HCUP is a group of databases that includes longitudinal data related to care provided to all hospitalized patients, regardless of payment source, in 38 states across the nation representing more than 1,000 hospitals, and 8 million patient admissions annually.[37] Although distinct drug data are not available, ICD-9-CM codes are included, which may be useful in identifying medication-related diagnoses. MEPS is a large survey of individuals and families. Each year the survey identifies a sample of participants, called a panel, and follows them for a period of 2 years, allowing examination of longitudinal changes within that panel. Over the course of the 2-year period, there are five rounds of surveys. Because of the design of MEPS, participant panels overlap such that in any given year one panel is finishing their participation in MEPS while another panel is just beginning. There are various components included in MEPS. The Household Component contains data from individuals and families and is freely available to the public. The Insurance Component includes information from employers about the types of insurance options offered to their employees. This component is available in various summary formats on the MEPS web site or through limited access at the AHRQ Data Center. The Medical Provider Component supplements

Table 4-2. Federal data sources of potential use in pharmacoepidemiology.

Data source	Description
Medication Expenditure Panel Survey (MEPS)	Large representative survey of U.S. households and medical providers; includes information on costs and utilization of health care, including prescription drugs. Web site: www.meps.ahrq.gov
Health Care Utilization Project (HCUP)	Consolidation of hospital discharge abstract information and charges from across the United States; includes individuals regardless of payer or insurance coverage; information on medication usage is not available, but hospitalizations related to overdoses or poisonings are included; various software tools to aid in analysis are available. Web site: www.hcup-us.ahrq.gov
National Ambulatory Medical Care Survey (NAMCS)/National Hospital Ambulatory Medical Care Survey (NHAMCS)	Nationally representative survey to examine the use of ambulatory care services in the United States; includes basic clinical information and medication therapy; NHAMCS focuses on ambulatory care provided at hospital emergency departments or outpatient clinics. Web site: http://www.cdc.gov/nchs/ahcd.htm
Medicare/Medicaid data	Administrative claims data for patients enrolled in Medicare or Medicaid plans throughout the United States, including Medicare Part D data; accessed through the Research Data Acquisition Center (ResDAC) Web site: www.resdac.umn.edu/Available_CMS_Data.asp or www.cms.hhs.gov/home/rsds.asp
Medicare Current Beneficiary Survey (MCBS)	Nationally representative survey of the Medicare population to determine the expenditures and sources of payment for all services used by Medicare beneficiaries, including drugs; conducted via in-person survey with administrative claims data; accessed through the Research Data Acquisition Center (ResDAC) Web site: www.resdac.umn.edu/MCBS/data_available.asp or www.cms.hhs.gov/home/rsds.asp
Long-Term Care Minimum Data Set (MDS)	Screening and assessment tool for residents in all long-term care facilities that participate in Medicare and Medicaid; full assessment data are obtained on all residents at admission, annually, and upon a significant change in status with data reviewed at least quarterly; information on the number of drugs given and certain important drugs in the elderly population (e.g., antipsychotics or hypnotics) are required by CMS, but some states require more detailed drug information. Web site: www.resdac.umn.edu/mds or www.cms.hhs.gov/home/rsds.asp
Adverse Event Reporting System (AERS)	FDA's repository of adverse events from approved drug and therapeutic biologic projects; includes mandatory manufacturer reports and voluntary reports from providers and patients through the MedWatch program Web site: www.fda.gov/cder/aers
Vaccine Adverse Event Reporting System (VAERS)	Similar to AERS except it contains information on approved vaccines. Web site: vaers.hhs.gov
National Electronic Injury Surveillance System (NEISS)	Reporting system of emergency room visits for product-related injuries from a nationally representative sample of hospitals across the United States; expanded to include drug-related injuries in 2000; Cooperative Adverse Drug Event Surveillance System (NEISS-CADES) begun in 2002 to examine all prescription and nonprescription medications, vaccines, immunizations, vitamins, and herbals/dietary supplements. Web site: www.cpsc.gov/library/neiss.html

and clarifies information in the Household Component by contacting physicians, pharmacies, hospitals, and home health care providers identified by respondents to the Household Component. Although the Medical Provider Component is not available to the public, information from this component is incorporated into the Household Component files by updating and clarifying information provided by participants in the survey panels. As MEPS is a panel survey, the public use data files can be obtained to represent each panel (i.e., data from the 2-year period for that panel) or to represent all participants from the two overlapping panels in a given year (i.e., the full-year consolidated data files).[38]

The National Center for Healthcare Statistics (NCHS) also maintains a set of health-related surveys of the U.S. population. Two frequently used surveys are the National Ambulatory Medical Care Survey (NAMCS) and the National Hospital Ambulatory

Medical Care Survey (NHAMCS).[39] Both of these surveys are representative samples of the U.S. population and collect data regarding the administration and prescription of drugs during the respondent's visit or as a result of the visit. Information about chief complaints, diagnoses made, and other services provided are also included in the data. In addition, the Centers for Disease Control and Prevention (CDC) also have large datasets available that may be used for pharmacoepidemiologic research (e.g., the National Health and Nutrition Examination Survey [NHANES] or the National Health Insurance Survey).[40]

Outside the United States, there are several important data sources that have been used in the study of drug-related issues. The General Practice Research Database (GPRD) is a database of general practitioners in the United Kingdom. Data in the GPRD represent more than 10 million patients from more than 450 primary care practices throughout the United Kingdom. Research-quality data are available on more than 6.5 million patients. The GPRD is administered by the Medicines and Healthcare Products Regulatory Authority, which serves a similar role in the United Kingdom as does the Food and Drug Administration (FDA) in the United States.[41] In a similar fashion, the Population Health Research Data Repository, which is administered by the Manitoba Center for Healthcare Policy, provides data for individuals residing in the Canadian province of Saskatchewan.[42]

▷ Adverse Event Reporting Systems

Pharmacoepidemiologic methods play an important role in postmarketing surveillance of approved drugs. Reports of adverse events associated with, or thought to be associated with, the use of drugs can be an important source of data for medication safety studies. In the United States, adverse event data are gathered by a spontaneous event reporting system known as MedWatch. This FDA-maintained system gathers reports from manufacturers, health care providers, and patients.[43] Although the FDA conducts its own analyses, data are made available for external analysis through the Adverse Event Reporting System (AERS) database.[44] The Vaccine Adverse Event Reporting System (VAERS) is a separate system maintained by the

FDA in cooperation with the CDC to monitor safety issues involving vaccines.[45] As with adverse events, there are also efforts to collect medication error reports at the national level, such as the MEDMARX Advent Drug Reporting program[46] administered by Quantros.[47] Adverse event reporting systems also exist in other parts of the world,[48] such as the Yellow Card Scheme in the United Kingdom.[49]

One of the primary drawbacks to using these spontaneous reporting systems is the level of underreporting that is associated with adverse events. Some reports suggest that less than 1% of suspected serious adverse reactions are actually reported to the FDA.[50] In the United States, this underreporting may be related to the fact that submission of adverse event reports is voluntary for patients and health care providers.[43] Although it is required of manufacturers, providers and patients may not report adverse events to the manufacturers. Another potential limitation is the amount of clinical detail that is submitted with reports that are included in databases. Sufficient information and clinical detail is usually not available in the report itself to make determinations of causality.[51] Adverse event and medication safety reporting data may also be available at the local institutional level. These local sources offer advantages over larger, national sources, as access to more detailed clinical information is available to the user.

▷ Other Sources

There are a variety of other data sources that do not fit into the previous categories that can be useful in pharmacoepidemiologic studies. Although RCTs are not commonly used in pharmacoepidemiology, data from these studies can be used for secondary analyses. Some large and/or government-sponsored RCTs may make data available for use upon approval of the initial research team. These datasets can be useful to answer questions that were not posed originally. For example, Reid et al.[52] examined the relationship between pravastatin use and bone fractures in data from the Long-Term Intervention with Pravastatin in Ischaemic Disease (LIPID) trial[53] (Case Study 4-1). Other epidemiologic, or observational, studies may also be available for secondary analysis, such as the use of the Nurses' Health Study data to examine the relationship between analgesic use and renal function[54] and the

CASE STUDY 4-1

Secondary Analysis of Randomized Controlled Trial Data

The Long-Term Intervention with Pravastatin in Ischaemic Disease (LIPID) study[53] was a double-blind, randomized controlled trial examining the effects of pravastatin on mortality due to coronary heart disease. Patients were randomized to pravastatin 40 mg or placebo and followed for an average of 6 years. Although the original study was related to coronary heart disease, Reid et al. used data from the original LIPID study to examine the effects of pravastatin on bone fractures.[52] Their motivation for the study was to explore further the hypothesis that statin drugs may reduce the risk of fractures. As discussed in the article, previous epidemiologic studies suggested that the effects of statins on fracture risk ranged from no effect to a 70% reduction in risk, with varying degrees of statistical significance. To overcome the limitations of these previous epidemiologic studies, Reid et al. used data from the LIPID study. This allowed them to examine the effects of pravastatin on fracture risk in a randomized setting without the expense and time associated with setting up a new study. The authors found that there was a 5% increase in the rate of fractures requiring hospitalization among those receiving pravastatin when compared to placebo. When they repeated the analysis to include patients with fractures that did not require hospitalization, there was actually a 4% reduction in the rate of fractures among those receiving pravastatin. In both analyses, the results were not statistically significant. The study findings revealed that there was insufficient evidence to support the hypoth-esis that statins can be protective against fractures. These findings contradicted the results of other observational studies. The authors offered some potential explanation for why there was not a statistically significant reduction in fractures among patients in the LIPID trial study who received pravastatin. There could have been other confounding factors for which observational studies reporting protective effects of statins did not control. For example, in the observational studies statin users may have been different from statin nonusers in their lipid profiles or other physiologic and lifestyle factors, all of which could be related to fracture risk and bone mineral density. By using data from the LIPID trial, Reid et al. were able to draw from the methodological strength of the original randomization so that these potentially confounding factors would be evenly distributed across the pravastatin and placebo groups, but this did not address another important limitation. In the original trial, the patients were not recruited on the basis of being at increased risk for fracture because the goal of the LIPID trial was to examine the effects of pravastatin on cardiovascular mortality. The enrolled patients were at relatively low risk for osteoporotic fractures with most being male. The fact that the original focus of the RCT was not the focus of the secondary analysis is an important consideration when using data from previous RCTs for a new study. Sufficiently different study goals between the original study and the planned secondary analysis can result in unexpected findings.

Cardiovascular Health Study to examine the relationship between statin use and new-onset dementia.[55]

Registries can also be useful data sources. These data sources can loosely be viewed as a collection of patient records on a particular topic.[56] Registries may be focused on a particular disease or the use of some drug. Some commonly used disease registries include the U.S. Renal Data System (USRDS)[57] and the National Cancer Institute's Surveillance, Epidemiology, and End Results (SEER) program.[58] Although disease registries vary in the amount of information included about drug use, some registries can facilitate collection of this data either by merging with another data source, such as administrative claims data,[59,60] or by survey or interview methods[61] for authorized projects. There are also various registries that have been created around the use of a certain drug or drug class. These are frequently used to monitor drug safety issues, such as the iPLEDGE program for isotretinoin[62] and the Antiepileptic Drug Pregnancy Registry.[63] There may also be population-based registries created for research purposes. Some of the previously mentioned national datasets, such as the Population Health Research Database in Saskatchewan, could also be viewed as registries.[42]

DEFINING OUTCOMES

The outcomes of interest in pharmacoepidemiology studies may include diseases or conditions, medical procedures (e.g., hemodialysis or mechanical ventilation), laboratory test values (e.g., hemoglobin A1c or blood glucose), or the use of a particular medication, including medication adherence. If data are being obtained by directly reviewing medical charts, the outcomes of interest can be identified somewhat easily, though prospective data collection can be time consuming. When data are obtained from a secondary data source, typically information will be recorded using some established codification scheme. Information on the particular coding schemes should be available in the documentation that accompanies any given data source. Table 4-3 provides an overview of selected codification schemes that will be useful for the following discussions about defining outcomes and exposure.

▶ Discharge Disposition

One of the most basic outcomes of interest is mortality. From the inpatient standpoint, this can be readily identified from the discharge disposition as

Table 4-3. Coding schemes for diagnoses, procedures, and drugs.

Coding scheme	Content	Comments
International Classification of Diseases (ICD)	Diseases and procedures	Clinical modification (ICD-9-CM) used for coding diseases and procedures; ICD-10 for coding causes of death; ICD-10-CM is under development; overseen by World Health Organization, maintained in the United States by the National Center for Health Statistics
Current Procedural Terminology (CPT)	Services and procedures	Includes services performed by the provider; updated annually by the American Medical Association
Healthcare Common Procedure Coding System (HCPCS)	Products, services, procedures, and drugs	Covers products, procedures, and services not contained in CPT, including drug products administered; maintained by the Centers for Medicare and Medicaid Services
National Drug Code (NDC)	Drugs	Contains information on manufacturer/packager, product, and package size; this is a drug identification system rather than an actual classification system; maintained by the Food and Drug Administration
American Hospital Formulary Service (AHFS) Pharmacologic-Therapeutic Classification System	Drugs	Hierarchical classification system of drugs that moves from broad categories (e.g., antiinfective agents) to specific chemical classes (e.g., third-generation cephalosporins); maintained by the American Society of Health-System Pharmacists
Anatomic Therapeutic Classification (ATC)	Drugs	Similar to the AHFS classification, but offers five levels of specificity where the fifth level is a unique chemical entity (e.g., ceftazidime); maintained by the World Health Organization

ICD-9-CM, International Classification of Diseases, Ninth Revision, Clinical Modification; ICD-10-CM, ICD-CM, Tenth Revision. Modified, with permission, from Ref. 35.

noted in the hospital discharge abstract. There are several discharge dispositions, but they can be collapsed into a "discharged alive" vs. "not discharged alive" dichotomy. Examples of other discharge dispositions include discharged to a skilled nursing facility, discharged to home health care, and discharged against medical advice. On an outpatient basis, identifying mortality may require more effort. If the patient's identity and location are known, then they could be cross-checked with the appropriate state vital records division to determine whether a death certificate is on record. Obviously, great care must be taken to ensure that the correct person's death certificate is identified. Ideally, the data sources would already include a mortality variable by cross-checking with death certificates.

▶ Diseases and Conditions

Diseases or conditions are frequently outcomes of interest (e.g., Was the patient admitted to the hospital with a myocardial infarction?). The International Classification of Diseases system is used to represent diseases and conditions in many data sources, such as automated health care databases or EMRs. The version being used currently for morbidity classification is the International Classification of Diseases, Ninth Revision, Clinical Modification (ICD-9-CM). The "clinical modification" is an important distinction because there is an "unmodified" version used to classify causes of death. Although the most recent version of the overall ICD system is the 10th revision (i.e., ICD-10), it is only used on death certificates at this time because the clinical modification (ICD-10-CM) is currently under development with implementation planned for 2013.[64] The ICD-9-CM is a hierarchical system that allows a significant amount of flexibility in determining the scope of the conditions identified by simply selecting the appropriate coding level. All ICD-9-CM codes are four or five characters in length (e.g., 008.45 Intestinal infection due to *Clostridium difficile*) and are grouped such that the highest level represents organ systems or disease processes (e.g., infectious and parasitic diseases, neoplasms, and circulatory system). Within each general group, codes allow increasing degrees of specificity. The coding for hypertension is shown as an example in Figure 4-1.

There are two important points to remember when defining disease or condition outcomes of interest. First, relevant codes should be used reliably within the data source. For example, an extremely uncommon condition that is documented infrequently by physicians in the medical record or coded unreliably by coding staff may not be a useful outcome of interest from a research standpoint.[7] The second consideration is that a disease or condition must be noted by the physician in the medical chart in order for it to be coded as a diagnosis by medical coding staff. In a related fashion, diseases or conditions may be more appropriate outcomes than symptoms would. For example, syncope or falling will probably not be frequently coded unless some significant event (e.g., a hip fracture) happened subsequently.[65]

For patients who have been admitted to the hospital, discharge diagnoses are the most likely source of information for diseases as outcomes of interest. The primary limitation of using discharge diagnoses is that they are not assigned until after the patient is discharged. Determining when a diagnosis occurred during the hospital stay can be very difficult because there is no date attached to a diagnosis given that it is assigned after discharge. Diagnosis dates for certain conditions can be estimated if appropriate data are available, such as the date of a positive culture or the start of an antibiotic to treat an infection.[66] The number of diagnoses recorded for patients may vary from institution to institution but generally ranges anywhere from 5 to 15 diagnoses with one code being identified as the *primary*, or *principal, diagnosis*. All other diagnoses are referred to as *secondary diagnoses*. As the reimbursements are tied to diagnosis codes, there can be an incentive to include codes that would increase the amount reimbursed for a given hospital stay. This must be kept in mind as those conditions that are likely to result in a higher reimbursement are more likely to be included as a discharge diagnosis.[16] Although admission diagnoses, or working diagnoses or problem lists, may be collected at the time of admission, these are not included in hospital discharge data, but they may be included in EMR data. The primary admission diagnosis will likely be similar to the principal discharge diagnosis, but this is not always the case with the true

```
390-459.9      Circulatory System
   401-405        Hypertensive Disease
      401            Essential Hypertension
                     401.0  Malignant Essential Hypertension
                     401.1  Benign Essential Hypertension
                     401.9  Unspecified Essential Hypertension
      402            Hypertensive Heart Disease
                     402.0  Malignant Hypertensive Heart Disease
                     402.1  Benign Hypertensive Heart Disease
                     402.9  Unspecified Hypertensive Heart Disease
      403            Hypertensive Chronic Kidney Disease
                     403.0  Malignant Hypertensive Renal Disease
                     403.1  Benign Hypertensive Renal Disease
                     403.9  Unspecified Hypertensive Renal Disease
      404            Hypertensive Heart and Chronic Kidney Disease
                     404.0  Malignant Hypertensive Heart and Renal Disease
                     404.1  Benign Hypertensive Heart and Renal Disease
                     404.9  Unspecified Hypertensive Heart and Renal Disease
      405            Secondary Hypertension
                     405.0  Malignant Secondary Hypertension
                            405.01  Malignant Renovascular Hypertension
                            405.09  Other Malignant Secondary Hypertension
                     405.1  Benign Secondary Hypertension
                            405.11  Benign Renovascular Hypertension
                            405.19  Other Benign Secondary Hypertension
                     405.9  Unspecified Secondary Hypertension
                            405.91  Unspecified Renovascular Hypertension
                            405.99  Other Unspecified Secondary Hypertension
```

▲ **Figure 4-1.** The International Classification of Diseases, Ninth Revision, Clinical Codification (ICD-9-CM) is commonly used to code diseases and conditions. The coding for hypertension is provided in the figure. ICD-9-CM codes are grouped by organ system and proceed to increasingly specific classifications. By selecting the appropriate number of digits, one can identify various diagnoses of interest. For example, selecting the code 401.XX would identify all patients with essential hypertension, whereas selecting 405.1X would identify all patients with benign secondary hypertension. When using ICD-9-CM codes, an "X" means that all numbers in that place were considered when selecting patients. Using benign secondary hypertension as an example, 405.1X would include 405.11 and 405.19.

degree of concordance between the admission diagnosis and primary discharge diagnosis being unknown.[67] The same ICD-9-CM system is used to code the primary presenting diseases or chief complains for medical office visits.

▶ Procedures and Services

The utilization of services may also be an outcome of interest. Measuring utilization may be as simple as counting the number of days in the hospital or determining whether a certain procedure was performed. Depending on the level of detail available in a data source, some types of length of stay variables (critical or intensive care days) may or may not be available. Procedures may also be outcomes of interest. For inpatient procedures or those that are billed through the hospital or facility, ICD-9-CM codes are used for identification of procedures. One interesting point to make is that ICD-9-CM procedure codes for hospitalized patients include a date of service provision, unlike the diagnoses codes. This can be useful to establish temporal relationships between the exposure of interest and the outcome. Medical office visits, office-based procedures, or those procedures that are billed directly by a provider, even if performed at a facility, are typically reported on provider claims using the Current Procedural Terminology (CPT) system and the related Healthcare Common Procedure Coding System (HCPCS). These codes represent services performed by health care providers.[68] Currently, there are codes included for medication therapy management services provided by pharmacists (codes 99605, 99606, and 99607).[69] CPT codes are nonhierarchical in nature but are loosely grouped on the effort involved in performing the procedure. The lack of a true hierarchy can make it difficult to identify clinically meaningful groups through the use of higher-level codes (e.g., all procedures relating to lung-function tests). Instead, the user must identify all codes of interest.[70]

Procedure codes can be particularly useful in the study of patient safety within hospitals. For example, a blood transfusion in a nonsurgical patient may be indicative of an overdose of an anticoagulant.[71] In a similar fashion, outpatient medical procedures can be useful to examine process-related outcomes like the extent to which monitoring is performed for various medications (e.g., aminotransferase levels and thyroid-function tests for amiodarone or the International Normalized Ratio for warfarin)[72,73] (Case Study 4-2). On occasion, the results of laboratory tests may be surrogates of the outcome of interest (e.g., meeting target hemoglobin A1c or serum lipid goals). The availability of these results will vary from source to source. Electronic medical records may include laboratory results. Although administrative claims data sources will typically have information about whether a laboratory test was ordered, they rarely include the results of those tests. If data are being obtained from medical record review or from local information systems, like the laboratory information system, it may be possible to gather useful laboratory information.[35]

▶ Drug Utilization

The use of a particular drug or class of drugs can be an important outcome in pharmacoepidemiology studies. Various coding schemes are used to identify drugs within secondary data sources and are discussed in greater detail in the next section. Certain

CASE STUDY 4-2
Identifying Outcomes with Administrative Claims Data

Although administrative claims data may not include actual laboratory test results, whether or not a specific laboratory test was performed (or billed) should be captured in the insurance claims submitted by the medical office. This type of information can still be useful in the measurement of process-related outcomes or the assessment of quality improvement programs through the use of claims data. Raebel et al. studied liver- and thyroid-function monitoring in a group of ambulatory patients being treated with amiodarone.[72] As discussed by the investigators, various recommendations exist surrounding the frequency of monitoring for any disturbances in thyroid or liver function when patients are on amiodarone therapy. The study was conducted in a group of 10 health maintenance organizations (HMOs). Although each HMO maintained its own administrative claims database, the standard coding system for procedures performed in the medical office and submitted for coding was used to identify laboratory tests of interest. Patients with eligible amiodarone use and medical office claims were identified. CPT codes were used to identify laboratory tests of interest. As mentioned in the text, CPT codes are nonhierarchical so multiple codes were necessary to identify the tests of interest. For example, there were five codes used to identify alanine aminotransferase (ALT) tests (CPT: 80050, 80053, 80058, 80076, 84460). This variety of codes relates to changes in coding over time (e.g., 80058 was for 1999, and 80076 was for 2000 and 2001) and differences in test names (e.g., 80053 is a comprehensive metabolic panel that includes ALT, and 84460 is for ALT only).

drugs can be used to identify potential adverse events and/or medication errors (e.g., sodium polystyrene for potassium toxicity or vitamin K infusions for warfarin overdoses or overanticoagulation). These uses have been the focus of significant research in the area of medication safety.[71] Drug utilization patterns can also be useful outcomes of interest. The addition of a new drug to an existing therapeutic regimen can represent therapeutic intensification and may be a marker of disease progression. Intensification can also result in improved outcomes as seen in a study of glycemic levels in type 2 diabetes patients by Davis et al.[74] In this study, intensification was associated with improvements in hemoglobin A1c levels and lipid profiles. Switching from one drug to another can be an indicator of therapeutic failure. Amidon et al.[75] examined patients who were part of a therapeutic interchange program of proton-pump inhibitors. In their study, therapeutic failure was defined as switching from the formulary agent to an alternate drug therapy for acid suppression in that study. *Adherence* and *persistence* associated with a given therapeutic regimen can also be important outcomes that involve drugs. Adherence, or compliance, and persistence are common measures of drug exposure when prescription claims or dispensing data are available. Methods for measuring medication adherence and persistence are discussed in greater detail in Chapter 8.

Another useful method of examining drug utilization, particularly when comparing drugs or drug classes, is the Defined Daily Dose (DDD) methodology. According to the World Health Organization (WHO), a DDD is "the assumed average maintenance dose per day for a drug used for its main indication in adults."[76] The DDDs that are developed by the WHO are specific to a drug and route of administration, so there can be an oral DDD and a parenteral DDD for the same drug. The number of DDDs for a given drug can be calculated by dividing the total amount (e.g., milligrams or grams) of drug dispensed or purchased during a specific time period by the WHO's assigned DDD for that drug and route of administration. Using enalapril tablets as an example, a patient may have received 3,600 mg of drug based on prescription fill records. The DDD for oral enalapril is 10 mg according to the 2009 Anatomical Therapeutic Chemical (ATC) DDD Index, so the total DDDs

received by the patient is 360 (3,600 mg ÷ 10 mg). The DDD methodology is particularly useful when comparing drug utilization at the group level, such as a hospital or drug plan, or when making state or international comparisons. When making these group-level comparisons, the utilization is usually normalized to produce some number of DDDs per 100 or 1,000 patient-days, admissions, discharges, health plan members, or population.[77] For example, a hospital wants to compare its use of ceftriaxone to the national average. The WHO DDD for ceftriaxone is 2 g. The hospital determines that it has dispensed 4,439.5 g of ceftriaxone over the previous calendar year. During the same time period, there were 69,052 patient-days representing 14,692 patients. The total DDDs of ceftriaxone per 1,000 patient days for the hospital could be calculated as follows.

$$(4{,}439.5 \text{ g ceftriaxone}) \times \left(\frac{\text{DDD}}{2 \text{ g}} \right)$$

$$= 2{,}219.75 \text{ DDDs of ceftriaxone}$$

$$\left(\frac{2{,}219.75 \text{ DDDs ceftriaxone}}{69{,}052 \text{ patient-days}} \right) \times 1000$$

$$= 32.1 \text{ DDDs of ceftriaxone per 1000 patient-days}$$

This hospital-specific value could then be compared to the national average or to peer hospitals to make standardized comparisons.

Although the DDD method is useful for making standardized comparisons and is promoted by the WHO, it does have some notable disadvantages. One of the most frequently cited disadvantages is that the DDD figures determined by WHO are somewhat arbitrary and may not be appropriate on a country-by-country basis due to practice variations. Researchers in various countries have adapted the DDDs published by WHO to more accurately reflect actual drug usage in their own countries.[78,79] The assigned DDD relates only to the primary indication as determined by WHO, but other indications may use different dosages. Also, the primary use of a drug in clinical practice may not be the same across all countries where the drug is approved. DDDs for combination products can be assigned using a "unit dose" (i.e., DDD of 1 for combination products given once a day or 2 for those given twice a day)[80] or may be based on specific rules developed by WHO. Some of these rules may systematically underestimate the true level of drug utilization.[76] As WHO's goal is to have the DDD serve as a finite quantity to generate standardized levels of drug usage, DDDs reflect a "standard" person (i.e., 70 kg if weight-based dosing is used). Furthermore, no adjustments in DDDs are made for renal or hepatic insufficiencies that may be necessary in the course of clinical practice.[81] This can be important if comparisons are being made across groups where the patient populations represented may include patients with conditions requiring dose adjustment. The WHO only assigns DDDs for adult patients,[76] so making standardized comparisons with respect to pediatric drug utilization can be difficult.

Several methods have been proposed to overcome the limitations of the DDD methodology. One method that is developed to be similar to the DDD is the Prescribed Daily Dose (PDD) method. This method is useful in that it can be calculated from the data at hand (e.g., hospital dispensing or ordering data) to reflect the actual average doses being prescribed to patients or from dispensing or ordering data reflective of national prescribing habits. Unfortunately, the PDD is not a standardized unit appropriate for international comparisons because it is by definition location specific. Although the PDD may be more reflective of local drug utilization patterns, it can be considerably different from the DDD as assigned by the WHO.[77] Another method is the Days of Therapy (DOT) method, which is simply a count of the number of days that at least one dose of the drug was taken or should have been taken.[81] This method overcomes issues with differing doses or required adjustments for renal or hepatic insufficiency. It does not, however, take into consideration the actual dose of the drug. For example, assume there are 3 patients receiving an antibiotic that is scheduled to be given 3 times a day. On the same day, the first patient receives one regular dose of the antibiotic because the order is started late in the evening, the second patient receives all three doses over the course of the day, and the third patient only receives two doses since he or she has reduced kidney function requiring a reduction in dose frequency. Under the DOT method, all three of these patients will be counted as having received one DOT. Although the DDD method and the DOT method may produce different quantities, they are frequently well correlated.[81]

DEFINING EXPOSURE

In pharmacoepidemiologic studies, the primary exposure of interest is often the use of some drug. There are two important issues in defining these exposures of interest. First, the drug, or drug class, must be identified within the data source. Second, the method of measuring the exposure must be selected. As mentioned previously, various coding schemes can be used to represent drugs (Table 4-3). Diseases, conditions, or procedures may also be exposures of interest in pharmacoepidemiologic studies. These can be particularly useful when examining compliance with practice guidelines (e.g., venous thromboembolism guidelines as studied by Yu et al.[82]). The principles related to disease and procedure coding discussed in the previous section apply when the exposure of interest is some disease, condition, or procedure.

▶ Drug Coding Schemes

When considering the ways to code drugs, especially within secondary data sources, there are two distinct concepts: identification and classification. *Drug identification* relates to the ability to uniquely identify the drug, or drug product, to which a given subject was exposed, whereas *drug classification* generally relates to placing drugs into various categories. Classification can be useful when a general drug group, rather than one particular drug, is of interest. This distinction is important because codes that are used to identify unique drug products may not effectively classify those same products (e.g., therapeutic or chemical classification), and vice versa. There may be situations where comparisons among unique drugs within a class are of interest (e.g., the relative effectiveness of various angiotensin-converting enzyme inhibitors in controlling blood pressure), so some system that could both classify and identify would be ideal. This requires some care when working with drug coding schemes. Some data sources may only use codes that identify drugs, leaving the user to derive the classifications; however, there are programs that can be used to facilitate the classification process. Other data sources use several coding schemes to allow more flexibility.

The most familiar drug coding scheme is probably the National Drug Code (NDC) system. The NDC is a drug identification scheme that is composed of three parts: a manufacturer (or packager) code, a product code, and a package size code.[83] These codes are used frequently by community pharmacies on pharmacy claims to identify the drug product being dispensed to a patient. One of the advantages of the NDC system is that it provides a great degree of specificity by allowing the identification of the drug product, manufacturer/packager, and package size. One of the drawbacks of NDCs is that they do not allow for classification of drugs. Although all products from one manufacturer can be identified through the manufacturer code, the NDC does not directly allow grouping of drugs into any therapeutically meaningful categories. Another drawback of NDCs is that there is a separate NDC for every product strength, manufacturer/packager, and package size combination. For example, simvastatin 20 mg tablets manufactured by Merck in a bottle of 100 will have a different NDC than a similar product produced by a generic manufacturer in the same package size. In a similar fashion, for simvastatin 20 mg tablets produced by Merck there will be one NDC for a bottle of 100 tablets and another NDC for a box of 100 tablets packaged in a unit dose form. Obviously, this can lead to extremely large numbers of NDCs for any given drug or drug product. To overcome this potential problem, other coding systems may be more appropriate when distinctions between unique drug products (e.g., two different strengths or manufacturers of the same drug) are not important. Other important limitations of NDCs include possible inconsistencies in the length of the code (10 digit vs 11 digit) and that some codes may be reused for a new product when an old one is no longer marketed.[70,83]

Two frequently used drug coding schemes that avoid some of the limitations associated with the NDC system are the American Hospital Formulary Service Pharmacologic-Therapeutic Classification System (AHFS)[84] and the Anatomic Therapeutic Chemical Classification System (ATC)[85] developed by the WHO.

The two schemes are similar in that they provide increasing levels of specificity with respect to classification. The primary differences are in the levels of specificity and the ability to identify unique drugs. The ATC system offers five levels of specificity compared to four in the AHFS system. Individual drugs can be identified within the ATC system. In contrast, all drugs in the same class (e.g., second-generation cephalosporins) would have the same code under the AHFS system. From this standpoint, the ATC system can be viewed as both a drug classification and a drug identification system. An example of the three drug coding systems discussed in this section is provided in Figure 4-2.

There are several other coding schemes that employ similar classification systems as AHFS and ATC. These can offer increased flexibility or specificity (e.g., distinguish between simvastatin 20 mg tablet and simvastatin 40 mg tablet). Some of these systems are maintained by companies that provide drug information to various health care organizations. These include the Generic Product Identifier system from Medi-Span, the Enhanced Therapeutic Classification System™ from First DataBank, and the therapeutic classifications within Cerner Multum's Lexicon.[35] The Veterans Health Administration also maintains its own drug classification system that is similar to the AHFS system. Sometimes drugs may be administered or provided to patients during the course of a medical office visit (e.g., cancer chemotherapy). In these situations, HCPCS codes are used to identify drugs for billing purposes (i.e., on the insurance claim).[86]

▶ Measuring Drug Exposure

Once the exposure of interest has been identified, some method of measuring the exposure is necessary. There are two general ways of measuring drug exposure. It can be categorized (e.g., yes vs. no) or measured in a continuous fashion (e.g., the actual number of doses received or the milligrams ingested). Categorical exposure may be used in preliminary exploration to provide a description of the extent of the sample that is exposed to the drug (e.g., 50% of patients received an antibiotic or 20% of patients received clopidogrel). Although this may seem relatively simple, categorical drug exposure must be carefully defined. For example, "exposure" could be defined as

National Drug Code (NDC)

60238-3130-*2 – Kefzol for injection (1 g single-dose vial in a package of 25)
60238-3135-*2 – Kefzol for injection (10 g multidose vial in a package of 6)
60505-0748-*4 – Cefazolin for injection (500 mg single-dose vial in a package of 10)
60505-0748-*5 – Cefazolin for injection (500 mg single-dose vial in a package of 25)
00781-3451-70 – Cefazolin for injection (1 g single dose vial in a package of 10)

Anatomic Therapeutic Chemical Classification System (ATC)

J – Anti-infectives for systemic use
J01 – Antibacterials for systemic use
J01D – Other beta-lactam antibacterials
J01DB – First-generation cephalosporins
J01DB04 – Cefazolin

Pharmacologic-Therapeutic Classification System (AHFS)

8:00 – Anti-infective agents
8:12 – Antibacterials
8:12.06 – Cephalosporins
8:12.06.04 – First Generation Cephalosporins

▲ **Figure 4-2.** Depending on which drug coding system is used, cefazolin could be represented in a variety of different ways. Notice that the NDC codes are product specific, so the same product by a different manufacturer or in a different dose/package size will have a different NDC. The ATC system can identify individual drugs but does not distinguish between manufacturers, doses, or package sizes. Although the AHFS system can identify varying levels of drug categories, it does not identify unique drugs.

one filled prescription for an outpatient or one dispensed dose for an inpatient, or the definition might require at least two filled prescriptions or dispensed doses. Taking basic therapeutic principles into consideration can be useful in developing these definitions (e.g., is one 30-day prescription of a lipid-lowering drug sufficient to reduce the 10-year risk of cardiovascular death?). The definition ultimately depends on the nature of the research question. Categorical drug exposure need not include only two levels, because there could be low, medium, and high classifications.

Sometimes it is desirable to quantify drug exposure. There are several general methods to accomplish this. The first method uses information about the actual amount of the drug prescribed. This information is usually available in pharmacy claims or dispensing data or potentially in the EMR. If the dosage documented in the EMR is used, it would need to be compared with prescription claims or dispensing data to verify that the drug was actually dispensed. The amount of drug can

be summed over the study period for a given patient to calculate the total exposure (e.g., in milligrams or grams) to the drug of interest. This same information could be used to determine the average amount of drug per day, or the *daily dose*. For example, a patient with diabetes is taking metformin at a dose of 500 mg 3 times daily would have a daily dose of 1,500 mg (500 mg per dose × 3 doses per day). This type of information could be calculated for individuals in the community or for hospitalized patients if the appropriate data are available. If comparisons between drugs or drug classes are being made, some method to arrive at a standardized dose, such as the previously described DDD methodology, is necessary.

In some situations, information about the amount of drug prescribed or dispensed is not available. In these instances, drug exposure can still be quantified from the perspective of time. One way to do this is to use the DOT methodology described previously. Another measure that is closely related to the DOT method is to measure the length (or duration) of therapy. The DOT and length of therapy will differ when a drug is prescribed less frequently than once daily (e.g., every other day or once a week). Calculating the length of therapy is as simple as determining the amount of time between the first dose and the last dose. Although the DOT and length of therapy methods are most appropriate when information about charges or administration for individual doses is available, outpatient drug data, such as prescription claims data, could be used to estimate the length of therapy by calculating the time between the filling of initial prescription to the time of the last prescription refill plus the days supply of the last prescription. This is quite similar to measuring persistence with a drug therapy. This assumes that the doses are taken as prescribed. Estimating DOTs with outpatient drug data is more difficult.

In addition to quantifying drug exposure, it is often useful to determine when exposure began. This is very important when the outcome must be determined to have occurred after exposure to the drug began. The concept of the index date as discussed in the previous chapter can also be applied to drug exposure. In this situation, the index date for drug exposure may be the date when the first prescription was filled for outpatients or when the first dose was dispensed or administered for inpatients. When conducting cohort studies (see Chapter 3), this index date for drug exposure would mark the beginning of observation time for the individual. Sometimes, drug exposure may be an outcome of interest (e.g., use of Drug X to treat a particular disease or as a marker of an adverse reaction). The index date would still be the date of initial exposure to the drug of interest. In this case, however, the study might involve looking retrospectively to determine whether some exposure (e.g., a disease or another drug) occurred within a specified time frame before the index date.

Prescription claims data or prescription dispensing data are often used when outpatient drug exposure is being measured. Adherence and persistence are common measures of drug exposure when claims or dispensing data are available, as further discussed in Chapter 8. Various studies have been conducted to look at drug adherence as predictors of outcomes, such as the relationship between adherence to bis-phosphonates and the risk of hip fracture by Rabenda et al.[87] or the relationship between medication adherence and the risk of hospitalization by Sokol et al.[88]

SPECIAL CONSIDERATIONS WHEN USING SECONDARY DATA

Using secondary data for research purposes offers several advantages over primary data collection, as described previously in this chapter. Some issues, such as research approval by the local institutional review or ethics board, are important regardless of whether primary or secondary data are being used. There are, however, several issues that are not typical considerations when using primary data. Two important issues are discussed here.

▶ Patient Privacy and HIPAA

The Privacy Rule enacted as part of the Health Insurance Portability and Accountability Act of 1997 (HIPAA) has made the safeguarding of *protected health information* (PHI) an important consideration for researchers using secondary data sources, especially administrative or transactional data. On the basis of the Privacy Rule, researchers may have access to *de-identified datasets* that have been stripped of specified pieces of identifiable and potentially sensitive information. As identifiable information has been removed, the resulting data are not PHI and may, therefore, be used without obtaining authorization from individuals. For projects requiring information that could potentially identify an individual (e.g., date of birth, ZIP code, and procedure dates), the information may be disclosed to researchers after obtaining an authorization from all individuals in the dataset. Obviously, obtaining an authorization from tens or hundreds of thousands of individuals is not practical. The Privacy Rule does provide a mechanism to waive the authorization requirement. By demonstrating that the use of the PHI results in minimal or no risk to the individuals, that the research could not be done without the waiver of authorization and that the PHI is necessary for the research question, an investigator can enter into an agreement with the data provider by signing a *data use agreement* (DUA) that specifies the appropriate use and further disclosure of the PHI that is being provided.[89]

Data Structure and Linkage

Sometimes the information necessary for a study may reside in separate databases. In order to bring the information together, the ability to identify the same participant across databases is vital. The process of identifying participants across databases and over time and matching their information is called data linkage.[19,90] The task of linking information requires a great deal of effort, given the potential issues with patient pri-

vacy, data security, and legal regulations associated with HIPAA. Fortunately, there are organizations that act as data aggregators. These organizations gather information from various sources and provide access to fully linked, HIPAA-compliant databases representing a wide range of information. These linked databases are typically available to researchers through licensing agreements; however, there may be considerable fees involved with using these data. Bringing information together at the local institutional level may be much easier, as you probably have access to medical record numbers and patient account numbers to facilitate linkage across sources from within the institution as

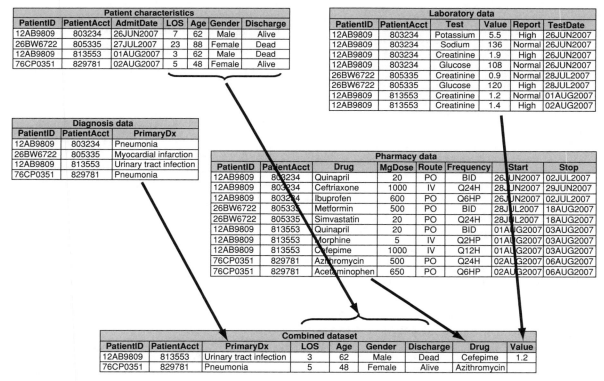

▲ **Figure 4-3.** Data from various sources can be linked together. This figure represents an example of linking data from separate sources within an institution. The medical record number (PatientID in the figure) can be used to identify patients, and the patient account number (PatientAcct in the figure), or some similar identifier, can be used to identify unique encounters within each patient. With these two pieces of information, the data from the various sources can be linked together. The figure might represent a query to identify those patients who received antibiotics no more than 1 day after admission and gather information on their first serum creatinine level, length of stay (LOS), age, gender, and discharge status. (Reprinted, with permission, from Ref. 35.)

shown in Figure 4-3. Similar principles apply when linking data from other sources (e.g., administrative claims data, and death certificates) except it can require more effort to ensure that the same patient's records are correctly linked across the multiple sources.

▼ SUMMARY

Although pharmacoepidemiologic research can be conducted on primary data, such studies frequently make use of secondary data. With the increased use of information technology in the provision of health care-related activities, tremendous amounts of data are routinely collected that can be useful from a research standpoint. It is important to be familiar with the various methods in which outcomes and exposures can be coded in order to use these secondary data sources effectively. When selecting a data source, special consideration must be given to the relative strengths and weaknesses of each particular data source and whether it might be able to address the research question. As with other forms of research, there are certain regulatory aspects that should be considered even though direct interaction with patients may not occur.

DISCUSSION QUESTIONS

1. What are the two general types of data sources that can be used in pharmacoepidemiologic studies? Give one advantage and one disadvantage for each type.

2. Briefly describe why pharmacoepidemiologic studies using secondary data can be viewed as being better suited to study drug effectiveness when compared to randomized controlled trials.

3. What is meant by the term "data linkage"? Why is it important in pharmacoepidemiology?

4. Using web sites or other resources, identify the appropriate ICD-9-CM code for the following conditions:
   a. End-stage renal disease
   b. Secondary diabetes mellitus without complication (regardless of controlled or uncontrolled status)
   c. Candidiasis (including all sites)

5. Briefly describe how a drug can be an exposure of interest in one study and an outcome of interest in another.

6. Discuss how the following exposures could be measured categorically and how they could be measured continuously:
   a. Hemodialysis
   b. Cefepime
   c. Intensive care unit admission

7. What is the difference between a drug classification system and a drug identification system?

8. In Case Study 4-2, one of the eligibility criteria for the study was that a patient was receiving amiodarone. There are several different coding schemes that could be used to identify this drug. For the following three drug coding schemes, list an advantage and a disadvantage of each:
   a. National Drug Code (NDC) system
   b. American Hospital Formulary Service (AHFS) system
   c. Anatomic-Therapeutic Classification (ATC) system

9. Using web sites or other appropriate resources, identify two (2) NDC codes, the appropriate ATC code, and the appropriate AHFS classification code for the following drugs:
   a. Fluconazole
   b. Dofetilide
   c. Paroxetine

REFERENCES

1. Sørensen HT, Sabroe S, Olsen J. A framework for evaluation of secondary data sources for epidemiological research. *Int J Epidemiol*. 1996;25(2):435-442.

2. Buring JE. Primary data collection: What should well-trained epidemiology doctoral students be able to do? *Epidemiology*. 2008;19(2):347-349.

3. Suissa S, Garbe E. Primer: administrative health databases in observational studies of drug effects: advantages and disadvantages. *Nat Clin Pract Rheumatol*. 2007;3(12): 725-732.

4. Schneeweiss S, Avorn J. A review of uses of health care utilization databases for epidemiologic research on therapeutics. *J Clin Epidemiol*. 2005;58(4):323-337.

5. Arana A, Rivero R, Egberts TCG. What do we show and who does so? An analysis of abstracts presented at the 19th

ICPE. *Pharmacoepidemiol Drug Saf.* 2004;13(suppl 1): S330-S331.

6. Gardner JS, Park BJ, Stergachis A. Automated databases in pharmacoepidemiologic studies. In: Hartzema AG, Tilson HH, Porta MS, eds. *Pharmacoepidemiology: An Introduction,* 3rd ed. Cincinnati, OH: Harvey Whitney Books,1998: 368-388.

7. Motheral BR, Fairman KA. The use of claims databases for outcomes research: Rationale, challenges, and strategies. *Clin Ther.* 1997;19(2):346-366.

8. Gandhi SK, Salmon JW, Kong SX, Zhao SZ. Administrative databases and outcomes assessment: An overview of issues and potential utility. *J Manag Care Pharm.* 1999;5(3):215-222.

9. Ary D, Jacobs LC, Razavieh A. *Introduction to Research in Education,* 6th ed. Belmont, CA: Wadsworth Group,2002: 287-288.

10. Rothman JK, Greenland S, Lash TL. Validity in epidemiologic studies. In: Rothman JK, Greenland S, Lash TL, eds. *Modern Epidemiology,* 3rd ed. Philadelphia, PA: Lippincott Williams & Wilkins, 2008:128-147.

11. Lau HS, De Boer A, Beuning KS, Porsius A. Validation of pharmacy records in drug exposure assessment. *J Clin Epidemiol.* 1997;50(5):619-625.

12. Glintborg B, Hillestrøm PR, Olsen LH, Dalhoff KP, Pulsen HE. Are patients reliable when self-reporting medication use? Validation of structured drug interviews and home visits by drug analysis and prescription data in acutely hospitalized patients. *J Clin Pharmacol.* 2007;47(11):1440-1449.

13. Kaboli PJ, McClimon BJ, Hoth AB, Barnett MJ. Assessing the accuracy of computerized medication histories. *Am J Manag Care.* 2004;10(11 Pt. 2):872-877.

14. Quan H, Parsons GA, Ghali WA. Validity of information on comorbidity derived from ICD-9-CCM administrative data. *Med Care.* 2002;40(8):675-685.

15. Peabody JW, Luck J, Jain S, Bertenthal D, Glassman P. Assessing the accuracy of administrative data in health information systems. *Med Care.* 2004;42(11):1066-1072.

16. Iezzoni LI. Coded data from administrative sources. In: Iezzoni LI, ed. *Risk Adjustment for Measuring Health Care Outcomes,* 3rd ed. Chicago: Health Administration Press,2003: 83-138.

17. Curtiss FR. Evidence-based medicine: Beware of results from randomized controlled trials and research with administrative claims data. *J Manag Care Pharm.* 2005;11(2):172-177.

18. Tierney WM, McDonald CJ. Practice databases and their uses in clinical research. *Stat Med.* 1991;10(4):541-557.

19. Dunn HL. Record linkage. *Am J Public Health.* 1946;36(12): 1412-1416.

20. Else BA, Armstrong EP, Cox ER. Data sources for pharmacoeconomic and health services research. *Am J Health Syst Pharm.* 1997;54(22):2601-2608.

21. Overview of Acute Inpatient PPS. Centers for Medicare and Medicaid Services Web site. http://www.cms.hhs.gov/ acuteinpatientpps. Accessed December 8, 2008.

22. Troiano D. A primer on pharmacy information systems. *J Healthc Inf Manag.* 1999;13(3):41-52.

23. Rose JS, Fisch BJ, Hogan WR, et al. Common medical terminology comes of age. Part One: Standard language improves healthcare quality. *J Healthc Inf Manag.* 2001; 15(3):307-318.

24. Ramick DC. Data warehousing in disease management programs. *J Healthc Inf Manag.* 2001;15(2):99-105.

25. Hashim R, Lewis TL, Rosenfeld SJ. Managing clinical research information: A case study in information access, presentation, and analysis. *J Healthc Inf Manag.* 2000;14(3): 5-18.

26. Aitken M, Berndt ER, Cutler DM. Prescription drug spending trends in the United States: Looking beyond the turning point. *Health Aff (Millwood).* 2009;28(1):w151-w160.

27. Wagner MM, Robinson JM, Tsui F, Espino JU, Hogan WR. Design of a national retail drug monitor for public health surveillance. *J Am Med Inform Assoc.* 2003;10(5):409-418.

28. Edge VL, Pollari F, Lim G, et al. Syndromic surveillance of gastrointestinal illness using pharmacy over-the-counter sales. *Can J Public Health.* 2004;95(6):446-450.

29. Jha AK, DesRoches CM, Campbell EG, et al. Use of electronic health records in U.S. hospitals. *New Engl J Med.* 2009;360(16): 1628–1638.

30. DesRoches CM, Campbell EG, Rao SR, et al. Electronic health records in ambulatory care–a national survey of physicians. *New Engl J Med.* 2008;359(1):50-60.

31. West SL, Blake C, Zhiwen Liu, McKoy JN, Oertel MD, Carey TS. Reflections on the use of electronic health record data for clinical research. *Health Informatics J.* 2009;15(2): 108-121.

32. Roth CP, Lim Y, Pevnick JM, Asch SM, McGlynn EA. The challenge of measuring quality of care from the electronic health record. *Am J Med Qual.* 2009;24(5):385-394.

33. Zweigenbaum P, Bouaud J, Bachimont B, Charlet J, Séroussi B, Boisvieux JF. From text to knowledge: A unifying document-centered view of analyzed medical language. *Methods Inf Med.* 1998;37(4-5):384-393.

34. Cios KJ, Moore GW. Uniqueness of medical data mining. *Artif Intell Med.* 2002;26(1-2):1-24.

35. Harpe SE. Using secondary data sources for pharmacoepidemiology and outcomes research. *Pharmacotherapy.* 2009;29 (2):138-153.

36. Research Data Assistance Center (ResDAC) Web site. http://www.resdac.umn.edu. Accessed April 20, 2009.

37. Databases and Related Tools from HCUP. Fact Sheet. AHRQ Publication No. 06-P022. May 2006. Agency for Healthcare Research and Quality Web site. http://www.ahrq.gov/ data/ hcup/datahcup. htm. Accessed April 18, 2009.

38. Survey Background. Medical Expenditure Panel Survey Web site. http://meps.ahrq.gov/mepsweb/about_meps/survey_ back.jsp. Agency for Healthcare Research and Quality. Accessed April 18, 2009.

39. About the Ambulatory Health Care Surveys. National Center for Health Statistics Web site. http://www.cdc.gov/nchs/ahcd/ about_ahcd.htm. Accessed April 19, 2009.

40. Available Surveys and Data Collection Systems. National Center for Health Statistics Web site. http://www.cdc.gov/nchs/ surveys.htm. Accessed January 25, 2010.

41. The Database. GPRD Web site. http://www.gprd.com/ products/database.asp. Accessed April 18, 2009.

42. Roos LL, Nicol JP. A research registry: uses, development, and accuracy. *J Clin Epidemiol.* 1999;52(1):39-47.

43. MedWatch: The FDA Safety Information and Adverse Event Reporting Program. US Food and Drug Administration Web site.

http://www.fda.gov/Safety/MedWatch/default.htm. Accessed May 2, 2009.

44. Adverse Event Reporting System (AERS). U.S. Food and Drug Administration Web site. http://www.fda.gov/Drugs/Guidance ComplianceRegulatoryInformation/Surveillance/Adverse-DrugEffects/default.htm. Accessed May 2, 2009.

45. Vaccine Adverse Event Reporting System Web site. http://www.vaers.hhs.gov. Accessed May 2, 2009.

46. Santell JP, Hicks RW, McMeekin J, Cousins DD. Medication errors: Experience of the United States Pharmacopeia (USP) MEDMARX reporting system. *J Clin Pharmacol.* 2003;43(7): 760-767.

47. Quantros acquires MEDMARX from United States Pharmacopeia (USP) [press release]. San Francisco, CA: Quantros, Inc., 2008.

48. Griffin JP. Survey of the spontaneous adverse drug reaction reporting schemes in fifteen countries. *Br J Clin Pharmacol.* 1986;22(suppl 1):S83-S100.

49. Yellow Card Scheme. Medicines and Healthcare Products Regulatory Authority Web site. http://www.mhra.gov.uk/Safetyin-formation/Howwemonitorthesafetyofproducts/Medicines/Th eYellowCardScheme/index.htm. Accessed May 3, 2009.

50. Goldman SA. Limitations and strengths of spontaneous reports data. *Clin Ther.* 1998;20(suppl C):C40-C44.

51. Burke LB, Kennedy DL, Hunter JR. Spontaneous reporting in the United States. In: Hartzema AG, Tilson HH, Porta MS, eds. *Pharmacoepidemiology: An Introduction*, 3rd ed. Cincinnati, OH: Harvey Whitney Books,1998:213-234.

52. Reid IR, Hague W, Emberson J, et al. Effect of pravastatin on frequency of fracture in the LIPID study: Secondary analysis of a randomised controlled trial. *Lancet.* 2001;357 (9255): 509-512.

53. LIPID Study Group. Prevention of cardiovascular events and death with pravastatin in patients with coronary heart disease and a broad range of initial cholesterol levels. *New Engl J Med.* 1998;339(19):1349-1357.

54. Curhan GC, Knight EL, Rosner B, Hankinson SE, Stampfer MJ. Lifetime nonnarcotic analgesic use and decline in renal function in women. *Arch Inter Med.* 2004;164(14):1519-1524.

55. Rea TD, Breitner JC, Psaty BM, et al. Statin use and the risk of incident dementia: The Cardiovascular Health Study. *Arch Neurol.* 2005;62(7):1047-1051.

56. Rabeneck L, Menke T, Simberkoff MS, et al. Use of the national registry of HIV-infected veterans in research: Lessons for the development of disease registries. *J Clin Epidemiol.* 2001;54 (12):1195-1203.

57. US Renal Data System Web site. http://www.usrds.org. Accessed June 1, 2009.

58. Surveillance, Epidemiology, and End Results Web site. http://seer.cancer.gov/index.html. Accessed June 1, 2009.

59. Wang PS, Walker AM, Tsuang MT, Orav EJ, Levin R, Avorn J. Antidepressant use and the risk of breast cancer: A non-association. *J Clin Epidemiol.* 2001;54(7):728-734.

60. Chubak J, Boudreau DM, Rulyak SJ, Mandelson MT. Colorectal cancer risk in relation to use of acid suppressive medications. *Pharmacoepidemiol Drug Saf.* 2009;18(7): 540-544.

61. Engels EA, Cerhan JR, Linet MS, et al. Immune-related conditions and immune-modulating medications as risk factors for non-Hodgkin's lymphoma: a case-control study. *Am J Epidemiol.* 2005;126(12):1153-1161.

62. Cheetham TC, Wagner RA, Chiu G, Day JM, Yoshinaga MA, Wong L. A risk management program aimed at preventing fetal exposure to isotretinoin: Retrospective cohort study. *J Am Acad Dermatol.* 2006;55(3):442-448.

63. Holmes LB, Wyszynski DF, Lieberman E. The AED (antiepileptic drug) pregnancy registry: A 6-year experience. *Arch Neurol.* 2004;61(5):673-678.

64. International Classification of Diseases, Ninth Revision, Clinical Modification (ICD-9-CM). National Center for Health Statistics Web site. http://www.cdc.gov/nchs/about/otheract/icd9/abticd9.htm. Accessed March 18, 2009.

65. Wray NP, Ashton CM, Kuykendall DH, Hollingsworth JC. Using administrative databases to evaluate the quality of medical care: A conceptual framework. *Soc Sci Med.* 1995;40(12): 1707-1715.

66. Schmiedeskamp M, Harpe S, Polk R, Oinonen M, Pakyz A. Use of International Classification of Diseases, Ninth Revision, Clinical Modification codes and medication use data to identify nosocomial *Clostridium difficile* infection. *Infect Control Hosp Epidemiol.* 2009;30(11):1070-1076.

67. Institute of Medicine. *Reliability of National Hospital Discharge Survey Data* (Report No. IOM 80–02). Washington, DC: National Academy of Sciences, 1980.

68. Overview HCPCS-General Information. Centers for Medicare and Medicaid Services Web site. http://www.cms.hhs.gov/MedHCPCSGenInfo. Accessed April 20, 2009.

69. Thompson CA. Pharmacists' CPT codes become permanent: Next step is to set valuation for each code. *Am J Health Syst Pharm.* 2007;64(23):2410-2412.

70. Rose JS, Fisch BJ, Hogan WR, et al. Common medical terminology comes of age. Part Two: Current code and terminology sets–strengths and weaknesses. *J Healthc Inf Manag.* 2001;15(3):319-330.

71. Resar RK, Rozich JD, Classen D. Methodology and rationale for the measurement of harm with trigger tools. *Qual Safety Health Care.* 2003;12(suppl 2):ii39-ii45.

72. Raebel MA, Carroll NM, Simon SR, et al. Liver and thyroid function tests in ambulatory patients prescribed amiodarone in 10 HMOs. *J Manag Care Pharm.* 2006;12(8): 656-664.

73. Javitt JC, Steinberg G, Locke T, et al. Using a claims-based sentinel system to improve compliance with clinical guidelines: Results of a randomized prospective study. *Am J Manag Care.* 2005;11(2):93-102.

74. Davis TM, Davis Cyllene Uwa Edu Au WA, Bruce DG. Glycaemic levels triggering intensification of therapy in type 2 diabetes in the community: The Fremantle Diabetes Study. *Med J Aust.* 2006;184(7):325-328.

75. Amidon PB, Jankovich R, Stoukides CA, Kaul AF. Proton pump inhibitor therapy: Preliminary results of a therapeutic interchange program. *Am J Manag Care.* 2000;6(5): 593-601.

76. DDD-Definition and general considerations. World Health Organization Collaborating Centre for Drug Statistics and Methodology Web site. http://www.whocc.no/ddd/definition_and_general_considera/. Accessed January 25, 2010.

77. Muller A, Monnet DL, Talon D, Hénon T, Bertrand X. Discrepancies between prescribed daily doses and WHO defined daily doses of antibacterials at a university hospital. *Br J Clin Pharmacol.* 2006;61(5):585-591.

78. Monnet DL. Measuring antimicrobial use: The way forward. *Clin Infect Dis.* 2007;44(5):671-673.
79. Rønning M, Blix HS, Harbø BT, Strøm H. Different versions of anatomical therapeutic chemical classification system and the defined daily dose–are drug utilisation data comparable? *Eur J Clin Pharmacol.* 2000;56(9-10):723-727.
80. Sketris IS, Metge CJ, Ross JL, et al. The use of the World Health Organisation Anatomical Therapeutic Chemical/Defined Daily Dose methodology in Canada. *Drug Inf J.* 2004;38(1): 15-27.
81. Polk RE, Fox C, Mahoney A, Letcavage J, MacDougall C. Measurement of adult antibacterial drug use in 130 US hospitals: Comparison of defined daily dose and days of therapy. *Clin Infect Dis.* 2007;44(5):664-670.
82. Yu HT, Dylan ML, Lin J, Dubois RW. Hospitals' compliance with prophylaxis guidelines for venous thromboembolism. *Am J Health Syst Pharm.* 2007;64(1):69-76.
83. National Drug Code Directory. U.S. Food and Drug Administration Web site. http://www.fda.gov/Drugs/InformationOn-Drugs/ucm142438.htm. Accessed May 1, 2009.
84. ATC-Structure and principles. WHO Collaborating Centre for Drug Statistics Methodology Web site. http://www. whocc.no/atc/structure_and_principles. Accessed January 25, 2010.
85. AHFS Pharmacologic-Therapeutic Classification System. AHFS Drug Information Web site. http://www.ahfsdruginformation.com/class/index.aspx. Accessed January 25, 2010.
86. Kruse GB, Amonkar MM, Smith G, Skonieczny DC, Savakis S. Analysis of costs associated with administration of intravenous single-drug therapies in metastatic breast cancer in a U.S. population. *J Manag Care Pharm.* 2008;14(9): 844-857.
87. Rabenda V, Mertens R, Fabri V, et al. Adherence to bisphosphonates and hip fracture risk in osteoporotic women. *Osteoporos Int.* 2008;19(6):811-818.
88. Sokol MC, McGuigan KA, Verbrugge RR, Epstein RS. Impact of medication adherence on hospitalization risk and healthcare cost. *Med Care.* 2005;43(6):521-530.
89. National Institutes of Health, U.S. Department of Health and Human Services. *Protecting Personal Health Information in Research: Understanding the HIPAA Privacy Rule* (NIH Publication Number 03–5388). Bethesda, MD: National Institutes of Health, 2003.
90. Selby JV. Linking automated databases for research in managed care settings. *Ann Intern Med.* 1997;127(8 Part 2):719-724.

Biostatistics and Pharmacoepidemiology

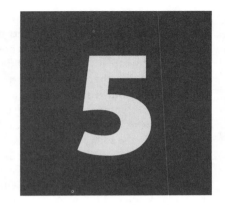

John P. Bentley

▼ OBJECTIVES

At the end of the chapter, the reader will be able to:

1. Explain what a variable is and differentiate between an independent variable and a dependent variable
2. Describe different approaches to classifying variables
3. Distinguish between descriptive and inferential statistics
4. Discuss different methods to summarize data and to describe the relationships between two variables
5. Distinguish between point estimation and interval estimation
6. Utilize key concepts related to hypothesis testing to arrive at statistical decisions and describe the relationship between hypothesis testing and confidence interval estimation
7. Discuss various statistical tests that can be used to describe the significance of group differences and appreciate the factors that are important in choosing an appropriate test
8. Describe how linear regression, logistic regression, and survival analysis (e.g., Cox regression) are used in pharmacoepidemiology and state the nature of the dependent variable as well as the commonly reported measure of association for each technique
9. Differentiate the concepts of confounding, mediation, and effect modification (interaction)
10. Appreciate the issues involved in estimating the sample size required for a pharmacoepidemiologic study

INTRODUCTION

In the conduct of a pharmacoepidemiologic study, large amounts of data are typically collected. Investigators are charged with appropriately summarizing these data to provide information and aid in decision making. Statistics provides a set of tools for performing these tasks, and the purpose of this chapter is to introduce the reader to the role of statistics, specifically biostatistics, in the analysis of data generated from pharmacoepidemiologic research. Many different statistical tests are available, and there are even different underlying philosophical schools of thought regarding statistical inference. While occasionally commenting on other approaches, this chapter will focus on commonly used methods, as it is not possible to cover the entirety of statistics in a single chapter. The intent is to enhance the statistical literacy of the reader; that is, the ability to understand statistics and to critically evaluate statistical issues in the pharmacoepidemiology literature. The focus is not about demonstrating how one conducts statistical analyses, but rather the interpretation of results from such analyses. While some formulas will be presented, these are only for illustrative purposes, and computational approaches for more complex techniques are avoided entirely. Coverage of more advanced techniques will primarily be based on a series of case studies that describe the use of these techniques in published studies.

THE ROLE OF BIOSTATISTICS IN PHARMACOEPIDEMIOLOGY

Biostatistics is the application of statistical methods to the medical and health sciences, including epidemiology. Although biostatistics reflects an application of statistics, biostatisticians have also advanced statistical theory and methods by addressing issues and concerns common in medicine and the health sciences. In defining the broader discipline of statistics, Barnett describes *statistics* as "the study of how information should be employed to reflect on, and give guidance for action in, a practical situation involving uncertainty."[1(p4)] Although this definition makes a number of interesting points, perhaps the most meaningful word in this definition is *uncertainty*. Pharmacoepidemiology is concerned with arriving at estimates, which may be descriptive (e.g., the prevalence of a disease or the extent of the use of a prescription drug), analytic (e.g., the extent of association between an exposure, such as medication use, and an outcome, such as an adverse event), or, in the case of causal analysis, the magnitude of an effect, such as a treatment effect in a randomized controlled clinical trial. Uncertainty in the process can distort the accuracy of an estimate. There are two general categories of error that affect the estimation process[2]:

- *Systematic error* or *bias*, which leads to estimates that depart systematically from true values (examples include confounding, selection bias, and information bias, as discussed in Chapter 6).

- *Random error*, which leads to estimates that depart from the true values due to chance alone, may be thought of simply as residual error after accounting for any systematic error.[2] As will become apparent, one common way to reduce the size of random error is by increasing the size of the study (this is not true for systematic errors).

The presence of these two types of error suggests that the primary roles of statistics (and biostatistics) in the analysis of data generated by epidemiologic research (one could easily argue pharmacoepidemiologic research as well) are[2]

- To produce estimates potentially corrected for biases such as confounding.

- To assess and account for variability in the data; in other words, to evaluate the impact of random error or chance in the estimation process.

REVIEW OF SOME IMPORTANT CONCEPTS

▶ Descriptive Statistics and Inferential Statistics

The definition of statistics stated earlier provides useful insight into the discipline of statistics as something concerned with providing information to guide action in the face of uncertainty. In an effort to further elaborate on meaning and function of statistics as a discipline, a distinction is often made between descriptive statistics and inferential statistics. *Descriptive statistics* are methods and procedures for summarizing and describing data, an important function, as large quantities of data are often collected and need to be condensed into more manageable information. As will be demonstrated in a subsequent section, different descriptive statistics are used to summarize different types of variables. Statistical methods that are used to make statements about populations based on information gathered from samples drawn from that population fall into the category of *inferential statistics*. Just like it is useful to make a distinction between the two general functions of statistics, descriptive and inferential, one can distinguish between two categories of statistical inference: estimation and hypothesis testing. The basics of these two activities will be discussed in a subsequent section, including a brief discussion of some of the controversies surrounding their use. In addition, some common statistical procedures will be discussed later in this chapter that perform both inferential functions, estimating population values while providing information to assist in drawing conclusions about a hypothesized population value.

▶ Classification of Variables

In epidemiology, investigators often collect data about characteristics of individuals.* Characteristics that take on different values or categories for different observations are called variables. The observations may vary across individuals, over time, or both. To understand the use of statistical methods, it is necessary to first understand different methods to describe and classify variables. There are numerous, useful ways to classify variables. Two categorizations attempt to classify variables by the values that they can take, whereas a third focuses on the conceptual roles played by the variables in defining relationships.

Discrete and Continuous Variables

What distinguishes *discrete* and *continuous variables* is that the former is comprised of distinct categories and the latter can take on any value within a defined range.[3] Examples of discrete variables include cigarette-smoking status (i.e., current smoker, past smoker, nonsmoker), eye color, treatment group assignment (i.e., active drug vs. placebo), the number of hospital admissions (sometimes called a count variable), and response to treatment measured as *much improved,*

somewhat improved, same, worse, or *dead* (sometimes called an ordinal variable). The terms "qualitative" or "categorical" are sometimes applied to discrete variables.[3] Examples of continuous variables include cigarette use defined as the number of cigarettes smoked in a day, serum drug concentration, and height. "Quantitative" variable is sometimes used interchangeably with continuous variable. Note from the cigarette-use example that an exposure variable can be either discrete or continuous depending on how it is measured.

Nominal, Ordinal, Interval, and Ratio Variables

Another way to classify variables according to the values that they can take addresses the level of measurement associated with a variable (i.e., nominal, ordinal, interval, ratio). Figure 5-1 defines different levels of measurement and provides examples of each level. Interval- and ratio-level variables are referred to as "numerical"[4] and although there may be some differences, statisticians basically treat and analyze interval and ratio variables the same way. Although this classification scheme provides more information than the discrete–continuous dichotomy, there is substantial overlap. For example, nominal variables are always discrete, and most would agree that interval and ratio variables can be considered continuous.†

Independent, Dependent, and Control Variables

A third variable categorization scheme focuses on the conceptual role played by the variable in defining relationships. A variable can be conceptualized as an independent variable, dependent variable, or control variable. The *dependent variable* (DV) is the response variable or the outcome of interest. It is what the investigator is attempting to describe in terms of other variables. *Independent variables* (IVs)

---

*The unit of analysis may also be at a higher level, such as groups of individuals. For example, one may examine the relationship between national rates of a disease, such as heart disease, and national rates of an exposure, such as the percent of the population that smokes cigarettes. Here the unit of analysis is countries rather than individuals. This is called an ecologic study.

†However, count data, such as the number of days in the hospital, are best conceptualized as interval and discrete and if some individuals spent zero days in the hospital, a true zero point, the variable would be ratio and discrete.

Nominal: Values indicate different named categories; one category is not higher or better than another
Examples: Country of birth, sex, eye color, marital status, primary mode of transportation

Ordinal: Finite number of categories with ordering
Examples: Response to treatment (much improved, somewhat improved, same, worse, or dead), socioeconomic status, cancer staging, different doses of a drug as a treatment variable

Interval: Variable with ordering but also a meaningful measure of the distance between categories
Examples: Temperature in Celsius or Fahrenheit, number of days stayed in the hospital, score on an IQ test, score on a quality of life measure

Ratio: Interval scale with a true zero
Examples: Temperature in Kelvin, height of a person, serum cholesterol, drug concentrations, most laboratory test values

▲ **Figure 5-1.** Levels of measurement.

or predictors are variables used to describe or explain the DV. IVs can be manipulated by the investigator (i.e., a treatment in an experimental design) or observed. Depending on the study objective, it is possible for a variable to be an IV or a DV. For example, a study with an objective of determining the effect of physical activity on serum cholesterol views physical activity as the IV and serum cholesterol as the DV, whereas a study with an objective of determining the effect of serum cholesterol on heart disease views serum cholesterol as the IV and the occurrence of heart disease as the DV. In the context of an experiment, such as a randomized controlled clinical trial, the IV is the treatment manipulation (e.g., new drug or placebo) and the response variable, such as blood pressure, survival, tumor size, is the DV. In analytic epidemiological studies, such as cohort and case-control studies, exposure to a risk factor is usually the IV and event status (i.e., whether or not a participant has the disease or the adverse drug event) is usually the DV. In other observational studies, the establishment of what is the DV and what is the IV may not be so straightforward. Control variables, sometimes called covariates, confounders, extraneous variables, or nuisance variables, are not the focal interest of the study but may affect relationships among other variables (more will be said about these different types of third-variable effects in a later section).

Univariate, Multivariate, and Multivariable Analysis

It is useful to distinguish among three other terms commonly used when describing statistical techniques. These terms are often not used consistently in the statistical literature or especially in the literature of specific content areas, such as the medical literature. *Univariate statistics* refers to the analysis of a single DV, even though there may be multiple IVs.[3] *Multivariate statistics* is used to describe methods in which several DVs are considered simultaneously. Many univariate methods have multivariate analogs or multivariate generalizations. For example, traditional analysis of variance (ANOVA; one DV) is extended to multivariate analysis of variance (MANOVA; multiple DVs) and multiple regression (one DV) is extended to multivariate multiple regression (multiple DVs). Most of the statistical techniques described in this chapter are univariate statistical techniques; however, there are many excellent resources for those interested in learning about the more advanced multivariate methods (e.g., see Refs. 3 and 22).

Multivariate is used by some to describe any statistical technique involving several variables, even analyses involving only one DV.[5] A more descriptive term for this type of an analysis (i.e., exploring the relationship between a number of factors, or IVs and a single outcome or DV) is *multivariable analysis*.[6] Multivariable analysis (also called multivariable adjustment) is one of several methods available to deal with confounding in data analysis.

DESCRIPTIVE STATISTICS

There are a variety of methods, including tabular, graphical, and numerical, to summarize data collected on a single variable as well as to describe the relationship between two variables. This section will primarily review numerical measures; however, tabular and graphical methods of displaying data are often discussed in introductory statistics textbooks. The decision of what method to use to summarize data is often based on whether the variable(s) can be classified as numerical (i.e., interval or ratio) or categorical.

▶ Summarizing Data
Numerical Variables

Several descriptive measures are available to summarize data on a single numerical variable, but researchers are generally concerned with measures of central tendency (measures of the middle) and measures of dispersion or spread. Measures of central tendency used most often in epidemiology include the mean, median, and mode. The *mean,* or more precisely the arithmetic mean, is simply the average. For a sample of observations the mean can be symbolized as:

$$\bar{X} = \frac{\sum_{i=1}^{n} X_i}{n}$$

Other measures of the mean, such as the geometric mean and the harmonic mean, are occasionally used in biostatistics; when used without qualification, *mean* refers to the arithmetic mean. The arithmetic mean should not be used as a summary measure for nominal variables, and generally should not be used for ordinal data, although it is not uncommon for some to treat ordinal data as interval and calculate a mean. However, the variable does not need to be continuous to compute a mean. Consider a count variable that only takes on integer values (e.g., the number of risk factors); the mean is an appropriate summary measure.

The *median* is the middle number or the value of a set of scores such that half of the data points are above it and half are below it. The median is the middle value for an odd number of scores, and it is defined as the mean of the two middle values for an even number of scores. It is generally less sensitive to extreme values than the mean; thus, it is generally preferred as a measure of central tendency when the distribution of observations is skewed, such as household income or cost data from a health economic evaluation. The median can also be used to describe the central tendency of an ordinal variable. The most frequently occurring value in a set of scores is called the mode. Although there can only be one mean and median for a set of data, a property called uniqueness, there can be multiple modes (e.g., bimodal or multimodal distributions). The mode can be used with all types of data, nominal through ratio.

Measures of dispersion are used to capture the amount of variability present in a variable and indicate how closely the data cluster around a central tendency. If all values of a variable are the same, there is no dispersion or variability. Some commonly used measures of dispersion are the range, the interquartile range, the variance, the standard deviation, and the coefficient of variation.

The *range* is the difference between the smallest and largest observed values on a single variable, a single value, although some provide the smallest and largest values, the minimum and maximum, to indicate the range. It can be used with ordinal data (as well as interval and ratio) and is often used with numerical data when one wishes to emphasize extreme values. The *interquartile range* is the distance between the first and the third quartiles of a set of scores and thus describes the middle 50% of the data. Like the range, the interquartile range can be used with ordinal-, interval-, and ratio-level data. The *variance* from a sample of observations is the sum of the squared deviations of the values from the mean divided by the sample size (n) minus 1. Smaller variances are associated with individual scores closer to the mean and vice versa. It can be symbolized as:

$$s^2 = \frac{\sum_{i=1}^{n}(X_i - \bar{X})^2}{n-1}$$

The variance represents squared units and thus is not expressed in terms of the original units. For example, if we are measuring height in inches, the unit of measurement for the variance is square inches. It is, therefore, somewhat limited in its usefulness as a descriptive statistic (but is very useful in inferential statistics). The positive square root of the variance is called the standard deviation and is an index of variability in the original measurement units. The standard deviation of a sample can be symbolized as

$$s = \sqrt{s^2} = \sqrt{\frac{\sum_{i=1}^{n}(X_i - \bar{X})^2}{n-1}}$$

The standard deviation (and the mean) is an essential part of many statistical tests. The standard deviation has other useful applications. For example, at least 75% of the values in a set of observations always lie between the mean ± 2 standard deviations, *regardless* of the underlying distribution of the observations.[‡] If we knew (or assumed) more about the distribution of the data, we could make more precise statements. For example, in a normal distribution (also called a Gaussian distribution), approximately 68% of the values fall within ± 1 standard deviation of the mean, 95% within ± 2 standard deviations, and 99.7% within ± 3 standard deviations. The standard deviation is also critical in the calculation of z scores (also called standardized or standard scores; the z score is a specific, and most common, type of a standard score):

$$z = \frac{X - \bar{X}}{s}$$

Such a score provides information on the relative status of a score in a distribution and describes how far

‡This is an application of Chebychev's inequality.[7]

an observation's value is from the mean in standard deviation units (i.e., tells us how many standard deviations away from the mean is an individual observation). The mean of a distribution of z scores is 0 and the standard deviation is 1. Such scores allow researchers to compare scores derived from different tests or measures (that have different means and standard deviations).

The standard deviation is very useful as a measure of variability for a given variable, but is less useful if we want to compare the variability of different variables measured in different units. Say we want to know whether, for a given sample, phenytoin plasma concentrations, measured in mg/L are more variable than body weight, measured in kilograms. A comparison of standard deviations makes little sense, as the two variables are measured on much different scales. The *coefficient of variation* adjusts the scales so that a sensible comparison can be made; it provides a number independent of the unit of measurement. The following is the formula for the coefficient of variation:

$$CV = \frac{s}{\bar{X}}(100)$$

It can also be used when one wants to compare the variability of a variable in two different sets of data, such as the older and younger individuals. It is used quite often in laboratory-testing and quality-control procedures, and whereas the variance and standard deviation can be used with variables classified as interval or ratio, the coefficient of variation is calculated only for ratio-level data.

Categorical Variables

Recall that the median and mode can be used as measures of central tendency for ordinal data, but the median (and mean for that matter) is not appropriate for nominal data. We can use the mode for nominal data, but we usually describe nominal data with ratios, proportions, and rates. A *ratio* is the value obtained by dividing one quantity by another. The numerator of a *proportion* is included in the denominator; thus, proportions are special types of ratios. For other types of ratios, the numerator and denominator are distinct quantities. A *percentage* is a proportion multiplied by

100. Like a proportion, a *rate* is also a special type of ratio, but includes a time component or some other physical unit (e.g., deaths per passenger mile can be used to compare modes of transportation in terms of accident rates). Rates provide information about the frequency of occurrence of a phenomenon. In epidemiology, specific proportions and rates are of interest, as discussed in Chapter 2.

▶ Describing Relationships Between Two Variables

Two Numerical Variables

The *correlation coefficient, r,* provides a measure of how two numerical variables are *linearly* associated in a sample; it offers information about the strength and direction of the linear relationship between two numerical variables. There are several measures of correlation; unqualified use of the term "correlation coefficient" generally refers to the Pearson (after Karl Pearson, a noted statistician) product–moment correlation coefficient. A correlation coefficient of 0 ($r = 0$) suggests that no linear relationship exists between two variables in a sample; there are tests available to assess whether the true correlation between two variables is significantly different from 0. It is important to keep in mind that $r = 0$ does not necessarily mean that two variables are independent or unrelated; it means they are not *linearly* related. Some basic properties of *r* can be found in Figure 5-2 and formulas for the calculation of *r* can be found in any basic statistics textbook.

A question commonly asked is "how large does *r* need to be to suggest a meaningful linear relationship?" In the physical sciences, the requirements for "meaningful" might be quite large (i.e., >0.9 or ≤0.9). An often-cited rule of thumb for medicine and the biological sciences is provided by Colton:

> Correlations from 0 to .25 [or −.25] indicate little or no relationship, those from .25 to .50 [or −.25 to −.50] indicate a fair degree of relationship, those from .50 to .75 [or −.50 to −.75] a moderate to good relationship, and those greater than .75 [or less than −.75] a very good to excellent relationship.[8, p. 211]

Similar rules exist for the social sciences, but generally with smaller values (e.g., see Ref. 9).

It is important to keep in mind that correlation does not imply causation. In other words, just because two variables have a meaningful correlation, this should not imply that they are causally related. Causation is a question best addressed through study design and theory rather than through statistics (see Chapter 6 for a more in-depth discussion of causality). This is true for any of the association measures presented in this section.

- *r* is a dimensionless quantity; that is, *r* is independent of the units of measurement of the variables.
- *r* is a number, always between −1 and +1.
- A positive *r* indicates a positive relationship (sometimes called a direct relationship) (as one variable's values increase, the other variable's values also increase): +1 describes a perfect positive linear relationship.
- A negative *r* indicates a negative relationship (sometimes called inverse relationship) (as one variable's values increase, the other variable's values decrease): −1 describes a perfect negative linear relationship.
- An *r* close to 0 suggests that there is little, if any, *linear* association between X and Y. By itself, *r* is usually not an appropriate measure of a curved relationship.
- *r* is *invariant* to linear transformations of one or both variables (e.g., the correlation between height measured in centimeters and weight measured in kilograms is the same compared with the correlation between height measured in inches and weight measured in pounds).

▲ **Figure 5-2.** Some properties of the Pearson product–moment correlation coefficient.

Table 5-1. Commonly used measures of association for categorical variables.

Measure of association	Minimum possible value	Maximum possible value	Value indicating no association
Odds ratio	0	$+\infty$	1
Risk ratio	0	$+\infty$	1
Rate ratio	0	$+\infty$	1
Risk difference	-1	$+1$	0
Rate difference	$-\infty$	$+\infty$	0

Another useful measure of association is derived simply by squaring the correlation coefficient. R-squared (r^2) is called the coefficient of determination and tells us the percentage of variation in one of the variables that is explained by, or is accounted for, by knowing the value of the other variable. Yet another measure of correlation is known as the *Spearman rank correlation*, sometimes called *Spearman's rho*. This measure is used to describe the relationship between two ordinal (or one ordinal and one numeric) variables. It can also be used with numeric variables that are skewed with extreme observations (it is less sensitive to outliers when compared to Pearson's r). Spearman's rho is called a nonparametric analog of Pearson's r.

Two Categorical Variables

It is fairly common in epidemiology and medicine to seek to explore the relationship between two variables, both of which are categorical. One variable is often an exposure variable (which may be hypothesized to have a negative effect, such as exposure to risk factor presumed to be a cause of a disease, or a positive effect, such as drug treatment), and the other variable is often the occurrence of a given outcome, such as a disease or an adverse drug event. Two characteristics on a nominal scale are often displayed in a *contingency table* (also called a cross-tabulation), in which observations are cross-classified according to their membership in the categories of the variables. The simplest contingency table is a 2 $\times$ 2 table, representing 2 dichotomous variables (an example of such a table can be found in Chapter 2). From the data

in a contingency table, especially a 2 $\times$ 2 table, several measures of association can be calculated to describe the relationship between the two variables. These include risk ratios, absolute risk reduction (or increase; sometimes called the risk difference[§]) relative risk reduction (increase), number needed to treat (or harm), and odds ratios (OR).[**] Chapter 2 provides examples of the calculation of these measures of association. If person-time is used rather than the number of participants at risk (i.e., incidence rates rather than incidence proportions are calculated), rate ratios and rate differences can be calculated. The term "relative risk" is sometimes applied to both risk ratios and rate ratios (and occasionally ORs) by some authors, which can lead to confusion. For short time intervals and for small risks, risk ratios and rate ratios are nearly equivalent, providing some justification for the use of the broader term "relative risk" to describe both risk ratios and rate ratios.[2]

It is critical for readers of the medical literature to understand whether effects are being stated in relative terms (i.e., based on ratio measures) or absolute terms (i.e., difference-based measures), as the overall size of the effect depends on the measure selected.[11] Table 5-1 provides information on the range of several measures of association as well as the value that suggests no

---

[§]This is also sometimes referred to as *attributable risk*, although this term is used to denote a number of other different concepts in epidemiology and is best avoided when describing the risk difference.[10]

[**]In some cases, it is possible to calculate an odds difference, but such a measure is rarely used.

relationship between the two variables (i.e., exposure is not associated with disease); as will be demonstrated in a subsequent section, it is possible to calculate whether there is a statistically significant relationship between two categorical variables using these null values.

Because of its considerable application in case-control studies, the OR deserves some additional consideration. Recall that in a case-control design, investigators begin by identifying cases (i.e., those with the disease or outcome of interest) and controls (i.e., those without the disease or outcome of interest). Because sampling occurred on disease status (or outcome status), it is not possible to calculate the risk of the disease (or the proportion of those with the disease) with data collected from a case-control disease. Therefore, technically, the risk ratio (or rate ratio for that matter) of interest (i.e., comparing the risk of the disease in the exposed and unexposed groups) cannot be calculated from the data collected in a case-control study. However, it is possible to assess the proportion of those who were exposed in each of the outcome categories (i.e., disease or no disease); therefore, it is possible to calculate an OR for exposure (i.e., the OR of exposure in the diseased and the not diseased). It can be shown (see Chapter 2) that the OR of exposure in the diseased and the not diseased equals the OR of disease in the exposed and unexposed (which is what we are really interested in when we do a case-control study). In other words, it is not necessary to classify one variable as the DV and the other as an IV in order to estimate the OR (this is not true for a risk ratio);[12] the OR is the same. So even though it is not possible to directly calculate a risk ratio or rate ratio of interest from a case-control study, it is possible to calculate the OR of interest because of the mathematical properties of an OR.

Although the OR is a good approximation of the risk ratio when the disease under study is rare (i.e., less than 10%), this "rare disease assumption" is not required for the OR from a case-control study to estimate risk ratio or the rate ratio, an idea that may be contrary to some references. The OR calculated from a case-control study actually estimates different measures of association, depending on how the controls are sampled. These differences in sampling schemes correspond to different variants of the case-control design. A type of case-control study design called a case-cohort study provides a valid estimate of the risk ratio and the density case-control study design provides a valid estimate of the rate ratio, even without the rare disease assumption.[2]

A Categorical Variable and a Numerical Variable

Measures of association have been presented for situations where there are two variables, when either both are numerical or both are categorical. When one variable is categorical and the other is numerical, a relationship between the two variables is suggested when there is a difference in mean values on the numerical variable for the groups that define the categorical variable. No differences in means among the groups would signify any relationship and the larger the difference, the stronger the relationship. Depending on the number of groups (and possibly other issues), different statistical tests can be used to assess whether or not the differences among the means can be considered statistically significant; this will be discussed in a subsequent section. Such an approach might be used in a randomized controlled clinical trial when two drugs (or a drug vs. a placebo) (i.e., the IV is categorical) are being compared to determine whether there are differences between the drugs in terms of ability to lower systolic blood pressure (i.e., the DV is continuous). It is also possible that the DV of interest is categorical and the IV is continuous, as observed in a cohort study designed to examine the relationship between a continuous-exposure variable and disease occurrence (categorical). Although it is possible to examine differences in mean exposure in the two groups, it is also possible to use techniques such as logistic regression, to examine the relationship between a continuous predictor and a categorical outcome (see later section for an explanation of logistic regression).

STATISTICAL INFERENCE

It is usually impossible (or at least practically infeasible) to study every case from an entire population (which would be called a *census*). In epidemiology (indeed, in most sciences) data are commonly collected from a sample of either an actual or conceptual population. Scientists then attempt to make inferences or draw conclusions about the population using information from the sample. Measures (i.e., related to a single variable such as measures of central tendency or related to two or more variables such as a measures of association) computed from the data of a sample are called statistics, whereas measures computed from the data of a population (or assumed to represent a population) are called parameters (usually symbolized by lower-case Greek letters).

We typically do not calculate population parameters, as we usually do not have access to data from an entire population; rather, in the process of analyzing data, we are interested in making estimates about population parameters from data obtained from a sample and also providing decision-making information about hypothesized values of an unknown parameters. These are the two critical functions of inferential statistics, estimation and hypothesis testing, and in the process of carrying out these procedures, we must take into consideration the possibility of error. Although bias or systematic error may be of concern, at this point, we are most concerned with random variation; a major contributor to this random error associated with inaccuracies is related to the selection of observations, known as sampling error.[††] This section explores the two major functions of statistical inference, estimation and hypothesis testing, and will use the OR to demonstrate how these procedures are conducted, used, and interpreted.

▶ Estimation Procedures, Including the Construction of Confidence Intervals

Data collected in a study are used to generate estimates of target parameters. The parameter of interest may be a descriptive measure for a population, such as the population mean or proportion, or may be an association measure, such as the population odds ratio or the difference in two population means (or even a logistic regression coefficient adjusted for other variables). When presented as a single computed value, the estimate is referred to as a *point estimate*. The rule for computing the point estimate is called an estimator.

There are many different methods of estimation (i.e., methods of finding estimators) used in statistics (e.g., maximum likelihood, method of moments, least squares),[7] and a review of the approaches to construct estimators is well beyond the scope of this chapter.

Although very useful, point estimates share a problem; namely, they do not provide information about random error, and as discussed earlier, random error is present in just about every estimation process. This leads to the concepts of *interval estimation* and a confidence interval. If point estimation is the process of finding a single value that is the best guess of the population parameter, then interval estimation is the process of associating with the point estimate a measure of statistical variation or random error. An interval estimate "consists of two numerical values defining a range of values that, with a specified degree of confidence, we feel [covers] the parameter being estimated."[13(p157)] These two numerical values are called the lower and upper confidence limits and the range of values, which are around the point estimate, is called a confidence interval. The confidence interval provides evidence of the precision of the estimate. Precision and random error have an inverse relationship; thus, the smaller the random error, the more precise the estimate and vice versa. Therefore, a wider confidence interval suggests lower precision and a narrower confidence interval indicates higher precision.[2] Just like we can arrive at a point estimate for many different population parameters, we can build confidence intervals for many different population parameters.

A confidence interval has the following general form:

$$\begin{pmatrix} \text{Point Estimate of} \\ \text{the Parameter} \end{pmatrix} \pm \begin{matrix} \text{(Reliability Coefficient)} \times \\ \text{(Standard Error)} \end{matrix}$$

Statistical theory is used to determine the distribution of the estimator (i.e., the sampling distribution), and this information can be used to determine both the reliability coefficient and the standard error (which is the standard deviation of the sampling distribution of the statistic). In essence, constructing a confidence interval requires us to make some assumptions about an underlying statistical model. The standard error is often estimated on the basis of sample data, and standard

---

[††]Sampling is not the only source of random error; for example, most epidemiologic studies (indeed, most studies in general) are also faced with random *measurement* error.

formulas are available for many estimators. A key component in standard-error calculations is the size of the sample; the larger the sample size, the smaller the standard error. Thus, more precision is associated with larger studies (i.e., the estimate is less subject to random error). The confidence level, together with knowledge of the theoretical distribution of the estimator, is used to determine the reliability coefficient (sometimes called a confidence coefficient) in the above general formula. The confidence level chosen is arbitrary, and it can be any value in the interval of 0% to 100%, but most scientific disciplines usually use values of 90%, 95%, or 99% (95% is the most common). There is a trade-off between precision and confidence—the higher the confidence, the wider the interval (and the lower precision).

Before calculating an example, it is worth noting a few issues about what a confidence interval actually tells us. For a 95% confidence interval, it suggests that if one collected many repeated sets of samples of the same size, about 95% of all such intervals calculated in this manner would be expected to contain the parameter. Although it is correct to say that one is 95% confident that the parameter of interest lies within the interval, it is not correct to say that the probability is 0.95 that the parameter lies within the interval. Thus, it is inappropriate to say that there is a 95% chance that the parameter lies between the lower and upper limits. The parameter is not random, the interval is.[‡‡]

Most examples of confidence intervals in the literature are generally based on large-sample (or asymptotic) theory. This means that such intervals are approximations, which are generally reasonable when the sample size is large enough. When data are sparse, readers should generally be skeptical; exact methods are available for such situations. Another important point is that when constructing confidence intervals, we are making an assumption about the appropriateness of the underlying statistical model and that no biases are operating. These assumptions are generally difficult to fully meet, especially with observational study designs

characteristic of epidemiologic research. For these reasons, confidence intervals should not be considered as "a literal measure of statistical variability but rather as a general guide to the amount of error in the data."[2(p115)]

To appreciate the calculation and subsequent interpretation of a confidence interval, let's construct a 95% confidence interval for an odds ratio (OR) using some data presented in Chapter 2 (Table 2-6) examining the relationship between stroke and systolic hypertension. The point estimate calculated for these data was 5.08. Rather than relying on the sampling distribution of the OR, we will use the sampling distribution of its natural logarithm, log(OR). This is because the sample log odds ratio, symbolized as $\log(\widehat{OR})$, has an approximate normal distribution as its sampling distribution with a standard error (SE) of:

$$SE = \sqrt{\frac{1}{a}+\frac{1}{b}+\frac{1}{c}+\frac{1}{d}},$$

where a, b, c, and d correspond to the cells from the contingency table.

Thus, a large-sample theory 100% (1-α) (or 95% when α = 0.05; the concept of α will be further discussed in the next section) confidence interval for log (OR) is:

$\log(\widehat{OR}) \pm z_{1-\alpha/2}(SE)$, where $\widehat{OR}$ is the point estimate and $z_{1-\alpha/2}$ is the percentile from the standard normal distribution (i.e., the value of z on a standard normal curve such that to the left of it lies $1-\alpha/2$ and to the right of it lies $\alpha/2$ of the area under the curve). For α = 0.05 (i.e., a 95% confidence interval), $z_{1-\alpha/2}$ = 1.96.

In our example,

$$SE = \sqrt{\frac{1}{417}+\frac{1}{744}+\frac{1}{83}+\frac{1}{752}} = 0.1308$$

Thus, the 95% confidence interval (95% CI) for log (OR) = 1.625 ± 1.96 (0.1308) or (1.369, 1.881). Exponentiating each limit (i.e., taking the natural antilogarithm), we find that the 95% CI for the OR is 3.93-6.56, suggesting that we can conclude with 95% confidence that the true OR of stroke comparing those with stage 2 systolic hypertension with those with normal blood pressure is between 3.93 and 6.56, indicating a positive association with fairly good precision.

[‡‡]Parameters are fixed, unknown quantities—at least in classical statistics, which is what we are dealing with in this chapter—you need to use Bayesian statistics to interpret interval estimates as the probability that the parameter is in the interval.[7]

A similar procedure allows one to calculate confidence intervals for many different parameters, including means, proportions, differences between two means, risk ratios, and regression coefficients.

The Basics of Hypothesis Testing

Hypothesis testing is the other major function associated with statistical inference and is used to provide information to assist in drawing conclusions about a hypothesized parameter. As will be shown later, it is possible to use information from a confidence interval to arrive at the same conclusion reached through hypothesis testing. Hypothesis testing (sometimes called significance testing[§§]) is a fairly complicated area of statistics that has a number of critics (for a review see Refs. 14–16). The purpose of the section is merely to introduce the reader to some of the terminology and procedures and caution against some misapplications.

Key to understanding hypothesis testing is the concept of a hypothesis, which can be thought of as a statement about one or more populations, frequently about some parameters from the populations. There are two complementary hypotheses used when conducting hypothesis testing: the null hypothesis (H_0) and the alternative hypothesis (H_A). Note that both are statements about a population(s), not the observed data. The null hypothesis is really the hypothesis to be tested. On the basis of our sample data, we will either reject or fail to reject the null hypothesis (statisticians generally avoid the word prove).

Many people believe that the "null" in null hypothesis refers to no difference, no relationship, or no association. It is important to note that the null hypothesis gets its name because it is the hypothesis to be "nullified" not because we are necessarily postulating no difference or no relationship. For example, it is possible to test null hypotheses of differences other than zero. In an attempt to clarify this, some refer to the null hypothesis of no difference (or no associa-

tion) as a nil hypothesis.[17] In most studies that you will come across, the null hypothesis is the nil hypothesis, but it does not have to be. The alternative hypothesis (sometimes called the research hypothesis) is what one chooses to believe if the evidence provided in the sample data lead to a rejection of the null hypothesis.

Alternative hypotheses can be stated in a directional or nondirectional manner, leading to one-sided (or one-tailed) or two-sided (or two-tailed) hypothesis tests, respectively. If we believe that only "sufficiently" large or "sufficiently" small values will lead to a rejection of the null hypothesis, a directional alternative hypothesis is warranted and a one-sided test can be used. However, if both large and small values (e.g., the difference could be either positive or negative; the association could be either positive or negative) lead one to reject the null (i.e., we are indifferent to the direction of the effect), then a nondirectional alternative is in order and a two-sided test is appropriate. Significant debate has occurred over the appropriateness of one-sided versus two-sided tests, especially in the clinical trials literature.[18,19] For a variety of reasons, scholars in the medical field may opine that two-sided tests are most appropriate unless there is a strong justification for using a one-tailed test.

In the clinical trials literature and occasionally in the epidemiology literature, you may see investigators who wish to show that a new intervention is not worse than a standard intervention or that the effects of two interventions are very similar. In the latter case, we might state our null hypothesis that the two treatments are not equivalent and the alternative hypothesis is that the two treatments are not different by more than some prespecified amount (usually some clinically insignificant amount). Such tests are referred to as tests for noninferiority and tests for equivalence.[20,21] The remainder of this chapter focuses on more conventional hypothesis tests.

Tests of hypotheses are inherently probabilistic, and there is a chance of being incorrect. Statisticians have labels for the different types of incorrect inferences. These, along with corresponding correct decisions, are often displayed in tabular form (Table 5-2). Thus, rejecting a null hypothesis when it is true is referred to as a type I error and failing to reject a false null hypothesis

[§§]Although there is technically a distinction between significance testing and hypothesis testing,[1] many authors use these terms interchangeably.

Table 5-2. Types of errors in hypothesis testing.

Decision about H_0	Population state ("Truth")	
	H_0 true	H_A true
Reject	Type I error	Correct result
Fail to reject	Correct result	Type II error

is referred to as a *type II error*. Probabilities are assigned to these errors, such that α refers to the probability of a type I error (sometimes called the significance level), and β refers to the probability of a type II error. Another term commonly used in hypothesis testing is "power," which is defined as the probability of correctly rejecting the null hypothesis when it is false (it equals $1 - \beta$). As outlined in Figure 5-3, several factors influence the power of statistical tests (or the ability of a test to correctly reject a false null hypothesis). Concepts related to power are often used in calculating necessary sample sizes *before* a study is conducted. This will briefly be explored at the end of the chapter.

But how does one go about making a decision about whether to reject or not reject the null hypothesis? One approach is to compute something called a test statistic from the observed data. The test statistic becomes our decision maker, as the decision to reject or not reject depends on the magnitude of the test statistic. The general form of a test statistic is:

$$\text{Test statistic} = \frac{\text{relevant statistic} - \text{hypothesized parameter}}{\text{standard error of the relevant statistic}}$$

What test statistic is calculated depends on what statistical test is being used. Some commonly used test statistics include the z statistic, the t statistic, the chi-square statistic, and the F ratio. Statistical theory, together with some basic assumptions, can be used to derive the sampling distribution of a test statistic under the assumption that the null hypothesis is true. Given such a distribution and on the basis of our desired level of significance (generally set at $\alpha = 0.05$), we can determine something called a critical value, which will define the rejection region (this will be demonstrated by an example later in this section). Our decision rule will be to reject the null hypothesis if the value of the test statistic calculated from the observed data is a value that appears in the rejection region (this is called statistical significance), and we will not reject the null hypothesis (i.e., the null hypothesis is said to be consistent with our data) if the computed value of the test statistic is a value in the nonrejection region.

The *P value* (sometimes called the observed significance level) is another way to arrive at the exact same conclusion, but has the potential to provide more information than the yes/no decision associated with hypothesis testing. The *P* value is often

---

Sample size
All other things being equal, the power of a test increases as sample size increases.

Variability or precision of the outcome variable
All other things being equal, the power of a test increases as variability decreases (i.e., more precision).

Magnitude of effect (or the degree of deviation from the value hypothesized in the null)
All other things being equal, the power of a test increases as the magnitude of the effect increases.

Level of significance (α)
All other things being equal, the power of a test increases as α increases. We often choose $\alpha = 0.05$ more by convention than design. Other values are allowed.

▲ **Figure 5-3.** Factors influencing the power of a statistical test.

The *P* value does not tell us about the probability of the null hypothesis being true. The *P* value, as we have defined it here, is a frequentist concept (i.e., classical statistics). Bayesian analyses can provide a probability that a hypothesis is true or false.

The *P* value does not indicate the "size of the effect." Statements such as "very highly significant" for small *P* value simply a certain magnitude of effect and are misleading. *P* values can be made small by simply increasing the size of the sample.

The *P* value does not tell us whether something is practically or clinically significant. Such decisions usually do not fall in the realm of statistics.

▲ **Figure 5-4.** The *P* value: misinterpretations.

misinterpreted (Figure 5-4). What it actually tells us is the probability of obtaining, *when the null is true,* a value of the test statistic as extreme or more extreme (in the direction supporting the alternative) than the one actually computed. It quantifies how unusual the observed results would be if H_0 were true. The general rule of thumb is that if the *P* value is less than or equal to α, we reject the null hypothesis (i.e., there is statistical significance); if the *P* value is greater than α, we do not reject the null. Given the same α, this will give us identical results to the hypothesis-testing procedure that uses a critical value and rejection region.

Let's return to the data from Chapter 2 (Table 2-6) used previously to calculate a 95% CI for an OR and instead conduct a hypothesis test. As described in Table 5-1, an OR indicating no relationship or no association (also called statistical independence between exposure and outcome) is 1. The Pearson chi-square test of independence (or association) can be used to test the null hypothesis that the OR summarizing the relationship between exposure to stage 2 systolic hypertension and the occurrence of stroke is 1 (i.e., no association, independence between exposure and event status). Formulas (there are several, including a shortcut formula) for calculating the test statistic, the Pearson chi-square statistic, from a 2×2 contingency table can be found in most introductory statistics books and will not be presented in this chapter.

For the data in Table 2-6, the Pearson chi-square statistic = 174.57. Under the null hypothesis, this test statistic has approximately a χ^2 distribution (chi-square distribution) with 1 degree of freedom (i.e., the number of values that are free to vary when computing a statistic). Assuming $\alpha = 0.05$, the critical value obtained from the χ^2 distribution is 3.841, and our decision rule suggests that we reject the null hypothesis if the calculated value of the test statistic is greater than 3.841; in this case it is, so we can reject the null hypothesis and conclude on the basis of these data that the true odds of stroke seem different for those with stage 2 systolic hypertension and those with normal blood pressure. The *P* value for this test is quite small (<0.0001), suggesting that given a true null hypothesis, the probability of observing a chi-square value of 174.57 or greater is quite small, leading to the same conclusion: reject the null hypothesis. Thus, we can say that the odds of having a stroke, given stage 2 systolic hypertension, are higher than the odds of having a stroke, given normal blood pressure.

One can also use the confidence interval to arrive at the same conclusion. The 95% CI calculated previously, 3.93-6.56, does not include the null hypothesized value of 1; therefore, we can reject the null hypothesis at the $\alpha = 0.05$ level of significance. If the 95% CI had included the hypothesized value of 1, we could say that 1 is a feasible candidate for the OR we are estimating; therefore, we would fail to reject the null hypothesis at the 0.05 level of significance. Daniel concisely summarizes this point:

> In general, when testing a null hypothesis by means of a two-sided confidence interval, we reject H_0 at the α level of significance if the hypothesized parameter

is not contained within the $100(1-\alpha)$ percent confidence interval. If the hypothesized parameter is contained within the interval, H_0 cannot be rejected at the α level of significance.[13, p. 223]

Because they do not lead to qualitative, dichotomous decisions and because they provide information on the strength of the relationship (i.e., the point estimate) and on the precision of the estimate, some argue that confidence intervals have certain advantages over hypothesis tests and that hypothesis tests should be avoided.[2] However, the use of P values and hypothesis testing is commonplace in the medical literature as well as many other disciplines, and the reader is encouraged to become more familiar with its basic precepts.

EXAMINING THE SIGNIFICANCE OF GROUP DIFFERENCES

A number of statistical methods are available for assessing whether there are statistically significant differences among groups. The groups may be defined on the basis of their exposure status, random assignment to treatment groups, or may even be the same group measured at two or more occasions. This section is designed to introduce the reader to some of the common statistical procedures for addressing such questions. Little attention is provided to the mechanics of performing the tests because such details are better addressed in statistics textbooks. As with the selection of descriptive statistics, the decision of what statistical test to use to assess the significance of group differences is often based on whether the outcome variable of interest can be classified as *numerical* (i.e., interval or ratio) or *categorical*. Several authors provide classification frameworks and flowcharts for assisting in the selection of an appropriate technique (e.g., see Refs. 3, 4, and 22).

▶ Numerical Outcome Variable

Independent Groups

The *t test* (also referred to as the independent-groups, two-sample, separate-groups, or unpaired *t* test) is the procedure used to test the null hypothesis that two different populations have the same mean; a statistically significant result provides evidence that the populations defined by the two groups have different means. It is common to provide a confidence interval for the difference between two population means; if this interval does not include 0, we can conclude that there is evidence of a difference in means between the two groups. Certain assumptions are made when using the *t* test. These assumptions are necessary to ensure the validity of the results of the hypothesis-testing procedure:

- The variable on which the two groups are being compared is *normally distributed* in each population.

- The variances of the variable in the two populations are equal (called homogeneity of variance).

- The observations within each group and between each group are *independent,* meaning that knowing the value of any one observation tells us nothing about the value of another observation.

Under certain conditions, the *t* test is said to be robust to violations of the first two assumptions, but the final assumption, independence, is critical. Violations of this assumption can lead to significant errors. There are other procedures available to address what is referred to as correlated data (i.e., when independence is violated).

Rather than comparing the means of two groups, one might be interested in comparing means from populations defined by three or more groups. ANOVA is a technique that can be used to achieve such a goal (the *t* test is actually a special case of ANOVA, used when there are only two groups). Although *means* are typically being compared in ANOVA, the primary tests of interest are actually made using estimates of *variance;* the test statistic employed in ANOVA is called the *F* statistic, which is actually a ratio of variance estimates. Hence the name, analysis of *variance.*

Nominal variables that comprise group membership (i.e., IVs) are called factors and the different categories of a factor are called levels. As with the *t* test, the DV is numerical. When the focus is on a single IV, it is referred to as one-way ANOVA. Thus, one may be interested in assessing whether the mean serum cholesterol levels differs among people on either drug A, drug B, or placebo or whether there are differences in systolic blood pressure among different categories of employees (with different levels of job stress).

The main analysis problem in fixed-effects (the most commonly used procedure) one-way ANOVA is to determine whether the population means are all equal or not. The test of this null is called an overall test or an omnibus test. The test statistic (i.e., the F statistic) used in ANOVA will have an F distribution when the stated null hypothesis is true and the basics of hypothesis testing covered earlier apply (i.e., critical values, rejection regions, P values, etc.). The assumptions required for ANOVA are quite similar to the t-test assumptions. If the null hypothesis is rejected, the next problem is to find out where the differences are. Such questions fall under the general statistical subject of multiple-comparison procedures (MCPs). Some commonly used MCPs are Tukey's HSD (honestly significant difference) test and the Bonferroni approach.

It is possible to incorporate additional IVs (or factors) when conducting ANOVA (e.g., analysis of two factors is referred to as two-way ANOVA). Such analyses allow one to assess questions such as, is the difference between an experimental group and a control group different for men and women? This is the basic idea of interaction and will be discussed in a subsequent section.

ANOVA and the t test are called parametric statistical techniques. Some statistical techniques test hypotheses that are *not* statements about population parameters (i.e., truly nonparametric procedures), whereas other techniques make little or no assumptions about the sampled population (i.e., distribution-free procedures). These techniques are generally referred to as *nonparametric statistical methods.**** Such techniques can be used when the outcome variable is ordinal (or lower) or when the outcome variable is interval or higher and there are assumption violations (e.g., the normality assumption). This is a large, vast, and important area of statistics, both at the theoretical and applied levels, and much

of it is beyond the scope of this chapter. It is important to recognize that there are nonparametric tests that are analogous to many parametric test procedures such as the Mann–Whitney U test (also called the Wilcoxon rank-sum test) for the unpaired t test and the Kruskal–Wallis test for one-way ANOVA.

Dependent Observations

For both the t test and ANOVA described thus far, the assumption is that there are independent groups. However, a researcher might be interested in:

- Comparing means on a variable measured at one time (pretest) and again 6 months later (posttest) on the same participants (or perhaps multiple time points)—this is sometimes referred to as longitudinal research.

- Having participants serve as their own controls, like when each one of them receives both the active drug and the control drug (or perhaps more than two treatment conditions), possibly with a sufficient washout period in between (this is called a crossover design[†††]) and you are interested in comparing the mean responses associated with both drugs.

- Comparing mean scores on some variable for two different groups in which individuals within each group have been matched on several criteria such as gender and age.

In each of these situations, it is not possible to assume independent observations. For example, we would expect a participant with a relatively low score at the pretest to have a relatively low posttest measurement as well. Procedures that appropriately account for the dependency in the set of observations include the paired t test (also called the dependent-groups t test or matched-groups t test) for comparing two means and repeated-measures ANOVA for comparing three or more means. There are actually several approaches to analyzing such data, and this remains an active area of research in the statistics community.

***Although technically distinct, the terms *distribution-free* and *nonparametric* are sometimes used synonymously, and this entire area of statistics is generally referred to as *nonparametric statistics.*[23]

[†††]The analysis of crossover designs is slightly more complicated than simply applying a paired t test, a technique often used to account for dependency in a set of observations. For more information, see Ref.[24]

▶ Categorical Outcome Variable

Independent Groups

Oftentimes, the goal of a researcher is to assess whether two categorical variables are associated. One variable may be a grouping variable as defined previously, whereas the other may be a categorical outcome, such as disease status. There are multiple approaches for assessing whether such a relationship is statistically significant (indeed, under certain conditions, such as an adequate sample size, these procedures generally provide the same answer), but the most commonly used approach is the *Pearson chi-square test of independence (or association)*. This test was demonstrated earlier in the chapter to test the null hypothesis that an odds ratio = 1 from a case-control study and can also be used to assess whether the risk difference is 0 (or the risk ratio is 1) based on data collected from a cohort study. The Pearson chi-square test of independence can also be used when one of the nominal variables (either the outcome or the grouping variable) has more than two categories (i.e., a contingency table that is larger than 2 × 2). Thus, it can be used when you want to compare proportions when you have more than two groups.

One of the assumptions when using the Pearson chi-square test of independence is that the sample sizes are "large enough" in each group. For a 2 × 2 contingency table, "large enough" usually means that the expected frequency of each cell (i.e., what is expected under the null hypothesis of independence) is at least 5. The Pearson chi-square test of independence (and other tests like it) relies on approximations, and this approximation is generally poor when this assumption is not met. In such cases, Fisher's (after the noted statistician, Ronald Fisher) exact test can be used instead to test the same basic hypotheses (i.e., two nominal variables are independent). It is called exact because we do not have to rely on approximations, but rather we can calculate the exact probability of obtaining the observed results or results that are more extreme.

Dependent Observations

As with numerical outcomes, a given research design might introduce dependencies in a set of data (e.g., participants were measured at different time points;

participants serve as their own control in a study; the use of matching). Indeed, using matching procedures is quite common in cohort and case-control studies. The Pearson chi-square test discussed earlier for nominal outcomes assumes independent groups and using such a procedure with nonindependent groups is not appropriate. But just like the paired *t* test or repeated-measures ANOVA can be used to appropriately account for dependencies in the set of observations when the outcome variable is numerical and one is interested in comparing means, the McNemar test and Cochran's Q test can be used to appropriately account for dependencies in the set of observations when the outcome variable is nominal and one is interested in comparing proportions. Alternative approaches for handing correlated data with a categorical outcome include the use of *conditional* logistic regression or logistic regression models estimated using a generalized estimating equations (GEE) approach (e.g., see Ref. 12). Conditional logistic regression will be discussed in Case Study 5-2.

EXAMINING RELATIONSHIPS BETWEEN PREDICTORS AND OUTCOMES

The statistical methods discussed thus far have focused on research questions involving the comparison of two or more groups. However, researchers are often interested in more general questions about relationships among IVs, control variables, and DVs. The IVs of interest may be grouping (categorical) variables or continuous and the relationships between the IVs of interest and the DV may or may not be adjusted for other variables, called control variables. We can generalize many of the techniques discussed earlier into a modeling framework that allows one to address a variety of possible research questions. These techniques are often labeled generally as *regression modeling techniques*. One can show that ANOVA and the *t* test are really special cases of *linear* regression. The term "regression" is used widely both in the statistical literature as well as in the literatures of many different content areas. When used without qualification, regression is generally referring to linear regression, a technique that is used for assessing relationships between one or more IVs (typically continuous, although in practice they can

Table 5-3. Examining relationships: different methods.

Nature of outcome	Statistical method	Association (or effect) measure
Continuous (numerical)	Linear regression	Regression Coefficient: β
Categorical (often dichotomous)	Logistic regression	Odds ratio: exp (β)
Time to event	Cox regression (and other methods of survival analysis)	Hazard ratio: exp (β)

be categorical) and a single, numerical DV. However, there are a number of different types of regression-modeling procedures, several of which will be described in this section and illustrated through case studies (there are many considerations when conducting such analyses most of which are beyond the scope of this chapter). Table 5-3 describes some differences among three popular approaches: linear regression, logistic regression, and Cox regression. A key difference among the three is how the outcome variable of interest (i.e., the DV) is measured. Although there are differences in how associations are described, the concepts of estimation and hypothesis testing still apply (i.e., one can calculate point and interval estimates for these measures as well as testing null hypotheses of no relationships between variables using these measures).

A common use of regression modeling is for the control of confounding (see Chapter 6 for a discussion of other methods for dealing with confounding and bias). This approach is generally referred to as multivariable adjustment or multivariable analysis, which is achieved by examining the relationship between the IV of interest (in epidemiology, often an exposure variable) and the outcome adjusted for potential confounding variables. Multivariable refers to the feature that the effects of many variables on the DV are being examined simultaneously. In the regression modeling, this is accomplished by adding predictors to a simple regression model that uses only the IV of interest as a predictor. Such models are called multiple regression models. The measure of association estimated without the potential confounders (or control variables) is called the crude (or unadjusted) estimate and the measure of association in the presence of the potential confounders is called the adjusted

estimate. The adjusted estimate can be thought of as the association between exposure and outcome while mathematically holding constant all of the observed confounding variables.

▶ Numerical Outcome: Linear Regression

Linear regression is used when the DV of interest is continuous (i.e., numerical), such as systolic blood pressure, health-related quality of life, or costs in a pharmacoeconomic study (although there are several issues involved when analyzing cost data, for example, see Refs. 25 and 26). The concept of correlation was discussed previously, and it can be shown that the correlation coefficient is closely related to linear regression. The primary measure of association (or effect) estimated in linear regression is the regression coefficient. In a simple linear model (i.e., only one predictor), the regression coefficient (i.e., the crude estimate) is simply interpreted as the slope of the best-fitting line that describes the relationship between the IV and the DV; thus, it describes the amount of change in the DV for a 1-unit change in the IV. In a multiple linear regression model, a regression coefficient for an IV refers to the amount of change in the DV for a 1-unit change in the IV holding all of the other variables in the model constant (the adjusted effect). As an illustration of the use of linear regression, Shrank et al.[27] used the technique to examine the relationship between several health belief and communication measures and the proportion of prescriptions filled with a generic drug over a period of time, a measure calculated for each individual in their data set and treated as a continuous variable (see Case Study 5-1).

CASE STUDY 5-1

The Use of Linear Regression

With ever-growing concerns about health care costs, the use of generic medications continues to receive attention. Although patients' preferences and perceptions about generic medications have been studied previously, Shrank et al.[27] add to the literature by using survey research as well as information captured in pharmacy claims data to explore whether (and how) certain patient beliefs, and self-reported communication with providers, about generic medications influence actual generic medication use behavior, as measured by the proportion of prescriptions filled with generics over a 17-month period. The generic proportion measure was calculated for each individual and linked to participants' survey responses. This measure was treated as a continuous variable (which is not uncommon) and served as the DV in a multiple linear regression. As discussed in the article, five different measurement scales were constructed from their questionnaire items and these scales were transformed to z scores (standard scores) and used as IVs in the analysis in addition to a set of control variables (e.g., age, gender, income, and education). Other noteworthy points concerning their analysis is the use of a technique called multiple imputation to address missing data on the set of IVs as well as the use of robust estimates of standard errors (i.e., Huber–White estimates) to adjust for an assumption violation (i.e., the assumption of homoscedasticity, which is conceptually related

to the assumption of homogeneity of variance discussed for the t test earlier in this chapter). We can use the results presented by the authors to examine the meaning of a linear regression coefficient, as well as demonstrate the application of confidence intervals and hypothesis testing using this linear regression. The scale intended to measure the extent that a patient communicates with providers about generics showed an estimated regression coefficient of 0.038 (95% CI = 0.009-0.068; P = 0.012) in a model that included the control variables as well as the other four scales. This was statistically significant at the $\alpha = 0.05$ level (notice that the 95% CI does not include 0) and suggests that after controlling for other variables, a 1-unit increase in this scale (which corresponds to a 1 standard deviation increase, as the scales were converted to z scores) is associated with a 3.8% increase in generic medication use. Thus, there is evidence that patients who talk more with their doctors and pharmacists about generic medications are more likely to fill prescriptions for generics than are patients who talk with their providers less about such issues. Of course, as pointed out by the authors, it is difficult to establish the order of causation from their study. Despite this limitation, the findings do suggest that educational programs encouraging patient–provider communications about generics may help to increase the utilization of generic drugs.

▶ Categorical Outcome: Logistic Regression

Logistic regression is used when the DV of interest is a binary (two-group, dichotomous) categorical variable rather than a numerical (or continuous) measure. For example, the DV of interest might be event occurrence (e.g., disease/no disease). Logistic regression can be generalized to the cases of a response variable with three or more categories (i.e., multinomial logistic regression) or when the response variable is ordered categories (i.e., ordinal logistic regression or

just ordinal regression). Logistic regression, especially its application to the case of a binary or dichotomous outcome, is one of the most commonly used techniques in medicine and epidemiology. This is because its parameter estimates have a fairly straightforward interpretation. With a little math and a basic understanding of the logistic regression equation, it can be shown that the natural antilogarithm of a parameter estimate from logistic regression is an OR (Table 5-3). Thus, the odds of the event multiply by the OR for every 1-unit increase in the IV (or we can use our previous understanding of an OR when we are comparing

The Use of Logistic Regression

Much of the information about drug–drug interactions in clinical practice comes from case reports. Until relatively recently, large population-based studies attempting to link drug–drug interactions and clinical outcomes were not available. Juurlink and colleagues[28] were one of the first research groups to undertake such an activity and examined possible outcomes associated with three potential drug–drug interactions in an elderly population: glyburide and cotrimoxazole, digoxin and clarithromycin, and angiotensin-converting enzyme (ACE) inhibitors and potassium-sparing diuretics. Each of these potential drug–drug interactions was evaluated with a separate design; thus, three different studies, all using essentially the same methodology, were conducted. All three used a nested case-control design. The authors appropriately describe how they defined continuous users of the study medications (i.e., glyburide, digoxin, or ACE inhibitors), how they identified cases among these continuous users (i.e., hospital admission with a most responsible diagnosis that is a presumed outcome of exposure to an interacting drug: hypoglycemia, digoxin toxicity, or hyperkalemia), how they attempted to find 50 matched controls for each case (controls were continuous users of the same medications, but did not experience a hospital admission with the diagnosis of interest), and how they measured exposure to the potentially interacting medications (i.e., use of cotrimoxazole, clarithromycin, or potassium-sparing diuretics in the

week prior to the index hospitalization) in both the cases and the controls. Because the authors used matching in their study design, they used a technique called conditional logistic regression to appropriately account for dependencies in their samples created by matching. To explore the meaning of an OR, as well as demonstrate the application of confidence intervals and hypothesis testing using logistic regression, we will examine the results examining the association between hospital admission for hypoglycemia and the use of cotrimoxazole in continuous users of glyburide. The authors report an adjusted OR (control variables included the use of other medications that could potentially cause such an admission and measures of previous hospital admissions and the total number of prescription drugs used) of 6.6 (95% CI = 4.5–9.7), indicating strong association with good precision. This was statistically significant at the $\alpha = 0.05$ level (notice that the 95% CI does not include 1) and suggests that after controlling for other variables, users of glyburide hospitalized for hypoglycemia were considerably more likely to have used cotrimoxazole in the week prior to hospitalization than users of glyburide who were not hospitalized for hypoglycemia. Adding credence to their findings, the authors also reported that there was no significant association between hospitalization for hypoglycemia and use of an antibiotic not believed to have a drug–drug interaction with glyburide, namely, amoxicillin.

two groups, such as exposed and unexposed groups). We can calculate both crude and adjusted ORs using logistic regression, and the advantages of OR for case-control studies described earlier still apply (i.e., for case-control studies, the OR is the primary association measure of interest and it can be estimated using logistic regression). As an example of the use of logistic regression, Juurlink et al.[28] conducted a case-control study to explore whether certain drug–drug interactions were related to cause-specific hospital admissions in the elderly (see Case Study 5-2). Since

these authors employed matching, they utilized a special kind of logistic regression called conditional logistic regression.

▶ Time Until Event Occurrence Outcome: Survival Analysis

Rather than focusing simply on whether or not an event occurs, the purpose of survival analysis (sometimes called time-to-event analysis) is to explore the occurrence *and* timing of events[29] and oftentimes evaluate what factors predict or explain the time to an event. Although survival analysis derives its name partially because the event of interest is often death (especially in medicine and epidemiology), the endpoint of interest can be relapse, adverse drug event, discontinuation of a medicine, or even cure of a disease. It is quite common that some participants will not reach the endpoint by the time a study concludes. It is not necessary for every individual to experience the event during the period of interest; those that do not experience the event are said to be censored. Survival analysis techniques are designed to address censoring.

An often confusing point about survival analysis is the sheer number of different methods. In medicine the two most common methods are the Kaplan–Meier method and proportional hazards regression (or Cox regression after the noted statistician David Cox). The Kaplan–Meier method produces plots of survival functions. Such plots are ubiquitous in the medical literature and often succinctly summarize the probability of survival over time for one or more groups. It is also possible to conduct statistical tests comparing the overall survival functions of different groups (i.e., does one group have significantly better survival times when compared to another group?). One of the most commonly used tests for this purpose is called the log-rank test. However, such procedures do not allow one to quantify the strength of the relationship between a variable and survival time (i.e., no parameter estimates are provided).

Cox regression models (proportional hazards models) provide such estimates and also allow adjustment for other variables (i.e., crude and adjusted estimates are possible). This approach has become the most commonly used method for survival analysis. Like logistic regression, the parameter estimates from Cox regression have a fairly straightforward interpretation. With a little math and a basic understanding of the Cox model, it can be shown that the natural antilogarithm of a parameter estimate from Cox regression is a hazard ratio (Table 5-3), which is conceptually identical to a rate ratio. Thus, the hazard (or rate) of the event multiplies by the hazard ratio for every 1-unit increase in the IV (or when comparing two groups, such as exposed and unexposed groups, it is simply the ratio of the hazard rates in the two groups). In the

standard Cox model, the relative effect remains constant over time. Crude and adjusted hazard ratios can be estimated. An adjusted hazard ratio describes the relationship between a variable and survival time, after controlling for appropriate covariates. An illustration of Cox regression is provided by Zuidgeest et al.,[30] who used Cox regression to explore predictors of the time until discontinuation of asthma medication in children who received asthma medications before the age of one (see Case Study 5-3).

AN OVERVIEW OF THIRD-VARIABLE EFFECTS

In the previous section, the concept of multiple regression (the inclusion of more than one IV in a regression model) was briefly considered. One potential role of such additional variables (i.e., confounder) was mentioned; however, variables added to a simple regression model may serve additional roles. When a third variable is added to a regression model, it can change the interpretation of the relationship between an IV (sometimes called the focal IV) and a DV, hence, the term "third-variable effects." The addition of a third variable to a model increases the possible relationships between the variables (and complicates the interpretation). Several types of third-variable effects are possible. Confounding, mediation, and moderation are three commonly examined third-variable effects. As with most of the material in this chapter the focus of this section is not on how to conduct such analyses, but rather on conceptual and definitional aspects.

Confounding

A confounder is a "variable that changes the relationship between an independent and DV because it is related to both."[31 (p7)] *Confounding* is said to exist if meaningfully different interpretations of the relationship between the IV and the DV result when the confounder is ignored or when it is included in the analysis.[5] This usually means that the inclusion of a confounder will reduce the magnitude of the relationship between an IV and DV (but it can increase it; something called negative confounding and occasionally called suppression). One approach for assessing confounding is to compare crude and adjusted estimates (i.e., regression coefficients) for the IV of

The Use of Cox Regression

Asthma medications are often prescribed to infants and young children with wheezing and other symptoms even though rarely is asthma definitively diagnosed in this patient population. Indeed, response to treatment with asthma medications is often used as a diagnostic tool; nonresponse followed by discontinuation of use suggests no asthma. Zuidgeest et al.[30] attempt to identify predictors of persistent use of asthma medication in preschool children as knowledge of such determinants might assist future practitioners in making decisions with respect to initiation of asthma medication therapy. Their analysis was conducted on a group of 165 children from the Prevention and Incidence of Asthma and Mite Allergy (PIAMA) study. Each child initially used an asthma medication before the age of 1. The primary outcome was time until discontinuation of asthma medication during a 3-year period following the initial prescription for asthma medication (the index date). Since the outcome variable was time until an event, Cox regression was used to arrive at crude and adjusted hazards ratios as well as 95% confidence intervals for a number of potential predictors classified as patient characteristics, severity of symptoms, familial predisposition, and environmental influences. In a multivariable model, only two factors were found to be statistically

significant: a prescription for inhaled corticosteroids (ICS) in the first year of life and doctor-diagnosed asthma. None of the other variables, including the environmental and familial predisposition variables, were statistically significant. In the multivariable model, the prescribed ICS variable had a hazard ratio of 0.59 (95% CI = 0.40-0.86; P < 0.05); this was statistically significant at the α = 0.05 level (notice that the 95% CI does not include 1). The finding suggests that after controlling for the other variables, at any point in time the hazard of discontinuing asthma medication for those children prescribed ICS in the first year of life is 0.59 times the hazard for those not prescribed ICS in the first year of life. What this means is that being prescribed ICS in the first year of life is associated with persistent use of asthma medication (i.e., these children are more likely to continue treatment with asthma medications). Although no objective measures that could be assessed prior to treatment initiation were found to be associated with persistent asthma medication use, the authors caution against relying entirely on "physician-decided" measures like prescribed ICS and doctor-diagnosed asthma to guide further asthma treatment decisions, as asthma is very difficult to diagnose in young children.

interest. If the change in the coefficient is substantial (often considered to be a 10% change[2]), there is evidence that the added variable is a confounder. Thus, a confounder accounts for all or part of the relationship between a predictor and an outcome. A number of techniques for addressing confounding (and other types of bias) are available and are explored in Chapter 6.

▶ Mediation (the Intermediate Endpoint Effect)

In their seminal piece, Baron & Kenny[32] define a *mediator* as a variable that accounts for all or part of

relationship between a predictor and an outcome (note that this definition implies that mediation and confounding are similar concepts). At its most basic level, mediation occurs when an IV causes an intervening variable, which in turn causes the DV. Although the terminology differs (and occasionally the assumptions and statistical tests), the concept of mediation, more broadly labeled the *intervening variable effect*, is prevalent in many different disciplines. MacKinnon et al.[33] note that psychology frequently uses the term "mediation," sociology uses "indirect effect," and epidemiology uses "surrogate" or "intermediate endpoint effect." MacKinnon, Krull, and Lockwood[34] note that mediation and confounding are mathematically equivalent concepts (at least in the context of a cross-sectional design analyzed with linear regression) and can only be distinguished conceptually. Confounding differs conceptually from mediation in that a confounder is not an intermediate in a causal sequence. Indeed, some criteria for defining a confounder explicitly state that the confounder must *not* be an effect of the IV—it cannot be part of the causal pathway.[2] Mediation continues to be a very active area of research, primarily in psychology.[‡‡‡]

Mediation models can fit in the context of linear regression, logistic regression in the case of a discrete outcome,[35] survival analysis,[36] and a variety of other techniques. Many studies of mediation use cross-sectional designs; the collection of longitudinal data adds potentially improved interpretation as well as additional considerations.[37,38]

▶ Moderation (Statistical Interaction or Effect Modification)

The concepts of *moderation* and *mediation* (and to some extent *confounding*) are often confused. A moderator variable alters the strength or direction of the relationship between the IV and the DV; in essence, the relationship between the IV and the DV is different at different levels (i.e., values) of the moderator.[32] Moderation involves the presence of a statistical interaction, whereas mediation implies that the effect of the IV is transmitted through the mediator. The *moderator effect* is commonly known as the *interaction effect,* and these terms are typically used interchangeably. In epidemiology, statistical interaction is often termed *effect modification,*[5] and moderator variables are called effect modifiers. Thus, the association between a predictor (i.e., exposure) of interest and a health outcome (i.e., disease status) is "modified" (i.e., is different) depending on the value of one or more effect modifiers (i.e., these variables modify the relationship between exposure and outcome). An important (and often confusing) point is that the

presence of effect modification may depend on the scale on which the researcher measures the association. For example, it is possible to find an interaction when one is examining risk ratios but not when evaluating risk differences.[39]

Moderation is often a question of interest in ANOVA (when you have two or more factors) and can also be assessed in the context of linear regression, logistic regression, and survival analysis (as well as other techniques). The concepts of mediated moderation and moderated mediation were also described by Baron and Kenny.[32] Several authors have recently discussed procedures to address these concepts.[40,41]

POWER ANALYSIS AND SAMPLE-SIZE PLANNING

In addition to its roles related to data description, estimation, error assessment, and hypothesis testing, statistics serves a related role in the conduct of research, namely, the calculating of necessary samples sizes for a study. It is important that researchers consider sample-size issues in the planning phase of their projects, as studies that are too large waste resources and studies that are too small are underpowered, leading to potentially erroneous conclusions regarding associations or effects. The concepts of type I and type II errors discussed previously are critically important when performing sample-size calculations. When estimation is a primary objective and the researcher is focused on determining a sample size necessary to achieve confidence intervals of a sufficiently narrow width, researchers use the techniques of precision analysis (e.g., see Refs. 42 and 43). Precision analysis is based in part of the desired probability of a type I error or α (recall, the selection of α determines the confidence level).

An alternative approach[§§§] is rooted in hypothesis testing rather than interval estimation and attempts to minimize the probabilities of type I and type II errors (α and β, respectively). In this approach, a

---

[‡‡‡]The reader is referred to MacKinnon[31] for an excellent discussion of many of the issues with respect to mediation analysis.

[§§§]It is important to note that these two approaches can be use in a complementary manner.[42]

researcher uses a predetermined α and attempts to achieve a desired level of β (or conversely power) by choosing an appropriate sample size to detect a clinically or scientifically meaningful effect. This method of sample-size determination is referred to as *power analysis*. Based on the principles of power analysis and some concepts described earlier in this chapter (Figure 5-3), one can show that the required sample size for a study increases with:

- Increasing variability of the effect of interest
- Decreasing type I error rate
- Increasing desired target level of power (recall, this is $1-\beta$)
- Decreasing size of the effect of interest

Sample-size planning using power analysis is more common in the medical literature (especially clinical trials; for example, see Ref. 44) and in the epidemiology literature (although to a lesser extent). Oftentimes, conducting prestudy power analyses forces researchers to consider in much more depth their planned statistical analyses, as conducting a power analysis requires consideration of issues such as: What type of data do I have (e.g., continuous, categorical, time to event)? What is a clinically meaningful effect? What do I know about variability? What are my targets for power and the probability of a type I error? Am I going to utilize groups of unequal size? The last issue may mean different things depending on the study design. In a clinical trial, it means having unequal number of participants receiving treatment and placebo; in a cohort study, it may mean having different number of exposed and unexposed individuals; and in a case-control study, it may mean having more controls than cases. Equal treatment allocation is generally used in clinical trials. Strom[45] outlines some reasons for using unequal group sizes in cohort and case-control studies and notes that rarely is there rationale for using ratios larger than 4:1.

A final note about power analysis is warranted. Researchers will sometimes use the principles of power analysis to estimate the power of a statistical test after data collection using the actual study data (this has been labeled *retrospective power analysis* or *post hoc power analysis*). Several commercial software packages facilitate such calculations. Such analyses do not add any information beyond what we already receive from performing the statistical test (e.g., see Refs. 46 and 47) and should generally be avoided.

▼ SUMMARY

Although not comprehensive in its scope, this chapter has attempted to provide relevant information concerning the role of statistics, specifically biostatistics, in pharmacoepidemiology. Statistics can be used to arrive at estimates of important concepts, whether descriptive, associational, or causal, as well as to provide information concerning uncertainty in the estimation process. Although it does not provide definitive information, statistics can and does provide information that individuals can use in making important decisions. It is important to recognize that statistics cannot "save" a poorly designed or executed study, but when misapplied, statistics can lead to erroneous conclusions even if a study has been well planned and conducted. Thus, it is important for readers of the pharmacoepidemiology literature to appreciate and understand not only features of study design and tools for translating study results into practice but also how statistics can be used to analyze data and generate information.

DISCUSSION QUESTIONS

1. Explain the relevance to statistics of the various variable classification schemes discussed in this chapter.

2. Name and describe four measures that can be used to describe the relationship between two categorical variables, both dichotomous.

3. What is the difference between the coefficient of variation and the coefficient of determination?

4. How are confidence intervals and hypothesis testing related? How are they different?

5. What is the difference between statistical significance and practical or clinical significance?

6. What is the difference between a paired t test and an unpaired t test? What situations would lead an investigator to choose one over the other?

7. What is the difference between one-way ANOVA and two-way ANOVA?

8. What is the difference between a paired t test and the McNemar test? What situations would lead an investigator to choose one over the other?

9. What is the nature of the DV for linear regression, logistic regression, and Cox regression and what association measure is associated with each technique?

10. Distinguish confounding and mediation.

11. In your own words, define the concept of a statistical interaction and give an example of a statistical interaction. Find a paper published in the biomedical literature where the investigators explored or described a statistical interaction. Provide your interpretation of their findings.

12. List the factors that are associated with the need for a larger sample size when conducting a study.

REFERENCES

1. Barnett V. *Comparative Statistical Inference*, 3rd ed. New York: John Wiley & Sons, 1999.

2. Rothman KJ. *Epidemiology: An Introduction.* New York: Oxford University Press, 2002.

3. Tabachnick BG, Fidell LS. *Using Multivariate Statistics,* 5th ed. Boston: Allyn & Bacon, 2007.

4. Dawson B, Trapp RG. *Basic and Clinical Biostatistics,* 3rd ed. New York: McGraw-Hill, 2004.

5. Kleinbaum DG, Kupper LL, Nizam A, et al. *Applied Regression Analysis and Other Multivariable Methods,* 4th ed. Belmont, CA: Duxbury, 2008.

6. Katz MH. Multivariable analysis: A primer for readers of medical research. *Ann Intern Med.* 2003;138:644-650.

7. Casella G, Berger RL. *Statistical Inference,* 2nd ed. Pacific Grove, CA: Duxbury, 2002.

8. Colton T. *Statistics in Medicine.* Boston: Little, Brown & Company, 1974.

9. Cohen J. A power primer. *Psychol Bull.* 1992;112:155-159.

10. Greenland S, Rothman KJ, Lash TL. Measures of effect and measures of association. In: Rothman KJ, Greenland S, Lash TL, eds. *Modern Epidemiology,* 3rd ed. Philadelphia: Lippincott Williams & Wilkins, 2008:51-70.

11. Barratt A, Wyer PC, Hatala R, et al. Tips for learners of evidence-based medicine: 1. Relative risk reduction, absolute risk reduction and number needed to treat. *CMAJ.* 2004;171:353-358.

12. Agresti A. *An Introduction to Categorical Data Analysis,* 2nd ed. Hoboken, NJ: John Wiley & Sons, 2007.

13. Daniel WW. *Biostatistics: A Foundation for Analysis in the Health Sciences,* 8th ed. Hoboken, NJ: John Wiley & Sons, 2005.

14. Rothman KJ, Greenland S, Lash TL. Precision and statistics in epidemiologic studies. In: Rothman KJ, Greenland S, Lash TL, eds. *Modern Epidemiology,* 3rd ed. Philadelphia: Lippincott Williams & Wilkins, 2008:148-167.

15. Harlow LL, Mulaik SA, Steiger JH, eds. *What If There Were No Significance Tests?* Mahwah, NJ: Lawrence Erlbaum Associates, 1997.

16. Nickerson RS. Null hypothesis significance testing: A review of an old and continuing controversy. *Psychol Methods.* 2000;5: 241-301.

17. Cohen J. The Earth is round ($p < .05$). *Am Psychol.* 1994;49: 997-1003.

18. Bland JM, Altman DG. One and two sided tests of significance. *BMJ.* 1994;309:248.

19. Moyé LA, Tita ATN. Hypothesis testing complexity in the name of ethics: Response to commentary. *J Clin Epidemiol.* 2002;55:209.

20. Norman GR, Streiner DL. *Biostatistics: The Bare Essentials,* 3rd ed. Shelton, CT: People's Medical Publishing House, 2008.

21. Blackwelder WC. "Proving the null hypothesis" in clinical trials. *Control Clin Trials.* 1982;3:345-353.

22. Hair JF, Black WC, Babin BJ, et al. *Multivariate Data Analysis,* 6th ed. Upper Saddle River, NJ: Prentice Hall, 2006.

23. Sprent P, Smeeton NC. *Applied Nonparametric Statistical Methods,* 3rd ed. Baco Raton, FL: Chapman & Hall/CRC, 2001.

24. Tabachnick BG, Fidell LS. *Experimental Design Using ANOVA.* Belmont, CA: Duxbury, 2007.

25. Manning WG, Basu A, Mullahy J. Generalized modeling approaches to risk adjustment of skewed outcomes data. *J Health Econ.* 2005;24:465-488.

26. Blough DK, Ramsey SD. Using generalized linear models to assess medical care costs. *Health Serv Outcomes Res Methodol.* 2000;1:185-202.

27. Shrank WH, Cadarette SM, Cox E, et al. Is there a relationship between patient beliefs or communication about generic drugs and medication utilization? *Med Care.* 2009;47:319-325.

28. Juurlink DN, Mamdani M, Kopp A, et al. Drug-drug interactions among elderly patients hospitalized for drug toxicity. *JAMA.* 2003;289:1652-1658.

29. Allison PD. *Survival Analysis Using SAS: A Practical Guide.* Cary, NC: SAS Institute, 1995.

30. Zuidgeest MG, Smit HA, Bracke M, et al. Persistence of asthma medication use in preschool children. *Respir Med.* 2008;102: 1446-1451.

31. MacKinnon DP. *Introduction to Statistical Mediation Analysis.* New York: Lawrence Erlbaum Associates, 2008.

32. Baron RM, Kenny DA. The moderator-mediator variable distinction in social psychological research: Conceptual, strategic, and statistical considerations. *J Pers Soc Psychol.* 1986;51:1173-1182.

33. MacKinnon DP, Lockwood CM, Hoffman JM, et al. A comparison of methods to test mediation and other intervening variable effects. *Psychol Methods.* 2002;7:83-104.

34. MacKinnon DP, Krull JL, Lockwood CM. Equivalence of the mediation, confounding, and suppression effect. *Prev Sci.* 2000;1:173-181.

35. MacKinnon DP, Lockwood CM, Brown CH, et al. The intermediate endpoint effect in logistic and probit regression. *Clin Trials*. 2007;4:499-513.

36. Tein JY, MacKinnon DP. Estimating mediated effects with survival data. In: Yanai H, Rikkyo A O, Shigemasu K, et al., eds. *New Developments in Psychometrics: Proceedings of the International Meeting of the Psychometric Society*. Tokyo: Springer-Verlag, 2003:405-412.

37. Cole DA, Maxwell SE. Testing mediation models with longitudinal data: Questions and tips in the use of structural equation modeling. *J Abnorm Psychol*. 2003;112:558-577.

38. Maxwell SE, Cole DA. Bias in cross-sectional analyses of longitudinal mediation. *Psychol Methods*. 2007;12:23-44.

39. Greenland S, Lash TL, Rothman KJ. Concepts of interaction. In: Rothman KJ, Greenland S, Lash TL, eds. *Modern Epidemiology*, 3rd ed. Philadelphia: Lippincott Williams & Wilkins, 2008:71-83.

40. Muller D, Judd CM, Yzerbyt VY. When moderation is mediated and mediation is moderated. *J Pers Soc Psychol*. 2005;89:852-863.

41. Edwards JR, Lambert LS. Methods for integrating moderation and mediation: A general analytical framework using moderated path analysis. *Psychol Methods*. 2007;12:1-22.

42. Kelley K, Maxwell SE. Sample size for multiple regression: Obtaining regression coefficients that are accurate, not simply significant. *Psychol Methods*. 2003;8:305-321.

43. Maxwell SE, Kelley K, Rausch JR. Sample size planning for statistical power and accuracy in parameter estimation. *Ann Rev Psychol*. 2008;59:537-563.

44. Chow S, Shao J, Wang H. *Sample Size Calculations in Clinical Research*, 2nd ed. Baco Raton, FL: Chapman & Hall/CRC, 2008.

45. Strom BL. Sample size considerations for pharmacoepidemiology studies. In: Strom BL, ed. *Pharmacoepidemiology*, 4th ed. Hoboken, NJ: John Wiley & Sons, 2005:29-36.

46. Hoenig JM, Heisey DM. The abuse of power: The pervasive fallacy of power calculations for data analysis. *Am Stat*. 2001;55:19-24.

47. Lenth RV. Some practical guidelines for effective sample size determination. *Am Stat*. 2001;55:187-193.

Other Methodological Issues

6

Qayyim Said

▼ OBJECTIVES

At the end of the chapter, the reader will be able to:

1. Identify the nature of causation and association in pharmacoepidemiology studies
2. Describe the key criteria to determine causation
3. Identify the main types and sources of bias in pharmacoepidemiology studies
4. Explain the concept of confounding
5. Describe and discuss methods to deal with bias and confounding
6. Explain the concept of risk adjustment
7. Describe the methods for adjusting for risk in pharmacoepidemiology studies

INTRODUCTION

One of the main objectives of the discipline of pharmacoepidemiology is to evaluate the use of and the effects of drugs in the postmarketing phase. In other words, pharmacoepidemiology is primarily concerned with the real-world usage and effects of drugs, as opposed to the use and effects in randomized controlled trials. In order to analyze pharmaceuticals in the postmarketing scenario, one must use large databases that are collected for either administrative claims processing or for the purposes of maintaining clinical records. These data are not collected and maintained for research purposes; therefore, they pose special challenges to researchers. Many of these

challenges emerge because drugs are used by or prescribed to patients on the basis of a host of patient, provider and societal factors. In addition, drug exposure may be related to factors that may also be associated with its outcome. Furthermore, patient outcomes are generally a result of not only the drug exposure but also a variety of patient and nonpatient characteristics.

More often than not, the treatment and control groups are different from each other in clinical and nonclinical characteristics. These differences can be a range of patient characteristics or risk factors that can influence outcomes. In order to arrive at correct estimates of association between treatment and outcomes, it is important to remove or mitigate the impact of these risk factors. Risk-adjustment measures are used to evaluate the outcomes by statistically controlling for group differences when comparing dissimilar treatment groups.

Analyzing large databases to evaluate associations between treatment and outcomes and interpreting results obtained from such analyses requires understanding of certain key methodological issues in the fields of epidemiology and statistics. In the following sections, several important methodological issues that need to be taken into consideration in investigations of drug treatment and outcomes are discussed.

This chapter begins with a discussion of causation and the criteria that may be used to distinguish causal association from a noncausal association. The next section deals with the issues of bias and confounding commonly encountered in pharmacoepidemiology studies that use large databases. The final section introduces the topic of risk adjustment and outlines some of the key measures and methods of adjusting for risk.

CAUSATION

In order to understand the concept of *causation,* it is important to distinguish it from the related concept of *association.* A scientific study of evaluation of the relationship between a treatment (i.e., intervention and exposure) and its outcome begins with a selection of participants who form the study sample. One gathers information for the study sample and draws a conclusion regarding the existence of a relationship between the treatment and its outcome, using appropriate statistical techniques. If the relationship is shown to be statistically significant then this conclusion may be generalized as existence of an *association* between the treatment and the outcome. Taking this process one step further, one may desire to generalize the results further by asking whether this association is causal or not. In order to establish causation, statistical inference is not enough. There must also be inference drawn on the theoretical, scientific, or biological basis. In such a case, the association may be concluded as *causal association.*

To further our understanding of the differences between association and causal association, we will take a look at three types of associations that are possible in epidemiological studies.[1,2] The first type is spurious or false association. Spurious association may occur by chance or by some type of bias. Association by chance is due to unsystematic or random variation, whereas association resulting from bias is due to systematic variation. Statistical techniques are used to estimate probabilities to ascertain whether an association is due to chance. Bias occurs when the groups under study are treated in a consistently different manner from one another. Existence of such a bias may represent an association where there is none or may disguise an association where there is one. Biases can be removed at the study design level or minimized at the analysis level by using appropriate methods.

The second type of association is called a *confounded association.* A confounded association may occur if a third variable is independently correlated with both the treatment and outcome variables. This correlation may create a spurious association or disguise a true association. Such a variable could be a confounder. As in the case of bias, confounding can be removed at the study-design level or controlled at the analysis level.[1,2]

The third and final type of association is the true causal association.[1,2] Following from the previous discussion on types of association, we find that there may be three types of errors that can possibly exist in a study: random error, error due to bias, and error due to confounding (i.e., systematic error). If all these three types of errors are removed, then what we get may be termed as *true causal association.*

▶ Criteria for Determination of Causation

Sir Austin Bradford Hill (1965)[3] proposed a set of "criteria" that can be used to differentiate causal from noncausal associations. These criteria were based on a list previously proposed in the landmark U.S. Surgeon General's report titled *Smoking and Health* (1964).[4] Following these early efforts, others have further developed the criteria for causation.[5] However, these criteria are neither necessary nor sufficient for the purposes of determining causation. It should be

Table 6-1. Criteria for determining causal associations.

1. Strength of association
2. Consistency in repeated analyses
3. Specificity of cause and effect
4. Time sequence of exposure and outcome
5. Biological gradient
6. Plausibility and coherence
7. Experimental evidence
8. Analogy with the existing literature

noted here that Hill used the word *viewpoints* rather than *criteria* for this list. Furthermore, meeting a greater number of criteria imply only a greater likelihood of causation.[6] The guidelines for establishing causation, as presented by Hill, are listed in Table 6-1 and further discussed in this section.

Strength

Strong associations generally present a more compelling case than weaker associations; however, it does not necessarily mean that weaker associations cannot be causal. For example, the association between smoking and cardiovascular disease is generally accepted as causal association but is considered weak.

Consistency

Repeated observation of an association in different conditions across different populations implies consistency. Therefore, an association that shows consistency may provide a strong case for a causal association. It should be mentioned that lack of consistency may not always imply lack of causal associations, as some effects resulting from a particular cause may only be apparent under certain conditions. When those conditions are not met, the effect will not be created. For example, transfusions can cause human immunodeficiency infections in patients if the HIV virus is present in the transfused blood. If no virus is present, then infections will not occur.[6]

Specificity

This is a very strong criterion and probably the most difficult to meet. The specificity criterion implies that a cause leads to a single effect or an effect has a single cause. In practice this requirement is almost never met. For example, not everyone who takes a second-generation antipsychotic has an increased level of triglycerides and not everyone who experiences an elevated level of triglycerides takes a second-generation antipsychotic.

Time Sequence

This criterion implies that a cause must precede the effect in a causal relationship. This may not always be easy to determine in cross-sectional studies. For example, if patients are asked on a survey whether they take acetaminophen and whether they are having headaches, a positive correlation is likely to result. However, this positive correlation does not imply a causal relationship. Does the drug cause the headache or does having a headache cause the person to take the drug? However, if a study is conducted with an appropriate time lag between having a headache and taking acetaminophen, then a causal relationship can be hypothesized between taking the drug and having a reduction in headache.

Biological Gradient

Biological gradient refers to dose–response and duration–response relationship. An investigator should observe whether there is an increase in the effect with an increase in dose. Furthermore, it is important to see whether the risk of outcome increases as the duration of treatment/exposure gets longer. If any of these phenomena occurs, then it provides evidence that there may be a causal association between treatment and outcome.

Plausibility and Coherence

This criterion refers to the existence of foundation of scientific theory in an association. This is an important consideration in establishing causation for an association. If there is no plausibility from the perspective of scientific theory of an observed association between a treatment and its outcome then the

CASE STUDY 6-1

Somnolence Effects of Antipsychotic Medications and the Risk of Unintentional Injury[7]

This study examined the relationship between antipsychotic medications, categorized by published somnolence effects, and unintentional injury (UI).[7] The study population included patients in the age group 18 to 64 years in a healthcare insurance database with claims from 2001 to 2004 and diagnoses of schizophrenia or affective disorder. A nested case-control design was used with cases defined by an E-code claim (a specified external cause of injury) for selected UIs. For cases, the index date referred to the first injury. For controls, the "control index date" was the date of claim if there was only a single medical claim; for patients with ≥2 claims, one was selected at random as the "control index date." Both groups had a prescription for a first-generation antipsychotic (FGA) or second-generation antipsychotic (SGA) overlapping the index date. Logistic regression models were used to estimate odds ratio (OR) and 95% confidence interval (CI) for UI, adjusted for gender, age, concomitant drug, and psychiatric diagnosis. Among 648 cases and 5,214 controls, high-somnolence SGAs were associated with risk of UI, as compared with low-somnolence SGAs. The study established causal association between the exposure to antipsychotic drugs and the outcome (UI) by invoking scientific plausibility, biological gradient, and time-sequence criteria.[7]

case for establishing causation becomes weak. However, in some cases, a hypothesis can be formed on the basis of some prior beliefs. This may happen when the existing base of science does not provide enough foundation to form a causal hypothesis.

Experimental Evidence

Experimental evidence refers to stopping exposure of a harmful treatment and then observing whether the risk of disease or outcome declines. If this occurs then it can be another consideration for establishing causation.

Analogy

As the name suggests, this criterion seeks to gain further insight to determine whether an association is causal or not by looking at analogies that may exist in the literature.

BIAS

Bias is related to systematic errors, as opposed to random errors, in performing a study.[2,5] A systematic error may occur when the study groups under investigation are selected in a manner that consistently treats one study group differently from the other group(s). In pharmacoepidemiology studies, interest is in estimating the relationship between exposure to a drug treatment or intervention and its effects on health status or outcomes. A challenge in this exercise is to arrive at an estimate of the effect that is unbiased. This is particularly true of postmarketing studies when many factors can affect the association between treatment and outcome. For example, prescribing by indication or patient adherence to treatment regimen could be important factors coming into play while evaluating the association between treatment and outcome. In this section we will briefly consider selection bias, information bias, and confounding bias. We will then describe the methods to deal with bias and confounding.

▶ Types and Sources of Bias in Pharmacoepidemiological Research

Selection Bias

Selection bias results when procedures followed in selecting study participants such that participants who get selected in the study are either more likely or less likely to experience the outcome than are those who are not in the study sample, even though they may have been theoretically eligible for inclusion in the study. Selection bias that may be present in pharmacoepidemiology studies in different forms is explained in this section.[2,5,8–13]

A type of selection bias that may be of concern is called *self-selection bias*. This type of bias may occur when participants themselves decide to participate in or drop out of a study. The decisions may be influenced by both exposure and outcome. This can occur in situations when particular types of patients are more likely to report a certain adverse drug event. For example, in studying the effect of second-generation antipsychotics on weight gain by using retrospective electronic health records, those patients who actually gain weight may be more likely to contact the clinic and report an increase in weight, whereas those who do not experience weight gain are less likely to report, even though they are taking second-generation antipsychotic medications. This type of self-selection bias should be reduced at the analysis level by using appropriate statistical techniques.

Another type of selection bias is called the *referral bias*. If a patient is referred to another provider (e.g., hospital, specialist) or referred to laboratory tests because of an exposure to a drug then referral bias may occur. For example, a patient taking a second-generation antipsychotic and having history of high glucose levels may be referred to the laboratory for glucose testing more frequently. This may result in overstating the association between the second-generation antipsychotics and the incidence of diabetes.

Information Bias

The logical next step after the selection of a sample for performing a pharmacoepidemiology study is to conduct an analysis to estimate the effect of the treatment/exposure variable. However, in order to do this one needs to collect information on the participants. Errors in measurement of such information on the study participants can cause bias. This type of bias is called *information bias*. A type of measurement error that occurs because of misclassifying exposed as unexposed (and vice versa) or when a diseased participant is classified as nondiseased (and vice versa) is termed as *misclassification*, which can lead to misclassification bias.[14] Misclassification may be divided into *nondifferential misclassification* and *differential misclassification*. In nondifferential misclassification, error occurs independently of the exposure–outcome relationship. The degree of misclassification is similar for all patients regardless of exposure or outcome. This type of misclassification may lead to the weakening of association between exposure and outcome and bias the results toward the null hypothesis.

Differential misclassification occurs when measurement error is related to or depends on exposure or outcome variables. When the information collected depends on whether the participant is exposed or unexposed or whether the participant is in the diseased or healthy group, differential misclassification may result. There are two types of situations that may lead to such a misclassification: *recall bias* and *detection bias*. Recall bias is more common in a case-control design and is likely to lead to situations where cases are more likely to recall their disease patterns than controls. Detection bias can occur when cases are given more importance than controls in collection of information, or when the exposed participants are followed more closely than the unexposed. For example, patients on second-generation antipsychotics may be followed more closely for elevated blood glucose (a side effect), and thus, more diagnoses of diabetes may be observed in the exposed/treatment group compared to the unexposed group.

Confounding Bias

The issue of confounding is especially concerning for observational studies. It occurs when the relationship between exposure or treatment and outcome is affected by another variable or a group of variables.[15–17] Specifically, a third variable called a *confounder* is a risk factor for the outcome of interest. The distribution of the confounding variable is different across different levels of exposure. A confounder is related to both exposure and outcome without being in the causal pathway of exposure and outcome (Figure 6-1). For example, in evaluating the effects of risperidone and olanzapine (second-generation antipsychotics) on lipid levels, age may be a confounder. This is possible because older age may be a risk factor for elevated lipid levels (outcome) and at

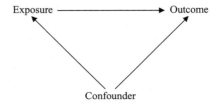

▲ **Figure 6-1.** Relationship of the confounder with exposure and outcome.

the same time may also affect prescribing patterns of second-generation antipsychotics (exposure/treatment). Specifically, participants from younger age groups are more likely to be prescribed risperidone because of its indication for children.

Confounding in pharmacoepidemiology can be of various types. Confounding by indication is probably the most common type found in pharmacoepidemiology studies.[6,18-21] This type of confounding is sometimes called *channeling bias* or *indication bias*. This arises when a physician prescribes drugs keeping in mind certain patient characteristics such as disease severity, age, or gender. There may also be other non–patient-related factors that are likely to influence physician prescribing and are not easily measurable, including the influence of sales promotion activities by drug manufacturers. Another type of confounding that is of concern is confounding by concomitant drug use. In the case of evaluating the effect of second-generation antipsychotics on weight gain, the use of a weight loss drug by a patient could present itself as a confounder that must be considered in the analysis.

▷ Methodologies Used to Address Potential Biases

Different types of biases can be corrected or reduced either at the study design level or at the analysis level. Following are some of the commonly used methods that are used to control for bias.

▷ Randomization

Randomization or random assignment is the process of assigning individuals to treatment or control group on the basis of an accepted mechanism (e.g., coin toss) that gives each individual the same probability of being in any given group (e.g., treatment or control). Such a mechanism is independent of any extraneous factors that can affect outcome. Therefore, any association between treatment group and extraneous factors can be considered as happening due to pure chance. Furthermore, randomization across treatment and control groups can remove selection bias because the objective is to make the exposed and unexposed groups as similar as possible in every respect except the exposure status.

▷ Restriction

Restriction involves defining certain characteristics that could be used to refine the study population, such as through *inclusion* and *exclusion* criteria. One purpose of restriction is to refine the study population in such a way that potential confounders are prohibited or "restricted" from varying and thus not produce the confounding effect. For example, a study investigating the effect of sedation caused by antipsychotic medications on the occurrence of unintentional injury would exclude patients with diagnoses for mental retardation, vision problems, epilepsy, hearing loss, muscular dystrophy, and stroke because these conditions could increase the risk of unintentional injury. Furthermore, to focus on the effects of antipsychotic medications, participants older than 65 years of age will be excluded because older age may be a confounding factor in the relationship between the treatment (antipsychotic exposure) and the outcome (unintentional injury).

▷ Blinding

Blinding is a strategy that is aimed at correcting information bias at the study-design level. Blinding refers to a situation where the patient or the data collector (the assessor of outcomes) is ignorant of the treatment assignment. Studies are termed as *double blind* if both the patient and the data collector are blinded to the treatment. It is important to keep the

Table 6-2. Methodologies used to address potential biases.

Methodologies	Key features
1. Randomization	• Controls for all known and unknown confounding factors. • Requires sophisticated statistical techniques to address in observational studies.
2. Restriction	• Easy to do was redundant. • May severely reduce sample size.
3. Blinding	• Only applicable in the case of experimental studies. • May not be possible in cases where drugs have known side effects.
4. Matching	• Provides tighter confidence intervals for the matching variable as opposed to directly controlling for in statistical modeling. • Does not allow the investigator to assess the effect of the matching variable itself. • May reduce sample size if participants cannot be matched, necessitating throwing out of the unmatched. • Costly and time consuming to perform.
5. Stratification	• Allows separate estimates of effects for the each stratum of the confounding variable. • Easy to perform at the analysis level. • Can be cumbersome if there are many strata of a confounder.
6. Multivariable modeling	• Very efficient way to control for more than one confounder simultaneously. • Requires advanced statistical modeling skills to perform. • May lead to misleading results and interpretation if not performed with proper knowledge of the techniques.
7. Propensity-score analysis	• Reduces treatment selection bias at the analysis level. • Only accounts for observable factors.
8. Instrumental variable estimation	• Reduces treatment selection bias at the analysis level. • Accounts for unobservable factors.
9. Inverse probability of treatment weighting	• Reduces treatment selection bias at the analysis level. • Accounts for time-dependent covariates. • Only accounts for observable factors.
10. Sensitivity analysis	• Powerful way to check the validity of model assumptions. • Can be used to assess the effect of unmeasured confounders.

data collector blind when the outcomes assessment is subjective, such as a specific diagnosis. On the other hand, the patient knowledge of assignment can affect adherence to the treatment. Both of these contingencies make blinding an important strategy to reduce bias. Sometimes the study can be termed as *triple blind* when the data analyst does not know which group of participants received the treatment and vice versa. On the other hand, it may not always be possible to have the parties blinded to the treatment assignment. Such a situation may be necessitated if a drug has specific and known side effects; thus, in such cases, the data collector or assessor of the outcomes needs to be aware of these possibilities. In this case, it may also possible for the patient to identify the treatment.

▶ Matching

Matching involves identifying some characteristic that is alleged to be a source of bias (i.e., a confounder) and matching cases with controls or exposed participants with unexposed ones in relation to that characteristic. For example, matching a case and a control on a 5-year age range or matching an exposed participant with a certain disease to an unexposed participant with the same disease. Matching the two groups (exposed vs unexposed or diseased vs nondiseased) on the confounding variable can be a useful strategy. Matching, however, is costly and time consuming at the study-design level. At the analysis level, matching may be constrained by sample size.

▶ Stratification

Stratification is used to control for variation driven by a confounder at the analysis level. Analysis is performed for each stratum defined by the levels of the confounder. For example, if gender is a confounder then analysis of the effect of treatment on the outcome may be performed by creating two strata, one for each gender. This strategy removes any variation emanating from gender differences.

Multivariable Modeling

An efficient way to control for confounding at the analysis level is to build multivariable mathematical models for controlling for multiple confounders at the same time. A model is specified and multiple regression techniques are used to calculate parameter estimates that provide information on the contribution of each individual confounder to the occurrence of the outcome. An advantage of this strategy is that it provides information on each confounder separately along with the estimates of effects of exposure on the outcome.

Propensity-Score Analysis

Propensity-score analysis is an advanced statistical approach that is designed to balance the treatment groups on all the observable characteristics so that they mimic a randomized trial.[22–25] In the first step, probabilities of being assigned to a treatment group are calculated on the observable characteristics. This is done using a logistic regression model in which the dependent variable is a dichotomous variable with two treatment categories. The independent variables are the characteristics that may have an impact on treatment assignment. Probabilities of being in a specific treatment group are then calculated for each patient. Those with similar probabilities or propensity scores are considered similar patients. These propensity scores are then used to either match patients on the scores before analysis, or used as a

covariate during regression analysis. This method of propensity scores has been used widely in pharmacoepidemiology and comparative effectiveness studies to control for selection bias.

Instrumental Variable Estimation

One weakness of the propensity-score analysis is that it does not account for unobservable factors that may be affecting treatment assignment. This issue is addressed by the instrumental variable approach.[26–28] Originated in the economics literature, this has now become an important approach to correct selection bias in pharmacoepidemiology studies. The basic idea is to find a variable, called an *instrumental variable* or *instrument* that is correlated with the treatment/exposure variable but not with the outcome. Once such a variable is found, regression analysis is used to predict treatment assignment for each patient. The predicted treatment assignment values by this instrumental variable are then used to estimate the effect of treatment on outcome. This approach reduces selection bias at the analysis level.

Inverse Probability of Treatment Weights

This is an advanced and relatively new method to address situations when covariates are time dependent and are both confounders and intermediate variables.[29] A new class of causal models, referred to as marginal structural models, is introduced in which the parameters are estimated using a new class of estimators called *inverse probability of treatment-weighted estimators.*[*]

Sensitivity Analysis

It is often the case that several assumptions are made while performing an analysis that seeks to examine the association between a treatment and its outcome. However, researchers are frequently required to check the robustness of those assumptions as to their effect on the outcome of interest. A common way to perform such checks is to conduct sensitivity analysis.[30] Sensitivity analysis is conducted by systematically repeating

---

*For further information on this topic, the reader is referred to Ref. 29.

CASE STUDY 6-2

Cardiovascular Outcomes and Mortality in Patients Using Clopidogrel with Proton-Pump Inhibitors After Percutaneous Coronary Intervention or Acute Coronary Syndrome[35]

The FDA has issued warnings about the reduced efficacy of clopidogrel when used concomitantly with proton-pump inhibitors (PPIs). Studies have been conducted to estimate this risk of reduced efficacy. Rassen et al.[35] speculate that previous studies may have overestimated the risk. The authors studied the potential for increased risk of adverse cardiovascular events, including myocardial infarction, hospitalization, death, and revascularization, among users of clopidogrel with and without concomitant PPI use between 2001 and 2005. Of the 18,565 participants, 2.6% of those with a PPI versus 2.1% of those without a PPI had a myocardial infarction hospitalization; 1.5% versus 0.9% died; and

3.4% versus 3.1% underwent revascularization. The authors used propensity-score analysis to adjust for selection bias and confounding. The rate ratio for the primary endpoint of myocardial infarction or death was found to be 1.22 (95% CI, 0.99–1.51). The authors concluded that there was no conclusive evidence of a clopidogrel–PPI interaction.[35] This result is contrary to those in the two recently published studies on the topic.[36,37] The authors compared their results with those two studies and suggested that the other studies did not adequately adjust for selection bias. The authors also mention the possibility of the existence of confounding by indication.[†]

the analysis by varying assumptions each time, in order to assess how sensitive the results obtained are to the variations in model assumptions and whether the results are consistent across the variations in assumptions. For example, often in studies of medication adherence a threshold for medication possession ratio (MPR) is specified for dichotomizing participants into adherent or nonadherent groups. It may be argued that the results are sensitive to the chosen threshold value and may require a sensitivity analysis by varying the threshold level, say from an MPR of 0.8 to 0.9. A further issue may be that the results are specific to a particular measure of adherence. In this case, a more general sensitivity analysis can be conducted by using an altogether different measure of adherence, such as Proportion of Days Covered (PDC) in place of MPR. Another example may be varying time windows or changing cutoff points in categorizing participants into various age groups.

Sensitivity analysis can also be classified as *one way* or *multiway*. In one-way analysis, only one variable is changed across a plausible range of values to study the impact on the outcome, keeping all other variables constant at their mean or baseline values. In a multiway analysis, values of two more variables are varied simultaneously to see the impact on the outcome.

Though less common, sensitivity analysis is also carried out to study the potential effects of various types of unmeasured biases, most notably confounding bias.[31,32] In order to perform this type of analysis, an estimate of the effect of confounding factor on the outcome and the prevalence of the confounding effect among treatment and control group should be available from the literature. Based on this information, confounding effects can be calculated for various levels of the potential confounder.[‡] A more advanced type of sensitivity analysis is called the *probabilistic sensitivity analysis*.[33,34] This type of analysis is derived from repeated Monte Carlo simulations to explore the impact on the outcome by allowing the variables to vary simultaneously across a reasonable range of values based on a predetermined probability distribution.[§]

[†]For a definition of "confounding by indication," see the earlier discussion on "Confounding Bias."

[‡]For further information on this topic, the reader is referred to Refs. 31 and 32.

[§]For further information on this topic, the reader is referred to Refs. 33 and 34.

Risk Adjustment

In observational studies, outcomes are developed as a result of a number of factors including the treatment. More often than not, the treatment groups are different from each other in clinical and nonclinical characteristics. These differences can be a range of patient characteristics or risk factors that can affect outcomes. In order to arrive at correct estimates of association between treatment and outcomes, it is important to remove or mitigate the impact of these risk factors. In other words, these group differences may confound the relationship between the treatment and outcome. The rationale for risk adjustment is to evaluate the outcomes by statistically controlling for group differences when comparing dissimilar treatment groups.[38–40] Risk adjustment is used to calculate an expected outcome measure based on risk factors considered and their relationship with outcomes.

Risk adjustment involves two main important steps.[40] First is to construct the measure used to define risk or severity, and second is to obtain outcomes adjusted for the constructed measure of risk or severity. The main factors that can be considered in risk adjustment are age, sex, principal diagnosis and its severity, extent and severity of comorbidities, physical functioning status, psychological and cognitive functioning status, quality of life, attitudes and preferences.[38] In the following expression, these risk factors may confound the relationship between the treatment and the outcome of interest.

Outcomes = f(treatment, age, sex, principal diagnosis and its severity, extent and severity of comorbidities, physical functioning status, psychological and cognitive functioning status, quality of life, attitudes and preferences, random chance).

For the purposes of this chapter, we will dwell upon only the risk arising from patient comorbidities. *Comorbidities* are defined as the concomitant medical conditions that exist in a patient, in addition to the medical condition under investigation. In pharmacoepidemiology, use of a composite *comorbidity index* or score is a common way to adjust for comorbidity risk. Several different types of comorbidity measures have been used in analyses conducted with administrative databases. These measures can be discussed under two main categories: diagnosis-based measures and pharmacy-based measures. In addition to these composite measures, researchers have also used simpler measures by directly including medical conditions or use of specific drugs as covariates. These measures are easy to use, and, in some cases, have been shown to be good predictors of outcomes of interest.[41] Furthermore, self-reported comorbidity assessment measures based on survey data have also been used in the literature.

In the following, we will outline the commonly used diagnosis-based and pharmacy-based measures developed for use in administrative data. Comorbidity measures can also be calculated by extracting information from patient charts or from electronic medical records. Most of the comorbidity risk-adjustment measures were developed to predict costs, resource utilization such as hospitalizations, or mortality. The main purpose for developing these measures was to set reimbursement levels for hospitals or managed care organizations. However, these measures were adopted for comorbidity adjustment in outcomes research and epidemiology studies. In view of this, a critical consideration is to determine whether a particular adjustment measure is likely to predict the outcome of interest in the pharmacoepidemiology study under investigation. For example, in a study that seeks to investigate the effect of second-generation antipsychotics on hyperlipidemia, the researcher must first assess whether a composite measure of risk is appropriate or needs to be modified to adequately control for confounding. This may be an issue if a general comorbidity adjustment measure is used and some of the conditions in the general measure may not have any impact on the outcome.

▶ Risk-Adjustment Models

Diagnosis-Based Models

The diagnosis-based models are based on codes from the International Classification of Diseases, Ninth Revision, Clinical Modification (ICD-9-CM). Some of these models are being updated using the International Classification of Diseases, Tenth Revision, Clinical Modification (ICD-10-CM).[42,43] Brief descriptions of some of the selected comorbidity risk-adjustment measures are presented in the following.

Charlson comorbidity index—The Charlson comorbidity index is the most commonly used measure to adjust for the risk arising from comorbidities in epidemiology research studies. It was primarily developed to predict 1-year mortality based on medical conditions extracted from hospital medical records.[44] The index calculates a comorbidity score by using 19 disease classifications that are weighted according to disease severity. Subsequently, several modifications and adaptations of the Charlson index occurred for the purposes of its use with administrative claims data.[45–48] These adaptations include Deyo/Charlson,[45] Romano (developed by the Dartmouth-Manitoba group),[46] D'Hoore,[47] and Ghali[48] adaptations and differ primarily on sets of diagnoses included in calculation of scores and the weights assigned to these diagnoses. The main difference between the Deyo/Charlson and Romano adaptations is that the latter interprets the comorbidity definitions less strictly than the former. Both collapse 3 items on the original Charlson index into 1 item to arrive at a total of 17 comorbid categories.[45,46] The Ghali adaptation uses a reduced set of diagnoses and new weights, as compared with the original Charlson index, to improve the prediction of inpatient mortality. The D'Hoore adaptation uses three-digit ICD-9-CM codes instead of the usual five-digit codes used in other adaptations. Schneeweiss et al.[49] examined the performance of the scores from each of the implementations to predict mortality and health care utilization. They concluded that Romano adaptations performed best among the various adaptations of the Charlson index.

Elixhauser index—This is a relatively recent diagnosis-based comorbidity index. The index uses 30 coexisting medical conditions to develop a risk score.[50] A feature of Elixhauser index is that it distinguishes between comorbidities and complications by considering only secondary diagnoses unrelated to the principal diagnosis through the use of diagnosis-related groups. A study performed by Farley et al.[41] that compared the performance of the Charlson comorbidity index with the Elixhauser index in predicting health care expenditures concluded that both performed similarly. Other studies have reported that Elixhauser index performed better in predicting mortality.[51]

Adjusted clinical groups (ACG)—ACGs were developed to predict ambulatory visits.[52] Originally, the index used outpatient diagnoses, but inpatient diagnoses were later incorporated into the calculation of the score. The model categorizes medical conditions into 32 groups mainly on the basis of severity of disease, likelihood of future specialty service use, and the duration of disease.

Diagnosis cost groups—hierarchical coexisting categories (DCG-HCC)—The DCG-HCC measure is used to predict health care costs and resource utilization for the Medicare population and is used to determine reimbursement to Medicare HMOs.[53] Initially, the calculation of scores was based on inpatient diagnoses, but outpatient diagnoses were included subsequently in calculating the score. The index categorizes diagnosis codes into about 800 groups, which are then further grouped into 184 condition categories. The categorization is based on clinical and resource use similarity. Finally, the 184 condition categories are ordered into roughly 100 hierarchical coexisting conditions.

Chronic illness and disability payment system (CDPS)—The CDPS is used to predict health care costs.[54,55] It mainly adjusts for risk of disabled populations in Medicaid. The model incorporates both inpatient and outpatient diagnosis codes in calculation of CDPS scores.

Global risk-adjustment model (GRAM)—The GRAM was developed to predict health care use and categorizes 350 diagnoses into 19 groups.[56] The groups are based on clinical attributes and expected responses to the disease.

Acute physiology and chronic health (APACHE)—The APACHE computes a variety of risk scores such as intensive care unit (ICU) mortality and length of stay for the ICU population, based on 17 acute physiologic parameters and other clinical information.[57]

Pharmacy-Based Models

Another source of adjusting for risk arising from comorbidities are the models based on pharmacy-claims data. Several models have been put forward in the past two decades using pharmacy data to develop risk score that would allow adjustment for coexisting conditions to evaluate outcomes of interest.[58–61] In the discussion below, two commonly used measures will be briefly described, namely, Chronic Disease Score and RxRisk Score.

Chronic disease score (CDS)—The Chronic Disease Score (CDS) employs outpatient pharmacy-dispensing data to assign patients to chronic disease groups.[62,63] Each of the 30 drug classes represent a comorbidity category, and a weight ranging from 1 to 5 is assigned to that category. An overall score is then obtained by summing all the weights. The CDS was originally developed at Group Health Cooperative of Puget Sound, using automated outpatient pharmacy data. One problem with CDS was that it was exclusively developed for an adult population and was not readily applicable to the adolescent and pediatric population. This is because children have a different set of chronic conditions than adults and may receive different pharmacologic treatment compared to adults. In order to address this shortcoming, a Pediatric CDS (PCDS) was developed. Attempts were made to unify the adult and pediatric risk measures in a single instrument. These attempts led to the development of RxRisk model that is described as follows.

RxRisk model—RxRisk score provides a measure for all ages. The model creates an individual patient's chronic-condition profile as measured by pharmacy-dispensing data and predicts both health care costs and mortality for that patient.[64] RxRisk score is calculated by including 28 chronic conditions among adults and 24 among children, based on outpatient prescription dispensing. It measures both comorbidity and disease severity. In addition to mortality and costs, RxRisk has been shown to predict health care resource utilization, including hospitalizations. Another version, called RxRisk-V, was developed specifically for the Veteran Affairs population.[65] Fishman et al.[64] have described in detail the steps in development of the model.

Comparison of Diagnosis-Based and Pharmacy-Based Models

Each of the two types of models has its relative strengths and weaknesses. Schneeweiss et al.[49] showed that diagnosis-based scores performed con-sistently better than the pharmacy-based scores, whereas the study by Farley et al.[41] found that RxRisk score outperformed both the Charlson and Elixhauser comorbidity indices. A brief description of strengths and weaknesses of both types of models will be provided in the following.

A weakness of the pharmacy-based measures is that patients already taking many medications are less likely to be prescribed additional medications for comorbid conditions. It has been found that medications with preventive effects are less commonly prescribed in very sick patients.[49] This situation makes these patients artificially healthy. Another issue with pharmacy-based indices arises when a prescription medication is used to treat more than one medical condition. In such a case, information regarding the prescribed drug alone will not be enough to identify the comorbid medical condition. An example is that of pain medications, which may be prescribed for several different underlying medical conditions. In such a case, information on diagnosis code will be necessary to identify precisely the coexisting medical condition. Another issue with pharmacy-based measures is that there are comorbidities where a drug marker is absent. An example is pregnancy, which is not identifiable through a drug. In all the above-mentioned situations, diagnosis-based measures are more appropriate and are likely to perform better. Another challenge with the pharmacy-based measures is the continuous updating of the algorithm by including new drugs, new uses of existing drugs, and discontinued uses of older drugs. Another problem is keeping abreast of changing prescribing patterns in light of new evidence. Finally, a pharmacy-based measure may underestimate comorbidities in less generous pharmacy-benefit plans.

On the other hand, comorbidity indices based on pharmacy data are likely to perform better in some cases as described in the following. Pharmacy data may be a better marker of disease severity as compared with the information on diagnosis alone. An example is asthma, where diagnosis alone is not a good indicator of disease severity. In this case, information in the prescription data is more valuable and may provide a more complete picture of disease severity. However, even in this case, pharmacy data again are not likely to provide information on the type of disease itself, as similar drug classes may be

CASE STUDY 6-3

Benzodiazepines and Injury: A Risk-Adjusted Model[66]

French et al.[66] used 3 years (1999–2001) of outpatient prescription data and inpatient and outpatient administrative data to develop a risk-adjusted model that investigated the association of benzodiazepine usage with the risk for an injury. Total number of benzodiazepine prescriptions analyzed were 133,872 for 13,745 unique patients for a VA medical center. Variables included in the analysis were Elixhauser comorbidity measures, hospital discharges, marital status, age, mean arterial pressure, and body mass index. In addition, drug dosage and duration of supply were included in the model. Variables that were found to be associated with an increased risk for injury were dose, duration, discharges, and various comorbidities. An increase in body mass index was also associated with increased injury risk. These findings shed light on the effects of various combinations of risk factors that may influence risk of an outcome, such as accidental injury risk in this case. This study provides a good example of diagnosis-based risk comorbidity adjustment in a pharmacoepidemiology study.

markers for both asthma and chronic obstructive pulmonary disease. Therefore, in many cases information on the diagnosis and prescription drug may be required to provide a complete picture of the disease profile. An advantage with using a pharmacy index is that pharmacy data are found to be more readily available and of higher quality as compared with the diagnosis data in managed care settings where capitation has affected data collection.[51] Under capitated payment systems, providers have less of an incentive to report diagnostic and procedure data. Furthermore, coding of diagnoses and procedures may be subject to gaming because of reimbursement issues.[64] Pharmacy data are less likely to suffer from this weakness and thus may be more reliable.

▶ Statistical Methods for Risk Adjustment

Comorbidity risk adjustment is important to control for potential confounding in the relationship between treatment and outcome. To accomplish this, the most common method is to perform multivariable modeling using statistical software. Typically, an appropriately selected comorbidity score is included as a covariate in the regression equation along with the treatment variable and other noncomorbidity-related risk factors. In addition to multivariable modeling, matched or stratified analyses can also be performed. The treatment groups can be matched on the confounding comorbidities to equate the risk across groups and then multivariable modeling can be conducted. In a stratified analysis, treatment groups can be stratified based on risk levels (e.g., low, medium, high) and then analysis for each stratum separately can be conducted. The key idea is to make the treatment groups as comparable as possible so that the a priori risk of occurrence of outcome is similar.

In addition to using a composite or a summary score of a comorbidity measure, potential comorbidities can be considered individually. In other words, potentially confounding medical conditions may be included as covariates in the analyses. Another strategy is to include medications specific to the conditions of interest as variables in the analysis.

▼ SUMMARY

This chapter introduced key methodological issues that are commonly encountered in performing analyses of use and effects of drugs during postmarketing phase. These issues are particularly useful in increasing precision and accuracy of estimates of treatment outcomes from analyses that are conducted using large databases. The chapter began with explanation of the important concept of causation and distinguished it from the concept of association in the context of treatment and its outcome. Next was the discussion regarding the crucial issue of various types and sources of biases arising in observational studies, including confounding bias. After an introductory discussion of various types of biases, the chapter elaborated on various methods to remove or mitigate those biases both at the study design and analysis levels. In the last part of the chapter, the issue of risk adjustment is presented. This issue has gained in importance in recent years but has not been given due attention in the context of pharmacoepidemiology. The chapter introduces major risk-adjustment measures developed using diagnosis codes and using pharmacy-dispensing information. A comparison of both types (diagnosis based and pharmacy based) is also provided.

DISCUSSION QUESTIONS

1. Distinguish between *association* and *causation*. Provide an example of each concept.

2. What are three different types of associations in pharmacoepidemiology? Provide examples.

3. Outline the criteria to determine causal nature of an association.

4. Define the term *bias*. Explain how it is related to systematic errors.

5. Define the term *confounding* with examples.

6. Discuss various methods that are used to deal with different types of biases in pharmacoepidemiology studies.

7. What is risk adjustment? Why is it important to incorporate in outcomes-research studies?

8. Discuss one diagnosis-based and one pharmacy-based comorbidity risk-adjustment measure. What are the strengths and weaknesses of each of the measures?

REFERENCES

1. Hernán MA. A definition of causal effect for epidemiological research. *J Epidemiol Community Health*. 2004;58(4):265-271.

2. Strom BL, Kimmel SE, eds. *Textbook of Pharmacoepidemiology*. Chicester, England: John Wiley & sons, 2006.

3. Hill AB. The environment and disease: Association or causation? *Proc R Soc Med*. 1965;58:295-300.

4. US Public Health Service. *Smoking and Health: Report of the Advisory Committee to the Surgeon General of the Public Health Service*. Washington DC: Government Printing Office, 1964.

5. Kaufman JS, Poole C. Looking back on "causal thinking in the health sciences". *Annu Rev Public Health*. 2000;21: 101-119.

6. Rothman KJ, Greenland S, Lash TL. *Modern Epidemiology*, 3rd ed. Philadelphia: Lippincott Williams & Wilkins, 2008.

7. Said Q, Gutterman EM, Kim MS, Firth SD, Whitehead R, Brixner D. Somnolence effects of antipsychotic medications and the risk of unintentional injury. *Pharmacoepidemiol Drug Saf*. 2008;17(4):354-364.

8. Hutchison GB, Rothman KJ. Correcting a bias? *N Engl J Med*. 1978;299(20):1129-1130.

9. Maldonado G, Greenland S. Estimating causal effects. *Int J Epidemiol*. 2002;31(2):422-429.

10. Szklo M0, Nieto FJ. *Epidemiology. Beyond the Basics*. Gaithersburg, MD: Aspen, 2000.

11. MacMahon B, Trichopoulos D. *Epidemiology. Principles & Methods*, 2nd ed. Boston: Little, Brown and Co, 1996.

12. Hennekens CH, Buring JE. *Epidemiology in Medicine*. Boston: Little, Brown and Co, 1987.

13. Gordis L. *Epidemiology*. Philadelphia: WB Saunders Co, 1996.

14. Greenland S, Robins JM. Confounding and misclassification. *Am J Epidemiol*. 1985;122(3):495-506.

15. Miettinen OS. Confounding and effect modification. *Am J Epidemiol*. 1984;100:350-353.

16. Greenland S, Neutra R. Control of confounding in the assessment of medical technology. *Int J Epidemiol*. 1980;9(4): 361-367.

17. Greenland S, Morgenstern H. Confounding in health research. *Annu Rev Public Health*. 2001;22:189-212.

18. Spitzer WO, Suissa S, Ernst P, et al. The use of beta-agonists and the risk of death and near death from asthma. *N Engl J Med*. 1992;326:501-506.

19. Strom BL, Carson JL, Morse ML, West SL, Soper KA. The effect of indication on hypersensitivity reactions associated with zomepirac sodium and other nonsteroidal anti-inflammatory drugs. *Arthritis Rheum* 1987;30:1142-1149.

20. Miettinen OS. The need for randomization in the study of intended effects. *Stat Med*. 1983;2:267-271.

21. Petri H, Urquhart J, Herings R, Bakker A. Characteristics of patients prescribed three different inhalational beta-2 agonists: An example of the channeling phenomenon. *Post-Mark Surveil*. 1991;5:57-66.

22. Rosenbaum PR, Rubin DB. The central role of the propensity score in observational studies for causal effects. *Biometrika*. 1983;70:41-55.

23. Joffe MM, Rosenbaum PR. Invited commentary: propensity scores. *Am J Epidemiol*. 1999;150:327-333.

24. Winkelmayer WC, Glynn RJ, Mittleman MA, Levin R, Pliskin JS, Avorn J. Comparing mortality of elderly patients on

hemodialysis versus peritoneal dialysis: A propensity score approach. *J Am Soc Nephrol.* 2002;13:2353-2362.

25. Grunkemeier GL, Payne N, Jin R, Handy JR, Jr. Propensity score analysis of stroke after off-pump coronary artery bypass grafting. *Ann Thorac Surg.* 2002;74:301-305.

26. Newhouse JP, McClellan M. Econometrics in outcomes research: The use of instrumental variables. *Annu Rev Public Health.* 1998;19:17-34.

27. McClellan M, McNeil BJ, Newhouse JP. Does more intensive treatment of acute myocardial infarction in the elderly reduce mortality? Analysis using instrumental variables. *JAMA.* 1994;272(11):859-866.

28. Greenland S. An introduction to instrumental variables for epidemiologists. *Int J Epidemiol.* 2000;29(4):722-729.

29. Robins JM, Hernán MA, Brumback B. Marginal structural models and causal inference in epidemiology. *Epidemiology.* 2000;11(5):550-560.

30. Greenland S. Basic methods for sensitivity analysis and external adjustment. In: Rothman KJ, Greenland S, eds. *Modern Epidemiology,* 2nd ed. Philadelphia: Lippincott-Raven, 1998:343-357.

31. Flanders WD, Khoury MJ. Indirect assessment of confounding: Graphic description and limits on effect for adjusting for covariates. *Epidemiology,* 1990;1(3):239-246.

32. Schlesselman JJ. Assessing effects of confounding variables. *Am J Epidemiol.* 1978;108(1):3-8.

33. Phillips CV. Quantifying and reporting uncertainty from systematic errors. *Epidemiology.* 2003;14(4):459-466.

34. Lash TL, Fink AK. Semi-automated sensitivity analysis to assess systematic errors in observational data. *Epidemiology.* 2003;14(4):451-458.

35. Rassen JA, Choudhry NK, Avorn J, Schneeweiss S. Cardiovascular outcomes and mortality in patients using clopidogrel with proton pump inhibitors after percutaneous coronary intervention or acute coronary syndrome. *Circulation.* 2009;120(23):2322-2329.

36. Juurlink DN, Gomes T, Ko DT, et al. A population-based study of the drug interaction between proton pump inhibitors and clopidogrel. *CMAJ.* 2009;180:713-718.

37. Ho PM, Maddox TM, Wang L, et al. Risk of adverse outcomes associated with concomitant use of clopidogrel and proton pump inhibitors following acute coronary syndrome. *JAMA.* 2009;301:937-944.

38. Iezzoni L, ed. *Risk Adjustment for Measuring Health Care Outcomes,* 3rd ed. Chicago: Health Administration Press, 2003.

39. Iezzoni LI. The risks of risk adjustment. *JAMA.* 1997;278(19):1600-1607.

40. Arcà M, Fusco D, Barone AP, Perucci CA. Risk adjustment and outcome research. Part I. *J Cardiovasc Med (Hagerstown).* 2006;7(9):682-690.

41. Farley JF, Harley CR, Devine JW. A comparison of comorbidity measurements to predict healthcare expenditures. *Am J Manag Care.* 2006;12(2):110-119.

42. Sundararajan V, Quan H, Halfon P, et al. Cross-national comparative performance of three versions of the ICD-10 Charlson index. International Methodology Consortium for Coded Health Information (IMECCHI). *Med Care.* 2007;45(12):1210-1215.

43. Li B, Evans D, Faris P, Dean S, Quan H. Risk adjustment performance of Charlson and Elixhauser comorbidities in ICD-9 and ICD-10 administrative databases. *BMC Health Serv Res.* 2008;8:12.

44. Charlson, ME, Pompei P, Ales KL, MacKenzie CR. A new method of classifying prognostic comorbidity in longitudinal studies: Development and validation. *J Chronic Dis.* 1987;40(5):373-383.

45. Deyo RA, Cherkin DC, Ciol MA. Adapting a clinical comorbidity index for use with ICD-9-CM administrative databases. *J Clin Epidemiol.* 1992;45(6):613-619.

46. Romano PS, Roos LL, Jollis JG. Adapting a clinical comorbidity index for use with ICD-9-CM administrative data: differing perspectives. *J Clin Epidemiol.* 1993;46(10);1075-1079.

47. D'Hoore W, Sicotte C, Tilquin C. Risk adjustment in outcome assessment: The Charlson comorbidity index. *Methods Inf Med.* 1993;32(5):382-387.

48. Ghali WA, Hall RE, Rosen AK, Ash AS, Moskowitz MA. Searching for an improved clinical comorbidity index for use with ICD-9-CM administrative data. *J Clin Epidemiol.* 1996;49(3): 273-278.

49. Schneeweiss S, Seeger JD, Maclure M, Wang PS, Avorn J, Glynn RJ. Performance of comorbidity scores to control for confounding in epidemiological studies using claims data. *Am J Epidemiol.* 2001;154:854-864.

50. Elixhauser A, Steiner C, Harris DR, Coffey RM. Comorbidity measures for use with administrative data. *Med Care.* 1998; 36:8-27.

51. Stukenborg GJ, Wagner DP, Connors AF Jr. Comparison of the performance of two comorbidity measures, with and without information from prior hospitalizations. *Med Care.* 2001;39(7):727-739.

52. Weiner JP, Starfield BH, Steinwachs DM, Mumford LM. Development and application of a population-oriented measure of ambulatory care case-mix. *Med Care.* 1991;29(5):452-472.

53. Ellis RP, Pope GC, Iezzoni L, et al. Diagnosis-based risk adjustment for Medicare capitation payments. *Health Care Financ Rev.* 1996;17(3):101-128.

54. Kronick R, Dreyfus T, Lee L, Zhou Z. Diagnostic risk adjustment for Medicaid: The disability payment system. *Health Care Financ Rev.* 1996;17(3):7-33.

55. Kronick R, Gilmer T, Dreyfus T, Lee L. Improving health-based payment for Medicaid beneficiaries: CDPS. *Health Care Financ Rev.* 2000;21(3):29-64.

56. Meenan RT, O'Keeffe-Rosetti C, Hornbrook MC, Bachman DJ, Goodman MJ, Fishman PA, Hurtado AV. The sensitivity and specificity of forecasting high-cost users of medical care. *Med Care.* 1999 Aug;37(8):815-23.

57. Knaus WA, Wagner DP, Draper EA, et al. The APACHE III prognostic system. Risk prediction of hospital mortality for critically ill hospitalized adults. *Chest.* 1991;100:1619-1636.

58. Lamers LM. Pharmacy costs groups: A risk-adjuster for capitation payments based on the use of prescribed drugs. *Med Care.* 1999;37:824-830.

59. Roblin DW. Physician profiling using outpatient pharmacy data as a source for case mix measurement and risk adjustment. *J Ambul Care Manag.* 1998;21:68-84.

60. Fishman P, Shay D. Development and estimation of a pediatric chronic disease score from automated pharmacy data. *Med Care.* 1999;37:872-880.

61. Gilmer T, Kronick R, Fishman P, et al. The Medicaid RX model: Pharmacy-based risk adjustment for public programs. *Med Care.* 2001;39(11):1188-1202.

62. von Korff M, Wagner EH, Saunders K. A chronic disease score from automated pharmacy data. *J Clin Epidemiol.* 1992;45(2): 197-203.

63. Clark DO, von Korff M, Saunders K, Baluch WM, Simon GE. A chronic disease score with empirically derived weights. *Med Care.* 1995;33(8):783-795.

64. Fishman PA, Goodman MJ, Hornbrook MC, Meenan RT, Bachman DJ, O'Keeffe Rosetti MC. Risk adjustment using automated ambulatory pharmacy data: The RxRisk model. *Med Care.* 2003;41(1):84-99.

65. Sloan KL, Sales AE, Liu CF, et al. Construction and characteristics of the RxRisk-V: A VA-adapted pharmacy-based case-mix instrument. *Med Care.* 2003;41(6):761-774.

66. French DD, Campbell R, Spehar A, Angaran DM. Benzodiazepines and injury: A risk adjusted model. *Pharmacoepidemiol Drug Saf.* 2005;14(1):17-24.

Evaluation of the Pharmacoepidemiology Literature

7

Douglas Steinke

▼ **OBJECTIVES**

At the end of the chapter, the reader will be able to:

1. Understand the importance of critically evaluating the pharmacoepidemiology literature
2. Understand key topics in evaluating the pharmacoepidemiology literature
3. Apply checklist questions in evaluating the pharmacoepidemiology literature

INTRODUCTION

The beginning of pharmacoepidemiology as a research area started in the late 1980s with crudely designed studies appearing in the literature. For example, Somerville et al.[1] published a brief report in *The Lancet*, quantifying the risk of gastrointestinal bleeding following nonsteroidal antiinflammatory drug (NSAID) use in elderly people; the report then sparked a flurry of studies trying to compare and contrast results. Since then, the research area has grown with pharmacoepidemiologists developing specialized methodologies and terminologies to describe the association between a medication exposure and an outcome. In fact, over the past few decades there has been an increase in the number of published articles in the field of pharmacoepidemiology.[2] Draugalis and Plaza[2] examined the trends in the use of epidemiology-related terminology over the past 20 years in 3 representative journals in phar-

macy, the *American Journal of Health-System Pharmacy*, *The Annals of Pharmacotherapy*, and *Pharmacotherapy*; in two medical journals, *The New England Journal of Medicine* and *JAMA*; and also the *American Journal of Public Health*. The authors found that there was a general increase in the proportion of epidemiologic terms used in these journals, with the most significant increase observed in *Pharmacotherapy*, from none in 1984 to 17.8% in 2004. This increase reflects the growing importance of population-based research of drug use and drug effects. More pharmacoepidemiology studies are being conducted and used by various stakeholders in the health care system.

Evidence-based medicine derives best practices for the management of patients from published clinical and epidemiologic research findings. For health care practitioners to practice evidence-based medicine and make informed decisions, it is critical that they understand and interpret the pharmacoepidemiology literature. By interpreting the

Rosiglitazone and Cardiovascular Risk

Rosiglitazone (e.g., Avandia) is a blood glucose–lowering drug in the thiazolidinedione (TZD) class.[3] Diabetes and heart disease are highly prevalent conditions, and rosiglitazone is a medication that is used to treat diabetes and, in theory, should reduce the risk of cardiovascular disease.[4] However, the initial clinical trials of rosiglitazone were not powered to determine its effects on diabetes-related micro- and macro-vascular complications, including cardiovascular morbidity and mortality.[4] This is important because a majority of deaths in the diabetes population are from cardiovascular causes.[4]

Nissen and Wolski[4] published a meta-analysis examining the effect of rosiglitazone on cardiovascular outcomes. This analysis specifically investigated the effect of rosiglitazone exposure on the risk of myocardial infarction (MI) and cardiovascular mortality.[4] This review pooled data from 42 clinical trials and provided data on 27,847 patients. Although the overall event rate for MI and cardiovascular mortality were low, the authors did document a 43% increase in the risk for MI [Odds Ratio (OR), 1.43; 95% confidence interval (95% CI), 1.03–1.98] among those using rosiglitazone relative to those using a comparator agent (either another oral hypoglycemic or placebo). There was also an increased risk of death from cardiovascular causes in the rosiglitazone group relative to the comparator group; however, this was not statistically significant (OR, 1.64; 95% CI, 0.98–2.74).[4]

The results of the meta-analysis were of interest to the medical profession, but even the authors of the study pointed out several important limitations, including small sample size and short duration to draw any definitive conclusions.[4] The study was also criticized for the controversial statistical methods used in the meta-analysis. Nissen and Wolski used the Peto analysis that provides a higher risk estimate than other alternative conventional methods, and the study combined several small trials with low numbers of events decreasing the heterogeneity between trials.[5] The regulatory bodies still had insufficient quality evidence to withdraw the medication from the mar-

ket. However, the media reported the results of this meta-analysis and informed the general public of the possible risk of MI for those who are taking rosiglitazone.[4] The sales of rosiglitazone dropped by $290 million in the United States in the months that followed the publication of the review, and new prescriptions of rosiglitazone significantly decreased.[6] Manucci and Monami[5] recently performed a comprehensive meta-analysis of all available trials with usual and valid statistical methods and ruled out any additional risk of MI or cardiovascular death associated with rosiglitazone, while confirming the well-known risk of hospitalization for cardiac failure. They found rosiglitazone-associated risk of MI was increased in trials with higher mean body mass index or greater proportion of insulin-treated patients. Lower blood lipids, particularly low triglyceride levels, were also associated with higher rosiglitazone-induced risk of congestive heart failure (CHF).[5] The Rosiglitazone Evaluated for Cardiac Outcome and Regulation of Glycemia in Diabetes (RECORD) trial[7] used interim trial data to determine cardiac risk associated with rosiglitazone use. Even though the RECORD trial was not sufficiently powered, the authors found rosiglitazone therapy was not associated with cardiovascular mortality or all-cause mortality, but was associated with an increased risk of heart failure.[8] A nested case-control analysis of a retrospective cohort used health care databases in Ontario to examine cardiovascular event rates in older patients with diabetes in relation to antidiabetic therapy. This study found that current treatment with a TZD (primarily rosiglitazone) as monotherapy was associated with a significantly increased risk of CHF (P < 0.001), acute MI (P = 0.02), and death (P = 0.03) compared with other oral hypoglycemic agent combination therapies.[9] The possible association between rosiglitazone use and increased risk of cardiovascular outcomes led the FDA to change the prescribing information for rosiglitazone in 2007.[10]

This case illustrates the need for health care professionals to be able to critically evaluate the pharma-

coepidemiology literature and be able to educate patients about evidence-based benefits and harms of medications. The review by Nissen and Wolski discussed that the meta-analysis was limited, by citing many trials that were small and short-term and having few adverse cardiovascular events or deaths.[4] The review also included studies that were not designed to examine cardiovascular safety.[4] Nissen and Wolski also excluded trials with no MI or cardiovascular deaths that could introduce bias to the study results.[4] With additional information from recent studies, a more informative picture of the risk associated with rosiglitazone use is made available to the decision-making process.

findings, health care practitioners can better understand the risks and benefits of a medication when used in a diverse patient population. A growing number of entities are also using the pharmacoepidemiology literature for a variety of reasons, including (a) regulatory bodies to ensure that newly marketed medications are safe and effective in large, "real-world" populations where adverse events can be monitored beyond randomized control trials; (b) marketing bodies to assess the impact of pharmacoepidemiology research findings on the market and identify groups of patients who would benefit the most from a medication; and (c) legal bodies to assess causality of negative outcomes in anticipation of possible legal issues. A description of how various stakeholders are using pharmacoepidemiology studies is provided in Case Study 7-1, thereby illustrating the importance of being able to critically evaluate the pharmacoepidemiology literature.

This chapter allows the reader to connect the concepts and methods presented in previous chapters and apply them in evaluating published pharmacoepidemiology studies. When evaluating a pharmacoepidemiology study, the study objectives, design, analyses, and results should be considered before drawing a conclusion. As evidenced from Case Study 7-1, people may interpret and apply pharmacoepidemiology findings differently. Most, if not all, studies have limitations that must be considered. Thus, it is important for users of the literature to be able to read and analyze the quality of a study before applying the results to their situation. This chapter provides a checklist for evaluating the pharmacoepidemiology literature and provides detailed explanations on how to apply the questions in the checklist in the evaluation of the pharmacoepidemiology literature.

CRITICAL EVALUATION OF THE PHARMACOEPIDEMIOLOGY LITERATURE

The pharmacoepidemiology literature provides research findings and information that helps one understand how drugs are used in populations and the effects of these drugs on people. Thus, it is critical that health care professionals and policy makers be able to evaluate the literature and interpret the findings appropriately. Table 7-1 presents a checklist for the critical evaluation of pharmacoepidemiologic studies. The checklist is composed of a series of elements in question format that the reader should expect to find in well-designed and well-conducted pharmacoepidemiology studies. It should be noted that individual studies are not expected to satisfy all of the elements in the checklist; rather, readers should use the checklist to identify and evaluate the strengths and weaknesses of each individual study. Later in this chapter, an illustration of the application of the checklist questions in evaluating a published pharmacoepidemiology study is provided.

▶ A Checklist for Evaluating a Pharmacoepidemiology Study

Most journals have set guidelines on the structure of published articles. The basic structure of a published paper in pharmacoepidemiology and other related fields includes the following: abstract, introduction or background, methods, results, discussion, and conclusions. An abstract is a short synopsis of the

Table 7-1. A checklist for evaluating pharmacoepidemiology studies.

A. The research questions, study design, and populations
1. Why was this study done and why is it important? Does the introduction section present any gaps in knowledge that the study addresses?
2. What were the objectives (or aims) of the study?
3. What was the hypothesis of the study?
4. What was the primary medication exposure of interest? Was this accurately measured? Was dose of the exposure medication accurately measured so that the dose–response characteristic can be evaluated?
5. What was the primary outcome of interest? Was this accurately measured? Was it a surrogate measure and was it appropriate?
6. What study design was used?
7. Was the source of study population, process of participant selection, sample size, and ratio of cases to comparison participants presented clearly?
8. Could there have been bias in the selection of study participants? How likely was the bias?
9. Could there have been bias in the collection of information? How likely was this bias?
10. What provisions were made to minimize the influence of confounding factors prior to the analysis of data? Were these provisions sufficient?

B. Data analysis
1. What methods were used to control confounding bias during data analysis? Were these methods appropriate and sufficient?
2. What measures of association were reported in the study? What measures of statistical stability were reported in this study?

C. Results and interpretation of study findings
1. What were the main results of this study?
2. How was the interpretation of the results affected by information bias, selection bias, and confounding? Consider both the direction and magnitude of any bias.
3. How was the interpretation of the results affected by nondifferential misclassification? Consider both the direction and magnitude of this misclassification.
4. Did the discussion section adequately address the limitations of the study?
5. What were the authors' main conclusions? Were they justified by the findings?
6. To what population can the results of this study be generalized?

Adapted with permission from: Monson RR. *Occupational Epidemiology.* 2nd ed. Boca Raton, FL: CRC Press; 1990:94.

study and its main results. An abstract is useful in identifying possible studies to critically evaluate; however, an abstract does not provide enough information on the study design, study population, and discussion for readers to evaluate the study properly and subsequently apply the study results in "real-world" health care decision-making. To help decision makers effectively assess the appropriateness and applicability of pharmacoepidemiology studies, published studies should be evaluated according to some guidelines. Some authors suggest reading the article twice before conducting a formal evaluation.[11] The first reading of a research article allows the reader to assess the contents, identify overall assumptions, and become familiar with the study in general. The second reading should be more specific and critical.

▶ Applying the Checklist Questions in Evaluating the Pharmacoepidemiology Literature

The Research Questions, Study Design, and Populations

1. Why was the study done and why is it important? Does the introduction section present any gaps in knowledge that the study addresses?—The authors, in the introduction of the article, should be able to convince the reader that there are specific gaps in the body of knowledge that the study intends to address.

The introduction should provide background information so that the reader knows why the study is conducted and why it is important.

2. What were the objectives of the study?—
Pharmacoepidemiology studies are regarded as useful tools in assessing population-based benefits and risks of drug use and assisting the decision-making process regarding the use and effects of medications. There are some important objectives for undertaking pharmacoepidemiologic studies in general, and there are specific aims for undertaking the specific study under review. The authors should state the study objectives (or aims).

3. What was the hypothesis of the study?—The
reader should identify statements that begin to form clear and quantifiable hypothesis for the study. For example, suggesting superiority if there is no quantifiable outcome leads to ambiguity and perhaps false pretenses of the results. Simply stating that "Drug A is a more effective medication for hypertension than Drug B" is insufficient; the reader needs to know by how much Drug A is more effective. The reader should find a quantifiable description that suggests superiority as in a hypothesis, such as "the use of Drug A will lower the blood pressure by 10 mmHg compared with Drug B." A specific hypothesis is more difficult to refute than a nonspecific one.[11]

4. What was the primary exposure of interest?—In
pharmacoepidemiology research, often the exposure of interest is a medication. Medications can cause, prevent, or treat the outcome of interest. There are several issues that the reader should consider while reading pharmacoepidemiology studies. First, the drug(s) under study should be considered. A particular drug may have different strengths, different formulations, and varying directions for use depending on the indication. The drug may be used for multiple indications. The study authors should clearly and explicitly define the drug or the therapeutic class of interest. The strength of a drug is another important consideration that should be defined appropriately. If a study evaluates the dose–response characteristic of the medication as a specific aim of the study, this should be clearly stated. For example, the researchers may be interested in the incidence of outcome at intermediate and high doses compared with low doses of a medication. In this way, a stratified exposure can be used in the study by defining low, intermediate, and high doses of medication and their effect on outcome.

5. What was the primary outcome of interest?—The
outcome of a study is the endpoint of interest. Examples of outcomes in pharmacoepidemiology studies include disease incidence or prevalence, the occurrence of an event, medication adherence and persistence, and mortality. The reader should consider whether the primary outcome of interest is clearly defined and appropriately measured. Simply choosing the development of disease as the primary outcome may not be sufficient. The outcome definition may need to include measurements that indicate the severity of disease, for example, stages of cancer or laboratory values of blood cholesterol. The identification and operationalization of the primary outcome of interest also affects the type of statistical analyses that should be performed.

Some outcomes may take longer to become evident, as most chronic conditions involve a preclinical (asymptomatic) phase. The reader should consider whether the medication has had enough time to establish a possible outcome and determine whether the temporal relationship between exposure and outcome has been taken into consideration. Some medications that are preventative of future disease or protective of a negative outcome may require long periods of time until an outcome can be identified. For example, cancer chemotherapy agents may be evaluated in terms of survival time; however, survival may be in the range of 10 to 30 years after the patient receives the medication therapy. In this example, the benefits of drug therapy would be underestimated because survival time would be censored at the end of the study period, usually shorter than the actual life expectancy of the patient. Another example is the benefits of post–myocardial infarction (MI) low-dose aspirin use in the prevention of a second MI. The second MI may occur sometime in the future; however, sometimes the only data available are 1-year worth of hospital claims data, which are insufficient to identify the outcomes of interest. Another factor to consider is that using time as a variable such as survival time requires specific, time-dependent, statistical analyses and graphing methods like Cox proportional hazards regression and Kaplan–Meier curves.

6. What study design was used?—Study designs used in pharmacoepidemiology are experimental designs (including randomized control trials) and observational study designs, which include case-control, cohort, cross-sectional, and ecological studies. It is important that an appropriate study design has been chosen for the study under review to ensure that the research questions of the study are correctly answered and that confounding and bias are minimized in the study. If a particular study is observing the use of a medication in a particular population, a simple descriptive design could be used to describe patients, place, and time of use. However, as the study hypothesis becomes more refined and the ultimate goal of the study is to establish causality linking a particular drug with an outcome, a large prospective trial may be needed to minimize confounding and bias in the study. The reader should consider study objectives while evaluating whether the study design is appropriate to address the research questions.

Experimental study designs provide the strongest evidence to establish causation because they minimize the effects of confounding and bias by randomization of the study population, ensuring that each group or arm of the study has an equal distribution of possible confounders. Trials with randomized controls are the study type of choice when the study objective is to evaluate the effectiveness of a treatment or a procedure. Disadvantages, however, include high cost and time needed to recruit enough people to participate and long follow-up times. Clinical trials are often sponsored by the pharmaceutical industry, which has to be considered when assessing and interpreting the results of the study.

Case-control studies offer an efficient approach to studying rare diseases, examining conditions that take a long time to develop (e.g., cancers) or conducting preliminary analysis of a possible association between a drug and an outcome. The case-control design is also the most vulnerable to confounding and bias, and the quality of a case-control study depends on the use of high-quality data. A study that uses a case-control study design has to be closely evaluated to make sure

that all possible confounding variables are identified and appropriate statistical analyses are performed to control for the confounders.

Cohort studies are the strongest study design for determining the incidence or natural history of a disease or when the temporal relationship between exposure and outcome becomes important. Cohort studies are also desirable when the exposure of interest is rare. In prospective cohort studies, following-up of a large population over time is often required, thus making these studies expensive to carry out; whereas in retrospective cohort studies participants can be identified from existing data (e.g., administrative claims data) and exposure can be defined based on a past single event or a period of exposure before the beginning of the study. The time needed to complete a retrospective cohort study is only as long as it takes to compile and analyze the data. However, because data are not originally collected to answer the research questions of interest, it is unlikely that all the relevant information would be available. When reviewing a cohort study, it is important to make sure all the possible confounders have been identified and that loss to follow-up has not damaged the power of the study to detect true differences in the comparison populations. The usefulness of retrospective cohort studies is illustrated in Case Study 7-2.

Cross-sectional and ecological (survey) studies are the most appropriate at determining the status of a condition in a population at a particular point in time. They are relatively less time consuming and easy to conduct; however, they do require specific skills, such as appropriate questionnaire design and suitable interviewing skills, to ensure that correct information is collected and the study is conducted appropriately. Because cross-sectional survey designs give a snap shot of the outcome at a point in time, they cannot provide information regarding the incidence of a disease in a population (both prevalent and incident cases are identified). In a cross-sectional study, data are usually more descriptive and no information on causality can be assessed.

7. Describe the source of study population, process of participant selection, sample size, and ratio of cases to comparison participants—Understanding from where (e.g., settings and location) and how the study

CASE STUDY 7-2

Where Have All the Cisapride Gone?

Cisapride entered the U.S. market in August 1993 as a gastrointestinal-tract promotility agent indicated for nocturnal heartburn.[12] The use of cisapride grew rapidly, and, in 2 years, approximately 5 million cisapride prescriptions were filled in the United States.[13] However, during this period, the FDA had received reports of 34 cases of torsade de pointes and 23 cases of prolonged QT interval among individuals using cisapride, including 4 death events.[13] A "black-box" warning was added to the cisapride label in 1995, contraindicating use in patients taking drugs that affected cisapride metabolism because it was found that many of these cases occurred in patients who were also taking drugs that inhibited cytochrome P450–3A4 enzymes that metabolized cisapride.[12,14] The manufacturer also sent a "Dear Health Care Professional" letter warning the risks associated with taking cisapride concomitantly with drugs that inhibited cytochrome P450–3A4 enzymes. Despite these efforts, use of cisapride continued to increase in the United States such that in 1998, there were 7 million prescriptions dispensed, which prompted the FDA to expand the black-box warning in June 1998.[13] The information regarding risks associated with cisapride use was also disseminated through the

FDA's press release and another "Dear Health Care Professional" letter distributed by the drug manufacturer in 1998.

Smalley et al.[13] conducted a retrospective cohort study, using population-based, pharmacoepidemiology research databases of two managed care organizations and a state Medicaid program, and found that there was no significant reduction in the number of prescriptions dispensed to patients with contraindications to cisapride in the year after the FDA's regulatory actions came into force in 1998.[13] They found that between 14% and 41% of the individuals in each of the insured populations were dispensed cisapride even though it was contraindicated on the label.[13]

This case shows the usefulness of retrospective observational studies in pharmacoepidemiology and changing drug use in populations. Observational study populations include a variety of patients with varying characteristics that are not usually involved in clinical trials where patient selection is more restrictive. A clinical trial of cisapride would have not included patients with contraindicated conditions or taking concomitant cytochrome P450–3A4 enzyme inhibitors.

population was selected allows the reader to determine whether there is any potential for bias, whether the sample size is powered to detect any statistically and clinically significant differences, and whether the study results can be generalized to other populations. For example, in a case-control study, the reader should be able to identify the underlying base population that the investigators used and the number of controls selected for each case. The ratio of controls to cases can vary from 1:1 to as high as 6:1. Increasing the sample size will generally increase the power of the study to detect differences; however, there is marginal gain in increasing power beyond a ratio of four controls to one case.[15]

8. Could there have been bias in the selection of study participants? How likely was the bias?—Selection bias is an error that arises from systematic differences in selecting the study cases and controls. Selection bias is more likely to occur in case-control studies because both the outcome of interest and the exposure to medication have already occurred. Selection bias can cause the true measures of association to be either over- or under-estimated depending on the degree of bias. Selection bias may also occur if the researcher follows each group for different periods of times (e.g., a cohort that receives Drug A was observed for 5 years, whereas the comparison cohort was observed for 2 years only). The reader should evaluate whether selection bias is present in a study, whether the investigators addressed such a bias, and whether the selection bias could alter the results significantly.

Another example of selection bias to consider is loss to follow-up, which may occur in studies that require a lengthy follow-up time. Loss to follow-up occurs when the participants can no longer be located or when participants wish not to participate in the study any longer. It can bias the study results with respect to exposure and outcome when participants who are lost to follow-up are different from those remaining in the study. When evaluating a study, it should be alarming if a large number of participants are lost to follow-up (greater than 20%).[11]

9. Could there have been bias in the collection of information? How likely was this bias?—Information bias is an error that arises from systematic differences in the way that information on exposure and disease is obtained from the study groups. It results in incorrect classification of participants as either *exposed* or *unexposed* or as *diseased* or *not diseased*. Again, the reader should consider this when assessing the quality of the study and interpreting the results.

10. What provisions were made to minimize the influence of confounding factors prior to the analysis of data? Were these provisions sufficient?— Confounding is a bias that affects the crude measure of association between an exposure and an outcome caused by a third factor that is associated with the exposure and is an independent risk factor for the outcome. Confounding can bias results either toward or away from the null hypothesis. Methods to control for confounding prior to data analysis include randomization, restriction, matching, and use of the same source population for the comparator groups. Confounders are usually identified prior to the initiation of the study, on the basis of extensive literature review and clinical knowledge. If the reader identifies major missing confounders in a study, the study results should be interpreted with caution because confounding factors not accounted for in the study may influence study results.[11]

One type of confounder that particularly affects pharmacoepidemiologic studies is confounding by the severity of disease or patient comorbidities. Sicker patients may respond differently to medications than would patients who have a mild or moderate disease or patients who have fewer competing comorbidities. Various comorbidity scores can be used for risk adjustment, as described in Chapter 6. These scores should be identified as possible confounders, and analysis should be conducted to adjust for disease severity or increased comorbidities on the outcomes of interest.

Data Analysis

1. What methods were used to control confounding bias during data analysis? Were these methods appropriate and sufficient?—The major topic with appropriate data analysis is the use of multivariable analyses. The reader should ask: Are the analyses appropriate and have they been used correctly? For example, if time to death is the final outcome, has a Cox's proportional hazard model been developed to examine the difference in hazard ratio at a point in time and a Kaplan–Meier curve constructed to demonstrate the differences between the death-rate curves taking into account the probability of death over time? The readers should also evaluate whether other statistical techniques to control for confounding bias, as discussed in Chapter 6, were used.

2. What measures of association were reported in the study? What measures of statistical stability were reported in the study?—Journals are increasingly moving away from reporting the *P* value to indicate statistical significance. In pharmacoepidemiology, researchers determine associations using measures such as the odds ratio (OR), risk ratio (RR), and standardized mortality rate. These measures not only indicate the strength of association but also tell whether the association is protective or a risk for developing the outcome of interest. In the pharmacoepidemiology literature, the OR should be accompanied by the 95% CI, and these components together can give the reader a clear indication whether the association is a risk or protective factor, whether the association is significant, and whether there is an effect of sample size. For example, study investigators may report that the OR between the use of sulfonylurea medications and lower limb amputation is 1.59 (95% CI, 0.95–2.79) among patients with diabetes. This tells the reader that patients taking sulfonylurea medications are 59% more likely to have a lower limb amputation. However, the 95% CI spans across 1.00, the null value, suggesting that the association is not statistically significant. If a 95% CI has a wide range, such as between 2.06 and 104.6, this may indicate that a larger sample may be needed to produce a more accurate estimate of the true association.

Results and Interpretation of Study Findings

1. What were the main results of this study?—The authors should provide the results of various statistical analyses and indicate whether the results are positive or negative. If the study results are vaguely stated, the reader should question the validity of the overall study design and study results.

2. How is the interpretation of these results affected by information bias, selection bias, and confounding? Discuss both the direction and magnitude of any bias—After gathering and reviewing all the critical information from other sections, the reader should determine the overall effect that bias and confounding factors may have on the study. It is important to assess bias and confounding in terms of both magnitude and direction. A small amount of bias and confounding usually does not have a major impact on the true association between exposure and outcome; however, if there is a large amount of bias and confounding, the true association may be altered significantly.

In studies where there is some uncertainty in some variables, the reader may consider whether a sensitivity analysis was conducted to evaluate the robustness of the study results in the presence of such uncertainty. For example, the likelihood that a patient may experience nausea and vomiting after a chemotherapy treatment is variable. In this case, a sensitivity analysis could be used to compare the worst- and best-case scenarios to determine whether there is a difference in outcomes between those who are more likely to experience nausea and vomiting and those who are less likely to experience such side effects.

3. How is the interpretation of these results affected by nondifferential misclassification? Discuss both the direction and magnitude of this misclassification—Nondifferential misclassification is a common form of bias that affects the association by "pulling" the results toward the null value. Null results should be carefully examined for nondifferential misclassification to determine whether mismeasurement or miscoding caused the findings. Nondifferential misclassification affects the final results by making the two comparison groups more similar than they truly are.[11]

4. Did the discussion section adequately address the limitations of the study?—The reader should note whether the investigators have identified any limitations of the study, especially those that affect the conclusions drawn from the study. It is at this point in the discussion that any research questions that have arisen from the study or questions that remain unanswered are discussed.

5. What were the authors' main conclusions? Were they justified by the findings?—Conclusions are a synopsis of the overall results of the study and should be presented in a few sentences at the end of the article. The reader should be given some indication of the importance of the study to public health policy or clinical practice, or some recommendations for future research at this point, relating back to the findings in the study. The reader should consider these recommendations as well as their own interpretation of the study findings. The reader should then connect all of the information and draw their own conclusions.

6. To what larger population can the results of this study be generalized?—The internal validity of a study must be established before the study results can be generalized to populations beyond the study participants. If a study is invalid, its results cannot be generalized to any populations. The evaluation of generalizability or "external validity" requires review of the study methods (e.g., was restriction used to control for confounding?), the composition of the study population (e.g., were minorities included?), and subject matter knowledge such as the biological basis of the association (e.g., would the same results be expected among men and women?). Before implementing the knowledge from pharmacoepidemiology studies into action, the reader may want to consider whether he or she should change his or her clinical practice or make recommendations to others on the basis of the study results. Should they make a recommendation to a formulary committee? Should they prescribe differently? Should a new policy be developed to influence medication use in this institution?

▶ Critical Evaluation of a Published Pharmacoepidemiology Study

In the following section, we present an example of a brief evaluation of a published pharmacoepidemiology study.[16]

The Research Questions, Study Design, and Populations

1. Why was this study done and why is it important? Does the introduction section present any gaps in the knowledge that the study addresses?

   The study was conducted to examine the association of acid-suppressive medications and acquired pneumonia in the hospital setting. This association is important because acid-suppressive medications are utilized quite often for stress ulcer prophylaxis in the hospital setting, yet research does not support this use. Other research suggests that current users of acid suppressors in the outpatient setting had an increased risk for community-acquired pneumonia. No large prospective study on the association between acid-suppressive medication and hospital-acquired pneumonia had been published prior to this study.

2. What were the objectives (or aims) of the study?

   The stated objective of the study was "to examine the association between acid-suppressive medication and hospital-acquired pneumonia."

3. What is the hypothesis of the study?

   The overall hypothesis is that acid suppressors are related to hospital-acquired pneumonia. The hypothesis was not specifically stated in the article, but it was implied.

4. What was the primary medication exposure of interest? Was this accurately measured? Was the dose of the exposure medication accurately measured so that dose–response characteristic can be evaluated?

   The primary medication exposure of interest was acid suppressors, namely, proton-pump inhibitors and histamine-2 antagonists. The medication exposure was measured as any pharmacy order for one of the medications of interest, regardless of dose, during the admission.

5. What was the primary outcome of interest? Was this accurately measured? Is it a surrogate measure and is this surrogate appropriate?

   The primary outcome of interest was the occurrence of hospital-acquired pneumonia. The outcome was directly measured as any discharge code (ICD-9-CM code) for bacterial pneumonia listed as a secondary discharge diagnosis. The authors provided detailed explanations of how the outcome of interest was measured, which appears appropriate.

6. What study design was used?

   A prospective cohort design using hospital claims data was used for the study. This study design is appropriate to address the study objectives.

7. Describe the source of study population, process of participant selection, sample size, and ratio of cases to comparison participants.

   The authors provided a thorough description of the inclusion and exclusion criteria for patient selection. The study population was comprised of all patients admitted to a large, urban, academic medical center in Boston, MA, from January 2004 through December 2007, with a stay of 3 or more days. All patients younger than 18 years of age were excluded. All patients admitted to the intensive care unit (ICU) were also excluded. The criteria resulted in a total cohort of 63,878 admissions representing 42,093 unique patients. A total of 2,219 (3.5%) admissions were classified as cases with hospital-acquired pneumonia.

8. Could there have been bias in the selection of the study participants? How likely was the bias?

   There does not appear to be selection bias in the study because all adults admitted to the hospital were included. The length of time that the participants were followed appears appropriate for the study.

9. Could there have been bias in the collection of information? How likely was this bias?

Because the information was collected from claims, there may be a bias related to the temporal relationship between the treatment (acid suppressor) and outcome (pneumonia). The study assumes that patients are given an acid-suppressive medication before they acquire pneumonia, but not the other way around. The bias is likely and may affect the results as revealed in the sensitivity analysis.

10. What provisions were made to minimize the influence of confounding factors prior to the analysis of data? Were these provisions sufficient?

To minimize the influence of potential confounding and bias, the authors used inclusion and exclusion criteria to refine the study population. Patients with any stay in the ICU were excluded to restrict the study to nonventilated patients only. Nonventilated patients with a stay of 3 or more days were included on the basis of the assumption that 72 hours (3 days) are necessary to relate cases of pneumonia to both hospital exposure and medication exposure. The tactic appears sufficient, so as to not overstate the treatment effect in the study.

Data Analysis

1. What methods were used to control confounding bias during data analysis? Were these methods sufficient?

Covariates for acid-suppression medication use and for hospital-acquired pneumonia were identified and included in the testing model. The covariates included demographics, seasonality, hospital admission and stay descriptors, medications, and comorbidities. In addition, propensity score–matched analysis was performed to make the group exposed to acid-suppressive drugs similar to the unexposed group. These approaches appear sufficient to control confounding bias.

2. What measures of association were reported in the study? What measures of statistical stability were reported in this study?

Odds ratio (OR) was the primary measure reported. Unadjusted, adjusted, and propensity-matched ORs were reported with 95% confidence intervals (CI).

Results and Interpretation of Study Findings

1. What were the main results of this study?

The authors presented the study results adequately. The main result was that patients receiving acid-suppressive medication had 30% greater odds of hospital-acquired pneumonia than patients not receiving acid suppressors (OR, 1.3; 95% CI, 1.1–1.4). In the subset analyses, the association between acid-suppressive medication and hospital-acquired pneumonia was statistically significant for proton-pump inhibitors (OR, 1.3; 95% CI, 1.1–1.4) but not for histamine-2 antagonists (OR, 1.2; 95% CI, 0.98–1.4).

2. How is the interpretation of these results affected by information bias, selection bias, and confounding? Discuss both the direction and magnitude of any bias.

Selection bias and confounding are not likely to affect the interpretation of the results because they were considered and accounted for. Information bias may have caused the authors to overstate the effect of the treatment. Because the source of information was claims, the temporal relationship between acid suppressor and pneumonia could not be verified.

3. How is the interpretation of these results affected by nondifferential misclassification? Discuss both the direction and magnitude of this misclassification.

The results should not be affected by misclassification. The authors performed sensitivity analyses, assuming misclassification for hospital-acquired pneumonia and for exposure to acid-suppressive medication.

4. Did the discussion section adequately address the limitations of the study?

Yes, the authors considered that they may have excluded important confounders and that the histamine-2 subgroup may have been underpowered in order to detect an effect, meaning that the lack of a significant effect in this subgroup may have been driven by sample size that is needed to detect the effect, if any. The authors also considered the possible effect of the amount of time exposed to the treatment (acid suppressors) on the risk of hospital-acquired pneumonia.

5. What were the authors' main conclusions? Were they justified by the findings?

The main conclusion was that acid-suppressive medications are associated with increased odds of hospital-acquired pneumonia, and the finding is significant for proton-pump inhibitors. The conclusions are supported by the findings of the study.

6. To what population can the results of this study be generalized?

Unless a location (e.g., hospital-specific and geography) effect exists, the results may be generalized to all adult patients hospitalized without a stay in the ICU.

SUMMARY

The importance, principles, and methods for evaluating the pharmacoepidemiology literature were discussed in this chapter. As the discipline of pharmacoepidemiology grows, it is important for health care professionals and policy makers to be able to critically evaluate the literature in pharmacoepidemiology and apply knowledge of pharmacoepidemiology in making health care decisions.

DISCUSSION QUESTIONS

1. Explain why it is important for health care professionals and policy makers to be able to critically evaluate pharmacoepidemiology literature.

2. Critically evaluate a published pharmacoepidemiology study using the checklist questions.

3. Give an example of how pharmacoepidemiology has impacted clinical practice or public policy.

REFERENCES

1. Somerville K, Faulkner G, Langman M. Non-steroidal anti-inflammatory drugs and bleeding peptic ulcer. *Lancet.* 1986;i:452-454.
2. Draugalis J, Plaza C. Emerging role of epidemiologic literacy. *Ann Pharmacother.* 2006;40(2):229-233.
3. Campbell IW. The clinical significance of PPAR gamma-agonism. *Curr Mol Med.* 2005;5(3):349-363.
4. Nissen SE, Wolski K. Effect of rosiglitazone on the risk of myocardial infarction and death from cardiovascular causes. *NJEM.* 2007;356(24):2457-2471.
5. Mannucci E, Monami M. Is the evidence from clinical trials for cardiovascular risk or harm for glitazones convincing? *Curr Dia Rep.* 2009;9(5):342-347.
6. Rabi DM, Lewin AD, Brown GE, et al. Lay media reporting of rosiglitazone risk: Extent, messaging and quality of reporting. *Cardiovasc Diabetol.* 2009;8:40.
7. Home PD, Pocock SJ, Beck-Nielsen H, et al. Rosiglitazone evaluated for cardiovascular outcomes—An interim analysis. *NJEM.* 2007;357(1):28-38.
8. Krentz A. Thiazolidinediones: Effects on the development and progression of type 2 diabetes and associated vascular complications. *Diabets Metab ResRev.* 2009;25(2):112-126.
9. Lipscombe LL, Gomes T, Levesque LE, Hux JE, Juurlink DN, Alter DA. Thiazolidinediones and cardiovascular outcomes in older patients with diabetes. *JAMA.* 2007;298(22):2634-2643.
10. FDA Alert. Information for Healthcare Professionals Rosiglitazone maleate (marketed as Avandia, Avandamet, and Avandaryl). Food and Drug Administration Web site. http://www.fda.gov/Drugs/DrugSafety/PostmarketDrugSafetyInformationforPatientsandProviders/ucm143349.htm. Accessed February 7, 2010.
11. Aschengrau A, Seage GR. *Essentials of Epidemiology in Public Health,* 2nd ed. Sudbury, MA: Jones & Bartlett Publishers, 2008:359.
12. Van Haarst AD, van't Klooster GAE, van Gerven JMA, et al. The influence of cisapride and clarithromycin on QT intervals in healthy volunteers. *Clin Pharmacol Ther.* 1998;64(5):542-546.
13. Smalley W, Shatin D, Wysowski DK, et al. Contraindicated use of cisapride: Impact of food and drug administration regulatory action. *JAMA.* 2000;284(23):3036-3039.
14. Hennessy S, Leonard CE, Newcomb C, et al. Cisapride and ventricular arrhythmia. *Br J Clin Pharmacol.* 2008;66(3):375-385.
15. Hennekens CH, Buring JF, eds. *Epidemiology in Medicine.* Boston, MA: Little, Brown & Company, 1987:142.
16. Herzig SJ, Howell MD, Ngo LH, Marcantonio ER. Acid-suppressive medication use and the risk for hospital-acquired pneumonia. *JAMA.* 2009;301(20):2120-2128.

Medication Utilization Patterns

David J. McCaffrey III

"Drugs don't work if people don't take them."[1]

"Why would someone who has gone to the trouble and expense of seeking out a physician, of undertaking arduous or uncomfortable tests and other diagnostic procedures, and of purchasing drugs and devices on the advice of the physician, then fail to follow the recommendations?"[2]

▼ OBJECTIVES

At the end of the chapter, the reader will be able to:

1. Describe the optimal definition of suboptimal medication utilization
2. Compare and contrast compliance, adherence, concordance, and persistence
3. Compare and contrast initial compliance, partial compliance, compliance, and hypercompliance
4. Discuss the advantages and disadvantages associated with the different methods of measuring medication utilization
5. Describe the essential elements for calculating adherence and persistence from administrative claims data
6. Calculate adherence/persistence from information contained in administrative claims data.
7. Recognize challenges to using administrative claims data to measure adherence/persistence
8. Recognize the elements that define a quality adherence and persistence study using administrative claims data

INTRODUCTION

The effectiveness of a therapy depends on only two elements. First, the prescriber, with or without consultation with another health care provider (e.g., a pharmacist), must select a therapy that is appropriate in all aspects.[3] In other words, assuming a correct diagnosis, the therapy must be the right drug, by the right route, in the right dose, at the right time, for the right duration, for the right patient.[4] The second consideration is the extent to which the patient consumes the medications as recommended.[3(p950)] In terms of patient care, the detection of suboptimal medication utilization is a prerequisite for adequate treatment.[5] Although the importance of proper diagnosis, medication selection, and treatment efficacy are not being debated, patient utilization of medication is the sole focus of this chapter.

Patients commonly fail to take their medications as directed, leading to additional diagnostics and treatments, unnecessary hospitalizations, avoidable nursing home admissions, and even death; estimates of the direct and indirect costs associated with suboptimal medication utilization exceed US$100 billion a year.[6] Many nursing home admissions are due to no cause other than the patient's inability to manage his/her medications.[7] When one considers the cost differences associated with patients living independently versus long-term care, the cost savings are tremendous. It is estimated that just over 5%[8] of hospital admissions and between 1% and 3%[9-12] of emergency department visits can be attributed to a patient's suboptimal medication utilization. Patients who exhibit better medication utilization (80%–100%) are significantly less likely to be hospitalized for disease-related reasons or for any other reason, compared with patients who exhibited suboptimal medication utilization.[13] It is a well-regarded fact that patients who consume their medications in a manner consistent with expectations experience positive health outcomes and decreased mortality.[14] However, in spite of increased knowledge and increased responsibility for their own care, patients still fail to follow the recommendations given by their health care providers about medication use.[15] This phenomenon continues to be studied; since the 1940s, the number of articles appearing in the peer-reviewed literature has increased from very few to many thousands, to such a degree that one may believe that suboptimal medication utilization is a disease itself with its own epidemiology.[16] Others have called suboptimal medication utilization "America's other drug problem."[17] Therefore, in an environment where the demand for health care dollars is exceeding supply and where a drug's effectiveness and safety is sometimes of concern, the utilization behaviors of patients require serious attention from pharmacoepidemiology researchers and health care providers among others.

THE TAXONOMY OF SUBOPTIMAL MEDICATION UTILIZATION

The extent to which patients take medications as prescribed by their health care providers is far more complex than many realize. There exist many known factors influencing the medication utilization behaviors of patients.[18] Moreover, it may be affected by more than one factor in any given moment. In fact, the complexity of this issue may begin with the very language used to describe it. Patient medication utilization behaviors have been referred to in the literature as compliance, adherence, concordance, fidelity, maintenance, and persistence to name but a few. Oftentimes confusion surrounds the application of these terms, for they have been used interchangeably and without consistency either in operationalization or in their application.

▶ "Optimal" Definition

Although the literature contains definitions that can be used to measure a patient's medication utilization behavior, what is it that constitutes the "optimal" definition of suboptimal medication utilization behavior? Ideally, any such definition would be tied to a biologic/physiologic outcome. In that vein, *suboptimal medication utilization* would be defined as the point below which the desired therapeutic effect is unlikely to be achieved.[19] Stated differently, suboptimal medication utilization would be the number of doses not taken or taken incorrectly that places the expected therapeutic outcome in doubt. Ultimately, researchers and clinicians alike are concerned most with how well a patient's medication utilization

Table 8-1. Relationship between medication utilization and treatment goal.

		Therapeutic goals	
		Achieved	Not achieved
Medication Utilization	High Low	Desired Inaccurate diagnosis or Over-prescribing?	Inadequate therapy ATTENTION

Adapted from Sackett DL. Introduction. In: Sackett DL, Haynes RB, eds. *Compliance with Therapeutic Regimens.* Baltimore, MD: The Johns Hopkins University Press, 1976:1-6. Adapted with permission of The Johns Hopkins University Press.

relates to the achievement of treatment goals (Table 8-1). However, weaving that consideration into a working definition of suboptimal medication utilization behavior is difficult, considering the many factors that may affect patient response to medication therapy.

The creation of an "optimal" definition of suboptimal medication utilization requires that some threshold utilization value be established. However, there are few instances where this cut point can be determined reliably. In addition, in instances where a utilization level is identified, the nonrandom pattern of poor utilization behavior may render the definition less than useful. Table 8-2 depicts four hypothetical patient's medication utilization patterns where it was determined that 50% utilization was the appropriate operationalization of *compliance*. By definition, each patient's utilization would be considered adequate; however, the differences in his/her actual patterns of utilization may determine whether he/she received any, some, or all of the therapeutic benefit.

For example, a patient may consume enough doses to be considered "good"; however, because of the pattern of that utilization, he/she may experience the same poor outcome that one would expect of a patient consuming less than the "recommended" amount.

Unless the researcher or clinician has access to reliable clinical definitions developed from valid sources of information (e.g., clinical trial), researchers and clinicians should rely on the cost-effective and reliable assessments of medication utilization patterns that produce continuous measures of medication usage.[20] This is an important issue in not only the design and execution of studies but also in the interpretation of the literature and the design of interventions. Determining the clinical sequelae of consuming medication at less than the recommended level is necessary before the labels of "good" or "poor" are attached to patients.[21] Despite the fact the 80% utilization is often used as the cut point of classifying patients as having

Table 8-2. Hypothetical utilization patterns of four patients.

Patient 1	+	+	+	+	−	−	−	−	−
Patient 2	−	−	−	−	+	+	+	+	+
Patient 3	+	−	+	−	+	−	+	−	+
Patient 4	+	−	+	+		+	−		+

Adapted from Gordis L. Conceptual and methodologic problems in measuring patient compliance. In: Haynes RB, Taylor DW, Sackett DL, eds. *Compliance in Health Care.* Baltimore, MD: The Johns Hopkins University Press, 1976:23–45. Adapted with permission of The Johns Hopkins University Press.

suboptimal medication utilization, simplistic dichotomies of medication utilization behavior should be avoided.[20(p416)]

▶ Compliance, Adherence, and Concordance

The term *compliance* is pervasive in medical science.[22] A popular term in the 1970s, compliance is defined as the extent to which a person's behavior (in terms of taking medications) coincides with medical or health advice.[23] The use of the term *compliance* to describe patient behavior received a great deal of criticism since its adoption, particularly due to its paternalistic overtones; the term *compliance* infers that the physician would develop the treatment plan devoid of input from the patient. In other words, the term implies a lack of involvement on the part of the patient, the person who is most likely able to affect medication utilization decisions. This belief has prompted many to consider its use obsolete or inappropriate in modern medical practice. *Adherence* is a term used oftentimes interchangeably with the term *compliance* to describe a patient's failure to consume medication according to the prescriber's directions. Whereas compliance is believed to denote actions on the part of the patient that conform or acquiesce to the demands of the health care provider, the term *adherence* suggests more self-motivated perseverance with the medication regimen.[24] In some circles, *adherence* has become the favored term with which to describe the medication utilization behaviors of patients due in part to the belief that it describes the outcome of a participative relationship between the patient and the health care provider as it relates to the patient's treatment. *Concordance,* the most recent term and used predominantly in the United Kingdom, is the "agreement between the patient and the health care professional, reached after negotiation, that respects the beliefs and wishes of the patient in determining whether, when, and how his medicine is taken . . . and the primacy of the patient's decision [is recognised]."[25] With concordance, it is believed that the patient and health care provider agree on all aspects of therapy before its initiation.[26] This "partnership" between the patient and health care provider extends beyond that described by the term *adherence*

and represents a relative ideal in the management of pharmacotherapy.

Because a number of common terms—*compliance, adherence, persistence,* and *concordance*—have been used concurrently, a report by the National Council on Patient Information and Education called on the public health community to reach agreement on standard terminology that will unite stakeholders around the common goal of improving the self-administration of medical treatments.[17(p25)] The Medication Compliance and Persistence Special Interest Group (SIG) of the International Society for Pharmacoeconomics and Outcomes Research (ISPOR), in an effort to reduce uncertainty surrounding the conduct and interpretation of studies of medication utilization and standardize the medical literature, evaluated the existing literature for the purpose of adopting medication utilization behavior terminology and developing definitions for compliance and persistence. Medication compliance is "the extent of conformity to the recommendations about day-to-day treatment by a provider with respect to timing, dosage, and frequency."[21(p46)] This definition is consistent with the existing definitions of compliance; however, it emphasizes the measurement of medication utilization beyond simply counting the number of doses consumed; it respects the pharmacokinetic parameters associated with medication use. Medication compliance can be calculated easily by comparing the number of doses consumed correctly to the number of doses expected to be consumed.

$$\text{Compliance} = \frac{\text{Number of doses consumed correctly}}{\text{Number of doses to be consumed}} \times 100\%$$

The choice of the moniker of compliance versus adherence is irrelevant largely within the context of measurement of suboptimal medication utilization. Each has involved with it an objective comparison of prescribed therapy against what was consumed by the patient. Others have noted similarities in deciding upon terminology by attaching a terminal phrase to definitions, "the extent to which the patient's behavior coincides with the clinical prescription, regardless of how the latter was generated."[27]

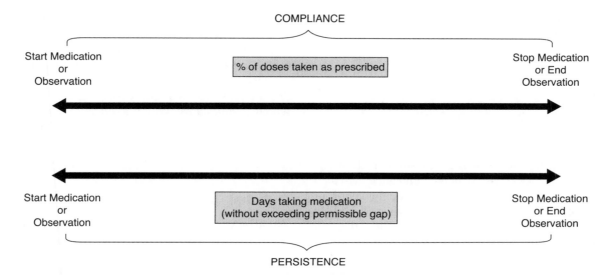

▲ **Figure 8-1.** Definitions of compliance and persistence. Reprinted from: Cramer JA, Roy A, Burrell A, et al. Medication compliance and persistence: Terminology and definitions. *Value Health.* 2008;11(1):44-47. Reprinted by permission of the International Society for Pharmacoeconomics and Outcomes Research. Copyright 2008. All rights reserved.

▶ Persistence

Persistence has been defined in the medical literature as the length of time of taking a medication, measured in days, weeks, months, and so on[28]; in other words, it is the act of conforming to a recommended therapy for the prescribed length of time. Although some argue that *compliance* and *adherence* are synonyms, *persistence* is a different concept altogether. Whereas compliance (adherence) is expressed as a percentage of doses consumed, persistence is measured by time (Figure 8-1). According to ISPOR's Compliance and Persistence SIG, persistence is the duration of time from initiation to discontinuation of therapy. As such, it is a continuous measure of the number of days for which medication was available.[21(p46)] In addition, persistence has been measured and reported as a dichotomous (persistent/nonpersistent) variable.[21(p46)] A patient who is persistent does not abruptly stop taking his/her medication, nor are there any long unexplained gaps (exceeding a permissible gap) in medication utilization during the time frame under investigation. The decision of what constitutes a permissible gap should be made on the basis

of the pharmacokinetic/pharmacodynamic characteristics of the medication and the treatment circumstances.[29]

Persistence can be viewed from either a therapeutic perspective or a product perspective. Some persistence studies focus on the measurement of persistence with only one therapeutic agent. In other words, these studies will report a persistence measure as the length of time taking a *specific* medication or as the percentage of patients remaining on a *specific* medication for a specified period. Although this may have clinical implications in that patient's failure to continue on an initially prescribed therapy could indicate that the product has associated with it some intolerable effects or unacceptable outcomes (e.g., subtherapeutic effect, interaction, or side effect), oftentimes, this perspective appears to be borne out of commercial interests. Persistence may also be calculated on the basis of a patient receiving any medication within the same therapeutic class or *any* appropriate medication for the disease/conduction. This view of persistence recognizes medication switching as a "normal" activity in pharmacotherapy and should be addressed in any medication utilization measure.

PATTERNS OF SUBOPTIMAL MEDICATION UTILIZATION

Although patient medication-taking behavior is often reported to be a dichotomous behavior (compliant vs. noncompliant), it is important to note that medication taking is rarely an all-or-none phenomenon. Medication utilization can vary along a continuum from 0% to 100%.[30] In fact, it has been argued that the continuum can extend beyond 100% in that some patients consume medications at a frequency greater than recommended.[31] In fact, viewing the medication utilization behavior of patients as a dichotomy is limiting, given the variety of different behaviors a patient may exhibit through the course of treatment. As such, it can be argued that patients should never be considered always compliant or always noncompliant. Rather patient medication-taking behavior can be plotted along a compliance continuum,[32] whereby patients may fall into one or several areas of medication-taking behaviors at any given time. This compliance continuum is composed of initial noncompliance, partial compliance, compliance, and hypercompliance.

▶ Initial Noncompliance

The patient's first decision, according to this continuum, is whether to follow a prescriber's treatment recommendation (i.e., prescription). *Initial noncompliance*, which would represent the far left anchor on the continuum, is the instance whereby patients do not receive the medication prescribed for them. Initial noncompliance is comprised of two different types of behaviors, the unpresented prescription and the unclaimed prescription.

Unpresented prescriptions are those prescriptions that are issued by the prescriber but never makes it to a pharmacy for fill.[33] Rather than arriving at a pharmacy by the patient or his/her caretaker or through some other means (e.g., phoned in, facsimile, electronic transfer, or mailed), this prescription remains "pocketed" or "pocketbooked" and the pharmacist remains ignorant to its existence and, therefore, making it difficult to intervene. Historical figures reveal that approximately 4%[34] of prescriptions that are issued fail to make it to the pharmacy.

Unclaimed prescriptions, by comparison, are prescriptions that have been presented in a pharmacy for fill but are either abandoned by the patient or his/her caretaker or are not delivered to the patient at home.[35] The literature shows that between 1% and 2%[35(p49)] of prescriptions that are presented to the pharmacy for fill remain unclaimed. With unclaimed prescriptions, the health care provider and researcher have accessible evidence that a noncompliance episode has happened. As such, intervention is more probable.

▶ Partial Compliance

Partial compliance, the next point along the continuum, is the instance whereby the patient receives his/her medication but does not follow the physician's orders on how this medication should be taken or used. Some examples would include errors in dose timing and self-regulation, underuse (skipping doses), stopping the medication too soon, or sharing medications with others. In fact, one study identified nine different partial medication utilization behaviors.[36] The majority of the literature on medication utilization is concentrated in this area, and it is the most frequently observed deviation from the prescribed regimen.[37] Estimates show that 20% to 80% of patients exhibit some level of partial compliance. Across 50 years of published studies and across multiple disease states, medication utilization was found to range from just under 5% to 100%, with an average utilization rate of about 75%. Although studies have demonstrated that "good" medication utilization is related to positive outcomes,[38] the failure to achieve desired outcomes due to poor medication utilization is pervasive and not unique to any one disease state or therapy. Many disease categories and their associated therapies have been shown to have compliance problems. Although studies of medication utilization in HIV disease have shown the highest levels of compliance, medication utilization across medical conditions is varied.[39] Table 8-3 presents compliance rates across various diseases/therapies.

▶ Compliance

Compliance is defined as the process of following a prescribed and dispensed regimen precisely as the prescriber and dispenser intended. Although it is believed

Table 8-3. Adherence rates across various diseases/therapies.

Disease/condition	Range of mean adherence (%)
Arthritis	72–89
Cancer	76–84
Cardiovascular diseases	73–80
Diabetes	59–76
End-stage renal disease	57–82
Gastrointestinal disorders	74–86
Genitourinary diseases and STDs	65–87
HIV disease	79–95
Infectious diseases	68–80
OB-GYN	64–84
Pulmonary diseases	61–76
Skin disorders	67–86
Sleep disorders	54–76

that few patients attain this behavior state, it is toward this goal that programs and interventions are designed.

▶ Hypercompliance

The rightmost point on the continuum, hypercompliance, occurs when the patient takes a prescribed medication at a level over and above the recommended dosing interval. Medication overuse or abuse has received some attention in the published literature, particularly focused on controlled substances. The potential for increases in adverse events and adverse health outcomes makes hypercompliance an issue of particular interest to pharmacoepidemiology researchers and heath care providers. For example, pharmacists have been integrally involved with the management of hypercompliance. Due to Federal and state laws, pharmacists practice due diligence when dispensing and refilling prescriptions for controlled substances. Online adjudication associated with third-party prescription plans also alerts pharmacists to the possibility of overuse at the time of dispensing.

MEASUREMENT OF MEDICATION UTILIZATION

Although solid definitions of medication-taking behavior exist, no one best and agreed-upon measure of patient medication utilization has been identified. As such, a variety of medication utilization detection/measurement methods have been reported in the literature, each having strengths and weaknesses and varying costs and applicability/feasibility in medical practice. In spite of the realization that no gold standard exists, some methods are clearly superior to others.[40] The choice of measure is important due to the ramifications of misclassification. Misclassifications in the clinic setting may result in changes in medication therapy, including adding medication therapies, additional diagnostic testing, and unnecessary referrals.[41] In pharmacoepidemiologic research, the risks associated with the inaccurate assessment of medication utilization include complicating the interpretation of a study's findings or possibly the underestimation of a treatment's effectiveness.[41(p259)] It is expected that the researcher/clinician understand the "ability" of the measure being used.

The methods used to measure medication utilization behavior are classified usually as being direct or indirect, although an objective-subjective dichotomy to describe these measures is used also. Direct methods are those that provide objective evidence that the medication was taken by the patient. Indirect methods rely on surrogate measures of utilization. In other words, utilization by the patient is assumed by the pharmacoepidemiologist or clinician.

▶ Direct Measures of Medication Utilization

Directly Observed Therapy

Directly observed therapy (DOT) simply means that a patient is observed consuming his/her medication(s). This method has been used in clinical trials and in certain public health initiatives (e.g., tuberculosis, HIV, and methadone) where high rates of relapse or resistance are expected to be associated with suboptimal medication utilization. DOT is considered impractical, hence its limited use. Therapy is typically dispensed at the site of utilization (clinic, residence, place of employment, etc.).[42] Patients enrolled in DOT may attempt to fool the observer by pretending to place the dosage in their mouth or by feigning consumption by "cheeking" the dosage and removing it when then they are no longer under observation.[30(p41), 43] This limitation notwithstanding, DOT, like other observational techniques, is valid in that it measures what it intends to measure.

Biological Fluids

Blood or urine samples have been used to detect medication levels, metabolites of medications, or markers/tracers (pharmacologically inert substances or low-dose medications) in order to assess medication utilization and offer objective evidence of medication utilization. Limitations to their use include cost, intrusiveness, and impracticality. These methods are sensitive to factors associated with the absorption, distribution, and elimination/metabolism characteristics of the patient as well as the susceptibility to interactions, all of which ultimately complicate the interpretation of the findings from these studies. In addition, assays measure medication utilization over relatively short time intervals and thus fail to provide information about consistency in medication adherence over extended periods. The use of serum or urine levels to detect medication utilization is highly susceptible to changes in behavior in the days leading up to evaluation.[44,45]

▷ Indirect Methods of Measuring Medication Utilization

Patient Self-Report—Interviews, Structured Instruments, and Diaries

The easiest strategy to assess medication utilization behavior is to ask the patient.[46] These reports are the most practical and, therefore, the most widely used in clinical practice.[47] Patient self-report of his/her medication utilization behavior is fast, inexpensive, and simple; it has applicability to many different settings within health care. Patient self-report of medication utilization behavior can include interview, the use of structured questionnaires, and completion of diaries. Despite the obvious advantages associated with the use of patient self-report, it is an often criticized technique for collecting medication utilization informa-

tion. Patients may not be able to recall their medication-taking behavior 30 days, 60 days, or 90 days in the past. Memory lapses aside, there is also a concern with patients overestimating their medication utilization. *Social desirability bias*, the tendency of respondents to respond in a manner that will be viewed favorably by others, is a common problem in survey research.[48] This problem affects all forms of self-report; however, its effect is more pronounced in interview surveys than it is in self-report techniques.[49]

Second, as an alternative to the patient interview, social scientists have developed standardized survey instruments to measure and predict suboptimal medication utilization. The Morisky Scale[50] was developed to be a simple tool to administer and assess medication utilization; thus, it could be used by clinicians at the point of care. This 4-item scale was developed with a yes/no response format with maximum possible score of 4 (suboptimal medication utilization) and lower scores (0 or 1) representing better utilization behaviors. Morisky Scale values, denoting proper medication utilization behaviors, have been associated with lower HbA1 c measurements[51] and higher medication and inhaler use in patients with asthma.[52] More recently, an 8-item self-reported measure of medication taking was developed from the Morisky scale.[53] The Brief Medication Questionnaire (BMQ) is another instrument developed for use in both research and in clinical practice.[54] This instrument focuses on the patient's regimen, his/her beliefs about the medication, and about potential difficulties remembering. It is expected that this instrument can not only predict nonadherence episodes but also, due to its construction, suggest helpful interventions. The ASK-12 (*Adherence Starts with Knowledge*) is a newer scale developed from the ASK-20[55] that assesses adherence behavior and barriers to adherence.[56]

Lastly, medication diaries are commonly used in health care and clinical research to assess patient experiences. As a patient consumes a medication, he/she is asked to record medication taking as it occurs (day and time) in the diary. This day and time information can be valuable in understanding drug action, hence the diary's use in clinical trial. The potential for patients to falsify medication utilization data is a common criticism of patient diaries; however, unlike the patient interview, diary completion should overcome or reduce the potential problem with overdemanding recall. Recently, electronic diaries have been put into use in clinical trials.[57]

Provider Estimates

Despite the importance of the role the health care provider plays in increasing the medication utilization behavior of patients, health care providers' estimates of patient medication utilization are believed to be unreliable. Physician estimates have been shown not to differ from patient self-report[58] and tend to overestimate medication utilization.[59–61]

Pill Counts

Pill counts long represented the standard "objective" method for measuring medication utilization. Pill counts are a straightforward, simple, and feasible method for detecting suboptimal medication utilization behavior in both research and clinical practice. Initially executed by having the patient or caretaker make a visit to the clinic, the feasibility of using pill counts has been enhanced by obtaining pill counts from patients or family members by telephone, e-mail, or other means of communication. Pill counts involve counting medications at two points in time (beginning of therapy and again at the end of observation). To calculate medication utilization, one would simply subtract the number of doses on hand at Time 2 from the number of doses received at Time 1, divide by the number of doses supplied and multiply by 100 to obtain a percentage of doses taken. "Pill count" activities can also be executed by a health care provider or researcher for liquids (measurement of volume remaining) and topical treatments[62] and inhaled therapies[63] (weight change).

Microelectronic Medication-Monitoring Devices (Electronic Event Monitoring)

Microprocessor technologies now have led to the development of electronic monitoring devices that can measure medication utilization behavior. These medication containers have integrated microcircuitry that records the time and date that the package is opened. As such the types of information available from these devices include chronology of dose administration, evidence of overuse (short-interval administration), and underuse (medication holidays).[64] These data can be downloaded from the device to a computer for subsequent analysis. One clear advantage of the electronic monitoring is that it collects information about the "utilization" of medication as well as the timing of such utilization.[65] Unfortunately, despite advances, this technology is costly, and it does not assure that the dosages have been consumed.

Administrative Claims Data

Administrative claims data are secondary sources of information; these are sources of data and other information collected by entities other than the researcher and archived in some form.[66] Administrative claims data oftentimes contain information on a very large population of patients (covered lives) and, as such, provide statistical power.[67] In addition, administrative claims data represent a cost-effective means to answer many important pharmacoepidemiologic research questions. This cost-effectiveness comes from the fact that collecting equivalent data using a primary data collection technique would involve a substantial time commitment and come at an incredible cost.[68] Given the nature of such data, it is believed that administrative claims data that include prescription claims information are well suited for pharmacoepidemiological studies. In fact, the use of administrative claims data to measure medication utilization has become increasingly common in the adherence and persistence literature.[69] In addition to reporting the measurement of adherence/persistence in populations[70,71] administrative claims data have been used to link suboptimal medication utilization to poor outcomes.[72–75]

Although administrative datasets have shown tremendous utility in the measurement of adherence and the association of suboptimal medication utilization with outcomes, administrative claims data may or may not contain information beyond prescription claims. Depending on the access that a researcher has to additional administrative data, it may be possible to combine data (data linkages) from prescription claims with basic demographic information, diagnoses, as well as information from ambulatory care visits and hospitalizations. These combined datasets offer the greatest amount of utility and represent a great opportunity for researchers to answer complex questions about medication utilization and associated outcomes (e.g., adverse drug events, hospitalization, or mortality). The remainder of this chapter will focus on measuring patient adherence and persistence with prescription medications using administrative claims data.

▶ Measuring Adherence and Persistence Using Administrative Claims Data

The measures that are used to assess medication utilization in administrative claims data are characterized by three parameters: dichotomous versus continuous distributions, the evaluation of single or multiple intervals, and the measurement of medication availability or gaps.[76]

Dichotomous Measures

Many examples of dichotomization (adherent/nonadherent) exist in the literature. The methods used for this classification scheme includes the anniversary method, the minimum refills method, and the threshold method. The anniversary method calls for defining a patient as *adherent* if he/she refills his/her prescription within a specific interval in the 1-year anniversary of the initial filling of the prescription.[28(p1413)] Although easy to calculate, this measure ignores any medication utilization behavior between the first and last fill and may significantly overestimate utilization. The minimum-refills method classifies a patient as being *adherent* if the number of prescriptions that he/she claims exceeds some a priori defined number of refills. The threshold method counts the number of days for which the patient had medication available. The patient is considered adherent if his/her proportion of days covered exceeds a predetermined threshold. This threshold is typically set to ≥80% within the period under observation. The establishment of cut points for determining adherence/nonadherence is an issue that generates a great deal of discussion. Oftentimes, it is the lack of credible information about medication

utilization and outcome attainment that causes researchers and scholars to advocate continuous measures rather than dichotomies. Using a Medicaid administrative dataset, it was determined that the optimal cut points for predicting disease-related hospitalization was 0.76, 0.85, 0.82, 0.81, and 0.58 for schizophrenia, diabetes, hypertension, hyperlipidemia, and congestive heart failure, respectively.[77] However, additional study is necessary in other disease categories, patient populations, and with other outcomes of interest.

Continuous Measures

Continuous measures of medication utilization can be determined by refill-sequence method and the proportion-of-days-covered method.[28(pp1419–1420)] Consistent with the ISPOR definition of persistence, the refill-sequence method is measured in days and represents the length of time between the initiation of pharmacotherapy and the appearance of a significant gap between subsequent fills. The determination of significant gap does vary by study. Some have considered gaps as small as 7 days as "significant," and others have considered permissible gaps based on 0.5 to 3 times the day's supply of the preceding fill of the prescription.[78] In the case of the 7-day permissible gap, it is essentially the equivalent of an 80% medication possession rate $[30/(30 + 7)]$.[29(p451)] An important note is that the greater the value that is chosen for the permissible gap, the higher the persistence values are likely to be. Rather than reducing the medication utilization data to the adherence/nonadherence dichotomy, the results of a proportion-of-days-covered technique can be reported as a continuous measure. This will avoid the possible misclassification associated with the choice of cut point.

▶ Calculating Adherence/Persistence

In studies of medication utilization, the measurement of adherence/persistence begins on the *index date*. The index date refers to the date of first fill of the medication and marks the beginning of the observation period. In studies of medication utilization using administrative datasets, despite patients' records being evaluated for the same length of time (e.g., 1 year), the beginning of observation period for each

Medication Possession Ratio (MPR)	$\dfrac{\text{Days' supply}}{\text{Days in evaluation period}}$
Continuous Measure of Medication Acquisition (CMA)	$\dfrac{\text{Cumulative days' supply of medication obtained}}{\text{Total days to end of observation period}}$
Continuous Measure of Medication Gaps (CMG)	$\dfrac{\text{Total days of treatment gaps}}{\text{Total days to end of observation period}}$
Proportion of Days Covered (PDC) *capped at 100%*	$\dfrac{\text{Total days supplied}}{\text{Total days evaluated}} \times 100\%$
Continuous Multiple Interval Measure of Oversupply (CMOS)	$\dfrac{\text{Total days of treatment gaps (+) or surplus (−)}}{\text{Total days in observation period}}$
Medication Refill Adherence (MRA)	$\dfrac{\text{Total days supplied}}{\text{Total days evaluated}} \times 100\%$

▲ **Figure 8-2.** Formulae for the calculation of adherence/persistence using administrative claims data.

patient will depend on the date of first fill. In other words, one study may have a patient who filled his/her first prescription days, months, or even years, before another in the same study. Once the initial fill has been identified, the patients record is evaluated over period of observation (index period). The length of time of the index period varies by study; however, it must be sufficiently long to provide stable estimates of medication utilization.

Many formulas exist for the calculation of medication adherence and persistence, and the choice of measure may vary depending on the patterns of utilization in the dataset.[29] In other words, it should not be assumed that all formulae are equivalent.[79–81] Commonly used adherence and persistence measures appear in Figure 8-2 along with its associated formula.

Figure 8-3 and Table 8-4 depict a hypothetical medication pattern for a patient. The prescription called for the patient to take 1 tablet twice daily and the quantity supplied was 60 (30 days supplied). In this example of simple medication use with no early fills, the measures that are based on medication availability (CMA, MRA, MPR, PDC) are identical. The measures that use gaps in the calculation of medication utilization (CMG, CMOS) are identical and are a complement of the availability measures (0.74 + 0.26 = 1.00) to the total of doses supplied.

The results from a direct comparison of several of the techniques used to measure adherence/persistence under different conditions revealed that CMA, CMOS, MPR, and MRA across several scenarios were identical in terms of measuring possession of medication across the evaluation period.[81(p1282)] It was

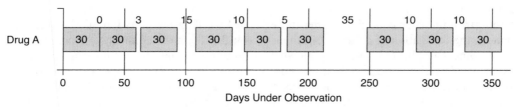

▲ **Figure 8-3.** Hypothetical patient's prescription-fill record.

Table 8-4. Hypothetical patient's prescription-fill record

Fill #	Fill date	Days supplied	CMA	CMG	CMOS	MRA	MPR	PDC
1	0	30	0.74[a]	0.26[b]	0.26[c]	74.0%[d]	0.74:1[e]	74.0%[f]
2	30	30						
3	63	30						
4	108	30						
5	148	30						
6	183	30						
7	248	30						
8	288	30						
9	328	30						
10	365	30						

[a]270/364.
[b]270/364.
[c]95/364.
[d]270/364.
[e]270:364.
[f]270/364.

suggested that MRA be the recommended measure of medication utilization using administrative datasets[81(p1286)] because of its relative simplicity of calculation when compared to the others. Although ease of use is an important consideration in choosing a measure, it is advisable to choose a measure that is consistent with the goals and objectives of the pharmacoepidemiology study.[70(p566)] Using a well-established, conservative measure of medication utilization is considered good practice. In the event that an atypical measure is used or a new measure is developed, it is necessary and appropriate that a detailed description of the measure be included in the study.

It is not unusual that in some disease states patients will receive a prescription for more than one medication to treat the same condition. Under those circumstances, the calculation of adherence/compliance can become complicated. For example if a patient is evaluated over a period of 90 days and possesses 70 days and 75 days of medication for Drug A and Drug B respectively, his/her MPR would be 145/90 = 1.61. The result for this patient, whose medication utilization was less than recommended, is an MPR value that makes it out that he/she consumed more doses than was expected. An alternative to this calculation would involve reinterpreting the days under observation. By doubling the value for period of observation the value for the MPR (145/180 = becomes equivalent to the average MPR for the two medications) may represent a more appropriate measure. Other ways to measure medication utilization for multiple medication therapy would be to calculate PDC for a class of medications.[82] Using the PDC the researcher will count all of the days that a patient had ANY of the study medications, in other words, no absolute gap in therapy. Using this technique, a patient who has nonoverlapping gaps in medication possession would still have a PDC value of 1.00. This interpretation may be questioned based on the intent of the therapy or the sensitivity of the combined therapy to missing doses. In those instances, it may be more advisable to compute an average utilization value for all medications.

Over the normal course of patient care, changing therapies can be expected. It is very important to

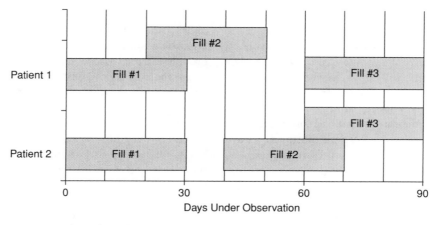

▲ **Figure 8-4.** Comparison of two hypothetical patients' prescription-fill records.

understand the measurement decisions made with respect to switching medications in the middle of an observation period. A switch is defined as an instance when a patient fills a drug product for one product, then at some time during the observation period fills a prescription for a drug in the same therapeutic class and does not refill the original prescription during the study period.[83(p89)] Patients who switch medications may be handled differently, on the basis of whether the switch was made to a medication in the same therapeutic category or a switch was made to another product in another therapeutic class that is recognized as being appropriate for the condition being treated. In fact, some researchers have labeled switching as "nonpersistence"—this is consistent with the definition of product persistence; however, this may serve to add confusion to the available literature in that persistence is a measure of the behavior of the patient[79(p7)] and not a measure of the adequacy of the medication therapy choices made by the physician.

The effect of oversupply on persistence measures will depend how it is handled in the calculation. It makes logical sense that if a patient fills a prescription early he/she will have medication on hand at the end of days-supplied period for that second fill. In other words, we do not evaluate gaps in coverage and ignore oversupply in previous prescription intervals. The net effect of this adjustment is that the duration

of the treatment gap is reduced. Using a simple example (Figure 8-4) where two patients are being evaluated for a 90-day period. The first patient had his/her prescription refilled on day 20 (early) and again on day 60 (late); his/her CMA and MPR would not be affected by this pattern of prescription filling (both 1.00), and his/her CMG would be 0/90 = 0.00 and the CMOS would be 0/90 = 0.00 because the oversupply (−10 days) matches the gap (+10 days).[83] However, if a second patient is evaluated for that same 90-day period and he/she refilled his/her prescription on day 40 (late) and again on day 60 (early) his/her CMG would be 10/90 = 0.11, but his/her CMOS would be 0/90 = 0.00. Even though CMG measures adjust gap measurement to adjust for oversupplies obtained in previous prescription fills (e.g., picking up a prescription before the last dose of the previous fill was consumed), the second example illustrates that the patient did not have supply on hand (surplus) when the gap occurred. The CMOS is negative, and the CMA is zero in situations where a cumulative oversupply exists.

Special Considerations of Using Administrative Claims Data to Measure Adherence and Persistence

A pharmacy claims database contains the records of thousands or more patients. However, not every patient whose data are contained within the dataset should be included in subsequent analysis. However, the decisions made at this stage can and do have an effect on the results of the study and, subsequently, how well the results will apply elsewhere (generalizability). A very basic, yet important, consideration when selecting patients for studies of adherence/persistence is whether the patient had continuous eligibility for prescription medications during the study period. Patients who fail to have prescription claims because of a change in eligibility (loss of coverage) will result in erroneous values on these measures (lower than actual).

When considering the measurement of medication utilization from administrative claims data, an important consideration is that the patients have enough data in order to make a valid inference about their utilization behavior. In addition, some of the calculations of medication adherence/persistence require at least two fills in order to calculate the measure. The calculation of medication utilization using administrative claims data is best determined across several refills. Although no hard-and-fast rule applies, it is probably best to include only patients for whom between 60 and 90 days of data are available.[84] Longer periods used for inclusion criteria, while improving the medication utilization measure, may result in too few cases remaining in the dataset for subsequent analysis.

Some studies measuring adherence/persistence with administrative claims data can use a washout period to control for experience with the drug. The washout period is a set period of time that the patient should be without treatment with the drug under investigation prior to the index date. This ensures that the patient is naïve to the medication under investigation, if that is an important consideration in the study.

Limitations of Using Administrative Claims Data to Measure Adherence and Persistence

In spite of significant advantages, the use of administrative claims data to assess medication utilization is not without limitations. Pharmacy claims records provide raw evidence of whether the patient obtained the medication; unfortunately, like other indirect measures of utilization, medication taking must be assumed. Prescription claims, therefore, provide the pharmacoepidemiology researcher only an estimate of the highest level of medication utilization.[86(p1169)] Moreover, researchers and clinicians are dependent solely on the data that is contained within the system; this information is limited to drug fills. As such, there may be discrepancies between the medical chart, pharmacy records, and verbal advice given to the patient.[85(p1169)] In other words, if a patient interview or chart review were possible, some instances of suboptimal medication utilization may be adequately explained. One such example would be medication samples (provided to the patient during the time under consideration but after first fill); the patient's utilization pattern may appear to be poor, whereas his/her actual medication utilization behavior may be "perfect." The distribution of samples will result in an MPR that is lower than actual (CMG would be higher than actual). A similar error can occur in calculations of adherence/persistence if a patient's stay in a hospital cannot be accounted for in the dataset. In situations where pharmacy claims records and other medical claims are available in the same dataset, medication utilization calculations can be adjusted for the period of hospitalization. However, in situations where the researchers possess only information about pharmacy claims, an artificially low value will be the result.

Because patients may receive prescriptions from more than one pharmacy,[85] it is best to secure data from prescription claims, rather than prescription records (available from pharmacies), if possible. It must be noted that by using a prescription claims database, the researcher will eliminate from consideration any patient without insurance (or that specific insurance) as well any data from an insured patient who chooses, for any reason, to pay for his/her prescription.

Data quality is another concern when using administrative data sets. The quantity dispensed and days supplied fields are essential to the successful use of administrative data sets to assess medication utilization; however, these fields are not always complete

CASE STUDY 8-1

Using Pharmacy Claims to Measure Adherence to Glaucoma Medications: Results from the Glaucoma Adherence and Persistence Study (GAPS)*

Data from administrative claims of more than 13,000 covered lives (available from managed care patients) and overlapping samples of patient charts and 103 physician interviews were used to determine the medication utilization behaviors of patients with glaucoma. Eligible participants needed to have a diagnosis code for open-angle glaucoma on a medical claim 6 months before their index date or 12 months after their index date. In addition, participants needed to be 40 years of age and have continuous enrollment in a health plan for 6 months prior to the index date and for at least 3 months after their index date. To assure that only newly treated patients were included in the study, participants were excluded if they had been treated with an ocular hypotensive medication during the 6 months prior to their index date (washout period), nor could they have a glaucoma-related surgical procedure during this same time.

In order to determine days supplied, using the literature, the researchers determined average bottle volume and drop count for the various glaucoma medications. MPR was the measure of medication utilization used in the study. The researchers assumed bilateral eye-drop use for all patients. The number of drops per day was determined by multiplying the daily frequency of administration by 2. Combination therapies were recognized in this study. The MPR denominator for combination therapies was the sum of the days supply for every medication in the regimen. For the measure of persistence, the permissible gap was variable (60 days for a 2.5 mL bottle, 90 days for a 5 mL bottle, and within 120 days for bottles with volumes that exceeded 5 mL). The observation period for the study was at least 1 year.

The retrospective pharmacy claims analysis of 13,956 persons found an average MPR of 0.64 (median 0.57). Only 10% of the sample had no gaps in refilling their prescriptions. Using patient interview (n = 343), it was discovered that 20% of the participants reported receiving samples on a regular basis (MPR = 62), 57% received samples 1 or 2 times (MPR = 0.64) and 23% reported never receiving samples (MPR = 0.76). Chart review (n = 300) revealed that 16.7% used the ocular hypertensive agent in only one eye.

or correct. If quantity dispensed or days supplied is unavailable or unable to be determined, the use of administrative claims data for the determination of adherence or compliance is difficult or impossible. In instances where missing or erroneous data are present, the researcher may be able to determine, using other available information (e.g., ICD-9 codes), the common directions for the drug supplied and complete or correct the days supplied field. However, it should be noted that error might be introduced if the

medication is being used off-label (e.g., frequency or indication).

Medication utilization patterns to PRN (as needed) therapies cannot be calculated accurately using prescription claims databases. In these instances, the days-supplied field may be present for the purpose of claims adjudication only, making its validity highly suspect. Other measurement considerations involve medications that are not tablets or capsules. In most cases, these products are packaged with overfill, resulting in wastage at the end of the period.[29(p7)] In addition, some patients may be able to "extract" additional doses from the overfill with the potential of creating small gaps in medication possession—methods for handling those unique measurement challenges are needed.

*Summarized from: Friedman DS, Quigley HA, Gelb L, et al. Using pharmacy claims data to study adherence to glaucoma medications: Methodology and findings of the Glaucoma Adherence and Persistency Study (GAPS). *Invest Ophthalmol Vis Sci.* 2007;48(11):5052-5057.

SUMMARY

It is clear that poor medication utilization on the part of patients reduces or negates any beneficial effects from pharmacotherapy. In addition, suboptimal medication utilization has associated with it a tremendous economic burden on the patient and society. Health care providers need to be apprised of the latest measurement possibilities and the associated strengths and weaknesses of their use. Furthermore, with the use of administrative claims databases becoming more commonplace, it is essential that pharmacoepidemiology researchers and clinicians understand the characteristics of a quality investigation. The ISPOR Compliance and Persistence Special Interest Group developed a checklist that is useful for both researchers producing these studies as well as those who are reviewing them and those consuming them (Appendix 8-1).

APPENDIX 8-1: CHECKLIST FOR ASSESSING/EVALUATING MEDICATION COMPLIANCE AND PERSISTENCE STUDIES USING RETROSPECTIVE DATABASES*

▷ Title/Abstract

- The title is descriptive and reflective of the purpose of the study.
- The abstract is a short, concise description, commensurate with the journal's standards.
- Abstract follows a structured format (as appropriate to the journal) and includes at least the following:
  - Objectives
  - Methods
  - Results
  - Conclusions

---

*Reprinted from Ref. 29 by permission of the International Society for Pharmacoeconomics and Outcomes Research. Copyright 2007. All rights reserved.

- The abstract accurately reflects the contents of the study, and there are no discrepancies.

▷ Introduction

- The author(s) clearly reviewed fundamental literature related to topic being addressed.
  - Appropriate clinical literature,
  - Appropriate compliance and persistence literature,
  - Appropriate health economic literature,
  - Other _____ (specify).
- Objective of study clearly stated.

▷ Objectives and Definitions

- The objective(s) of the study has been clearly stated and can be readily identified as one of the following:
  - Exploratory
  - Descriptive
  - Analytical
- There is an explicit definition of the compliance and persistence variable, and the definition used is based on a published, accepted definition.
- Compliance or persistence is the primary "outcome" of interest or
- Compliance or persistence is being used as an explanatory or control variable to explain variance in another outcome.

▷ Design and Methods

Design

- The design is clearly stated.
- The design matches the objectives.

Data Sources

- All of the data sources have been described adequately.
- The time frame for data has been clearly stated.
- The methods for sampling the population are well described.
- The data have been appropriately "cleaned" (i.e., erroneous data were fixed or removed).

- There is evidence for the reliability/accuracy of the data.

Inclusion/Exclusion Criteria

- The inclusion and exclusion criteria for the study are clearly stated.
- The rationale for these criteria is described.
- The method by which the researchers verified participants meeting the inclusion/exclusion criteria is stated and appropriate.
- Continuous eligibility for drug benefit during the study period was verified.
- Patients had sufficient data to make a valid estimate of compliance.
- For studies of patients who are newly initiated on a drug regimen, there was an examination of data from a sufficient preenrollment period to ensure that the participant was truly naive to the drug.
- The duration of the study period is appropriate to the objectives of the study.
- There is evidence for protecting the confidentiality of participants.
- The matching process, if appropriate to the study design, is well described.
  - Matching strategy minimizes the potential for bias.
  - Propensity scores used to control for selection bias.

Measurement of Compliance

- The methods for calculating the compliance or persistence variable are clearly described.
- The measurement matches the operational definition provided earlier.
  - Do the objectives indicate that the study is to measure compliance but persistence is actually calculated?
- Standard methods are used for calculating compliance.
  - Continuous measure of medication availability/medication possession ratio (MPR).
    - The researchers explained how they handled values greater than 1.
      - Were the values retained or converted to 1?

  - Gaps methods (continuous measure of medication gaps).
    - The researchers explained how they handled negative gap values.
    - Were the values retained or converted to 0 (no gap)?
  - Proportion of days covered.

Standard Methods for Calculating Persistence

- If an atypical method is used for calculating compliance, the rationale/formula for the new method is provided.
- The researchers provided an appropriate explanation for how patients who switched drugs within, or between, therapeutic classes were handled.
- If multiple medications were included within a single compliance or persistence estimate, the researchers provided a rationale and/or a formula for this variable.
  - The average of the MPR/gap across the different medications was used.
  - The analysis controlled for the influence of how many medications were combined into a single variable.
  - Was another variable created to indicate whether the patient was on one drug for diabetes versus multiple drugs for diabetes?
  - Is there a logical argument for combining the MPRs? It may be more appropriate to combine the MPRs for drugs that treat the same condition (e.g., combining the MPR for two drugs for diabetes) as opposed to combining the MPRs for drugs used for different conditions.

Statistical Analyses

In general, the use of continuous data to measure compliance and persistence is encouraged.

- If continuous data are converted to categorical data, the rationale for the selection of cut points should be provided and consistent with existing evidence for compliance in the selected population (e.g., cut point of 95% may be most appropriate for antiretrovirals, but 80% may be appropriate for hypertension).
- The tests are appropriate, given the objectives, design, and the nature of the data.

- Appropriate adjustments for multiple comparisons were conducted.
- Appropriate adjustments were made to the analyses if the data were not normally distributed.
- Power and/or sample size calculations are presented and appropriate.
- There was an attempt to control for selection bias (e.g., propensity scoring).
- If the researcher is evaluating an association between compliance or persistence and another variable, the researcher attempted to control for other variables that may confound the association being studied.

▶ Presentation and Discussion of Findings

Results

- The distribution of the compliance or persistence variable is presented.
- Test statistics and confidence intervals are appropriately presented in addition to P values.
- The number of participants is clearly identified in tables and graphs.
- Graphs were constructed with an appropriate scale.

Discussion/Conclusion

- The limitations are appropriately noted, and the implications of the limitations are discussed.
  - The influence of the decision to retain values or cap values is discussed.
  - Power and sample size limitations are addressed.
- The findings of this study are placed in the context of our existing knowledge of the participant.
  - Appropriate comparison of the current findings to that of similar studies is made.
- The findings and conclusions are related to the objectives of the study.

Disclosure of Potential Conflicts of Interest

- Potential conflicts of interest are disclosed.

DISCUSSION QUESTIONS

1. Compare and contrast the terms compliance, adherence, concordance, and persistence.
2. Which of these terms (*compliance, adherence, concordance,* and *persistence*) is best in terms of the measurement of suboptimal medication utilization? Why?
3. A community pharmacist wants to make compliance enhancement an integral part of the service mix at his/her pharmacy. Because he/she has access to patient pharmacy records, he/she expects that he/she can use these easily for the measurement of compliance and adherence. What cautions would you share with him/her about this technique?
4. What are the limitations of using administrative claims data for the measurement of compliance/adherence to medication regimens?
5. Define index date and period of observation.
6. Define washout period and describe the importance of using a washout period in studies of adherence/persistence using administrative claims data.
7. Using the following prescription-fill information from a patient being evaluated for 1 year, calculate CMA, PDC, CMG, and CMOS.

Fill #	Fill date	Days supplied
1	0	30
2	30	30
3	63	30
4	108	30
5	148	30
6	183	30
7	218	30
8	235	30
9	328	30
10	365	30

8. In light of the results of the case study presented, what comments do you have about the use of administrative claims data to measure compliance/adherence?

REFERENCES

1. Koop CE. *Keynote Address. Improving Medication Compliance: Proceedings of a Symposium. 1985*. Reston, VA: National Pharmaceutical Council, 1985:1-4.

2. Stone GC. Patient compliance and the role of the expert. *J Soc Issues*. 1979;35(1):34-59.

3. Epstein LH, Cluss PA. A behavioral medicine perspective on adherence to long-term medical regimens. *J Consult Clin Psychol*. 1982;50(6):950-971.

4. Hatoum HT, Valuck RJ. Drug use and the health care system. In: Knowlton CH, Penna RP, eds. *Pharmaceutical Care*. New York: Chapman & Hall, 1996:68-94.

5. Bond WS Hussar DA. Detection methods and strategies for improving medication compliance. *Am J Hosp Pharm*. 1991;48(9):1978-1988.

6. Berg JS, Dischler J, Wagner DJ, Raia JJ, Palmer-Shevlin N. Medication compliance: A healthcare problem. *Ann Pharmacother*. 1993;27(suppl 9):S1-S24.

7. Strandberg L. Drugs as a reason for nursing home admissions. *J Am Health Care Assoc*. 1982;10(4):20-23.

8. Sullivan SD, Kreling DH, Hazlet TK. "Noncompliance to medication regimens and subsequent hospitalizations: A literature analysis and cost of hospitalization estimate," *J Res Pharm Econ*. 1990;2(2):19-33.

9. Prince BS, Goetz CM, Rihn TL, Olsky M. Drug-related emergency department visits and hospital admissions. *Am J Hosp Pharm*. 1992;49:1696-1700.

10. Dennehy CE, Kishi DT, Louie C. Drug-related illness in emergency department patients. *Am J Health Syst Pharm*. 1996;53:1422-1426.

11. Schneitman-McIntire O, Farnen T, Gordon N, Chan J, Toy WA. Medication midadventures resulting in emergency department visits at an HMO medical center. *Am J Health Syst Pharm*. 1996;53:1416-1422.

12. Patel P, Zed PJ. Drug-related visits to the emergency department: How big is the problem? *Pharmacotherapy*. 2002;22(7):915-923.

13. Sokol MC, McGuigan KA, Verbrugge RR, Epstein RS. Impact of medication adherence on hospitalization risk and healthcare cost. *Med Care*. 2005;43(6):521-530.

14. Simpson SH, Eurich DT, Majumdar SR, et al. A meta-analysis of the association between adherence to drug therapy and mortality. *Br Med J*. 2006;333:15-18.

15. Falvo DR. *Effective Patient Education: A Guide to Increased Compliance*, 3rd ed. Sudbury, MA: Jones & Bartlett Publishers, 2004.

16. Koltun A, Stone GC. Past and current trends in patient noncompliance research: Focus on diseases, regimens-programs, and provider-disciplines. *J Compliance Health Care*. 1986;1(1):21-32.

17. National Council of Patient Information and Education. 2007. *Enhancing Prescription Adherence: A National Action Plan*. Bethesda, MD: National Council of Patient Information & Education, 2007.

18. Krueger KP, Berger BA, Felkey B. Medication adherence and persistence: A comprehensive review. *Adv Ther*. 2005;22(4):313-356.

19. Gordis L. Methodologic issues in the measurement of patient compliance. In: Sackett DL, Haynes RB, eds. *Compliance with Therapeutic Regimens*. Baltimore, MD: The Johns Hopkins University Press, 1976:51-66.

20. Dirks JF, Kinsman RA. Nondichotomous patterns of medication usage: The yes-no fallacy. *Clin Pharmacol Ther*. 1982;31(4):413-417.

21. Cramer JA, Roy A, Burrell A, et al. Medication compliance and persistence: Terminology and definitions. *Value Health*. 2008;11(1):44-47.

22. Lutfey KE, Wishner WJ. Beyond "compliance": Is "adherence" improving the prospect of diabetes care. *Diabetes Care*. 1999;22(4):635-639.

23. Haynes RB. Introduction. In: Haynes RB, Taylor DW, Sackett DL, eds. *Compliance in Health Care*. Baltimore, MD: The Johns Hopkins University Press, 1979:1-7.

24. Turk DC, Salovey P, Litt MD. Adherence: A cognitive-behavioral perspective. In: Gerber KE, Nehemkis AM, eds. *Compliance: The Dilemma of the Chronically Ill*. New York, NY: Springer Publishing Company, 1986:44-72.

25. Royal Pharmaceutical Society of Great Britain. 2007. *From Compliance to Concordance: Achieving Shared Goals in Medicine Taking*. London: Royal Pharmaceutical Society of Great Britain, 2007.

26. Cushing A, Metcalfe R. Optimizing medicines management: Form compliance to concordance. *Ther Clin Risk Manag*. 2007;3(6):1047-1058.

27. Sackett DL. Introduction. In: Sackett DL, Haynes RB, eds. *Compliance with Therapeutic Regimens*. Baltimore, MD: The Johns Hopkins University Press, 1976:1-6.

28. Caetano PA, Lam JC, Morgan SG. Toward a standard definition and measurement of persistence with drug therapy: Examples from research on statin and antihypertensive utilization. *Clin Ther*. 2006;28(9):1411-1424.

29. Peterson AM, Nau DP, Cramer, JA, Benner J, Gwadry-Sridhar F, Nichol M. A checklist for medication compliance and persistence studies using retrospective databases. *Value Health*. 2007;10(1):3-12.

30. Spilker B. Methods of assessing and improving patient compliance in clinical trials. In: Cramer JA, Spilker B, eds. *Patient Compliance in Medical Practice and Clinical Trials*. New York: Raven Press, 1991:37-56.

31. Osterberg L, Blaschke T. Adherence to medication. *N Engl J Med*. 2005;353(5):487-497.

32. Fincham JE, Wertheimer AI. "Elderly patient initial noncompliance: The drugs and reasons," *J Geriatr Drug Ther*. 1988;2(4):53-62.

33. McCaffrey III DJ, Smith MC, Banahan III BF, Juergens JP, Szeinbach SL. The financial implications of initial noncompliance: An investigation of unclaimed prescriptions in community pharmacies. *J Res Pharm Econ*. 1995;6(1):39-64.

34. Kennedy J, Tuleu I, Mackay K. Unfilled prescriptions of medicare beneficiaries: Prevalence, reasons, and types of medicines prescribed. *J Manag Care Pharm*. 2008;14(6):553-560.

35. McCaffrey III DJ, Smith MC, Banahan III BF, Frate DA, Gilbert FW. A continued look into the financial implications of initial noncompliance in community pharmacies: An unclaimed prescription audit pilot. *J Res Pharm Econ*. 1998;9(2):33-57.

36. Hill Z, Kendall C, Fernandez M. Patterns of adherence to anti-retrovirals: Why adherence has no simple measure. *AIDS Patient Care STDs*. 2003;17(10):519-525.

37. Kruse W. Patient compliance with drug treatment—new perspectives on an old problem. *Clin Investig*. 1992;70:163-166.

38. DiMatteo MR, Giordani PJ, Lepper HS, Croghan TW. Patient adherence and medical treatment outcomes: A meta-analysis. *Med Care*. 2002;40(2):794-811.

39. DiMatteo. Variations in patients' adherence to medical recommendations: A quantitative review of 50 years of research. *Med Care*. 2004;42(3):200-209.

40. Melnikow J, Kiefe C. Patient compliance and medical research: Issues in methodology. *J Gen Intern Med*. 1994;9(2):96-105.

41. Rand CS. "I took the medicine like you told me, doctor": Self-report of adherence with medical regimens. In: Stone AA, Turkkan JS, Bachrach C, Jobe JB, Kurtzman HS, Cain VS, eds. *The Science of Self-Report: Implications for Research and Practice. 1999*. Mahwah, NJ: Lawrence Erlbaum Associates, 1999.

42. Weis SE, Slocum PC, Blais FX, et al. The effect of directly observed therapy on the rates of drug resistance and relapse in tuberculosis. *New N Engl J Med*. 1994;330(17):1179-1184.

43. Farmer KC. Methods for measuring and monitoring medication regimen adherence in clinical trials and clinical practice. *Clin Ther*. 1999;21(6):1074-1090.

44. Feinstein AR. One white-coat effects and the electronic monitoring of compliance. *Arch Intern Med*. 1990;150(7):1377-1378.

45. Cramer JA, Scheyer RD, Mattson RH. Compliance declines between clinic visits. *Arch Intern Med*. 1990;150(7):1509-1510.

46. Fletcher SW, Pappius EM, Harper SJ. Measurement of medication compliance in a clinical setting: Comparison of three methods in patients prescribed digoxin. *Arch Intern Med*. 1979;139(6):635-638.

47. Rapoff MA, Barnard MU. Compliance with pediatric medical regimens. In: Cramer JA, Spilker B, eds. *Patient Compliance in Medical Practice and Clinical Trials. 1991*. New York, NY: Raven Press, 1991.

48. Sudman S, Bradburn NM. *Asking Questions: A Guide to Questionnaire Design. 1982*. San Francisco, CA: Jossey-Bass Inc., Publishers, 1982.

49. Dillman DA, Smyth JD, Christian LM. *Internet, Mail and Mixed Mode Surveys: The Tailored Design Method*, 3rd ed. Hoboken, NJ: John Wiley and Sons, Inc., 2009.

50. Morisky DE, Green LW, Levine DM. Concurrent and predictive validity of a self-reported measure of medication adherence. *Med Care*. 1986;24(1):67-74.

51. Krapek K, King K, Warren SS, et al. Medication adherence and associated hemoglobin a1 c in type 2 diabetes. *Ann Pharmacother*. 2004;38(9):1357-1362.

52. Brooks CM, Richards JM, Kohler CL, et al. Assessing adherence to asthma medication and inhaler regimens: A psychometric analysis of adult self-report scales. *Med Care*. 1994;32(3):298-307.

53. Morisky DR, Ang A, Krousel-Wood M, Ward HJ. Predictive validity of a medication adherence measure in an outpaitent setting. *J Clin Hypertens*. 2008;10(5):348-354.

54. Svarstad BL, Chewning BA, Sleth BL, Claesson C. The brief medicaiton questionnaire: A tool for screening patient adherence and barriers to adherence. *Patient Educ Couns*. 1999;37(2);113-124.

55. Hahn SR, Park J, Skinner EP, et al. Development of the ASK-20 adherence barrier survey. *Curr Med Res Opin*. 2008;24(7):2127-2138.

56. Matza LS, Park J, Coyne KS, Skinner EP, Malley KG, Wolever RQ. Derivation and validation of the ASK-12 adherence barrier survey. *Ann Pharmacother*. 2009;43(10):1621-1630.

57. Stone AA, Shiffman S, Schwartz JE, Broderick JE, Hufford MR. Patient Compliance with Paper and Electronic Diaries. *Control Clin Trials*. 2003;24(2):182–99.

58. Goldberg AI, Cohen G, Rubin AE. Physician assessment of patient compliance with medical treatment. *Soc Sci Med*. 1998;47(11):1873-1876.

59. Miller LG, Liu H, Hays R, et al. How well do clinicians estimate patients' adherence to combination antiretroviral therapy? *J Gen Intern Med*. 2002;17(1):1-11.

60. Bangsberg DR, Hecht FM, Clague H, et al. Provider assessment of adherence to HIV antiretroviral therapy. *J Acquir Immune Defic Syndr*. 2001;26(5):435-442.

61. Murri R, Antinori A, Ammassari A, et al. Physician estimates of adherence and the patient-physician relationship as a setting to improve adherence to antiretroviral therapy. *J Acquir Immune Defic Syndr*. 2002;31:S1568-S162.

62. Hess LM, Saboda K, Malone DC, Salasche Warneke J, Alberts DS. Adherence assessment using medication weight in a phase iib clinical trial of difluoromethylornithine for the chemoprevention of skin cancer. *Cancer Epidemiol Biomarkers Prev*. 2005;14(11):2579-2583.

63. Rand CS, Wise RA. Measuring adherence to asthma medication regimens. *Am J Respir Crit Care Med*. 1994;149(2):569-576.

64. Burke LE. Electronic Measurement. In: Burke LE, Ockene IS, eds. *Compliance in Healthcare and Research. 2001*. Armonk, NY: Futura Publishing Company, Inc., 2001.

65. Cramer JA. Microelectronic systems for monitoring and enhancing patient compliance with medication regimens. *Drugs*. 1995;49(3):321-327.

66. Stewart DW, Kamins MA. *Secondary Research: Information Sources and Methods*, 2nd ed. Thousand Oaks, CA: Sage Publications. 1993.

67. Crystal S, Akincigil A, Bilder S, Walkup JT. Studying prescription drug use and outcomes with medicaid data: Strengths, limitations, and strategies. *Med Care*. 2007;45(suppl. 10):S58-S65.

68. Sorensen HT, Sabroe S, Olsen J. A framework for evaluation of secondary data sources for epidemiological research. *Int J Epidemiol*. 1996;25(2):435-442.

69. Andrade SE, Kahler KH, Frech F, Chan KA. Methods for evaluation of medication adherence and persistence using automated databases. *Pharmacoepidemiol Drug Saf*. 2006;15(8)565-574.

70. Yeaw J, Benner JS, Walt JG, Sian S, Smith DB. Comparing adherence and persistence across 6 chronic medication classes. *J Manag Care Pharm*. 2009;15(9):728-740.

71. Briesacher BA, Andrade SE, Fouayzi H, Chan KA. Comparison of drug adherence rates among patients with seven different medical conditions. *Pharmacotherapy*. 2008;28(4): 437-443.

72. Huybrechts K, Ishak K, Caro J. Assessment of compliance with osteoporosis treatment and its consequences in a managed care population. *Bone*. 2006;38(6):922-928.

73. Monance M, Bohn RL, Gurwitz JH, Glynn RJ, Levin R, Avorn J. Compliance with antihypertensive therapy among elderly medicaid enrollees: The roles of age, gender, and race. *Am J Public Health*. 1996;86(12):1805-1808.

74. Pladevall M, Williams LK, Potts LA, Divine G, Xi H, Lafata JE. Clinical outcomes and adherence to medications measured by claims data in patients with diabetes. *Diabetes Care*. 2004; 27(12):2800-2805.

75. Weiden PJ, Cozma C, Grogg A, Locklear J. Partial compliance and risk of rehospitalization among california medicaid patients with schizophrenia. *Psychiatr Serv*. 2004;55(8):886-891.

76. Steiner JF, Prochazka AV. The assessment of refill compliance using pharmacy records: Methods, validity, and applications. *J Clin Epidemiol*. 1997;50(1):105-116.

77. Karve S, Cleves M, Helm M, Hudson T, West DS, Martin BC. Good and poor adherence: Optimal cut-point for adherence measures using administrative claims data. *Curr Med Res Opin*. 2009;25(9):2303-2310.

78. Sikka R, Xia F, Aubert RE. Estimating medication persistency using administrative claims data. *Am J Manag Care*. 2005; 11(7):449-457

79. Karve S, Cleves MA, Helm M, Hudson TJ, West DS, Martin BC. Prospective validation of eight different adherence measures for use with administrative claims data among patients with schizophrenia. *Value Health*. 2009;12(6):989-995.

80. Hess LM, Raebel MA, Conner DA, Malone DC. Measure of adherence in pharmacy administrative databases: a proposal for standard definitions and preferred measures. *Ann Pharmacother*. 2006;40(7-8):1280-1288.

81. Vink NM, Klungel OH, Stolk RP, Denig P. Comparison of various measures for assessing medication refill adherence using prescription data. *Pharmacoepidemiol Drug Saf*. 2009;18(2): 159-165.

82. Martin BC, Wiley-Exley EK, Richards S, Domino ME, Carey TS, Sleath BL. Contrasting measures of adherence with simple drug use, medication switching, and therapeutic duplication. *Ann Pharmacother*. 2009;43(1):36-44.

83. Morningstar BA, Sketris IS, Kephart GC, Sclar DA. Variation in pharmacy prescription measures by type of oral antihyperglycemic drug therapy in seniors in nova scotia, canada. *J Clin Pharm Ther*. 2002;27(3):213-220.

84. Christensen DB, Williams B, Goldberg HI, Martin DP, Engelberg R, LoGerfo JP. Assessing compliance to antihypertensive medications using computer-based pharmacy records. *Med Care*. 1997;35(11):1164-1170.

85. Polinski JM, Schneeweiss S, Levin R, Shrank WH. Completeness of retail pharmacy claims data: Implications for pharmacoepidemiologic studies and pharmacy practice in elderly patients. *Clin Ther*. 2009;31(9):2048-2059.

Medication Safety and Pharmacovigilance

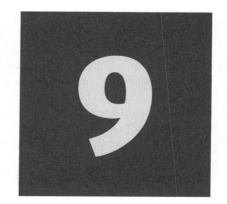

Benjamin F. Banahan III

INTRODUCTION

Pharmacovigilance is the science relating to the detection, assessment, and prevention of adverse effects of medicines. As such, pharmacovigilance is primarily involved in the identification and evaluation of safety signals that are identified for drug products. Proper management of drug safety risks has always been a major concern in health care systems worldwide and among pharmaceutical manufacturers. In fact, major drug safety events have served as the stimuli for many of the major changes that have occurred in drug regulation in the United States and other countries. As a result, drug regulations have evolved over time to address our growing understanding of drug safety and the evolution of the pharmaceutical industry. During the past few decades it has been stated that a

paradigm shift has occurred in the assessment and management of patient-related drug safety. Some of these changes, especially the most recent, have resulted in a significant increase in the importance of pharmacoepidemiology and its use in pharmacovigilance.

Some of the major changes during the past few decades have included:

- An evolution of the drug market from short-duration-use products used to treat acute diseases to long-term-use products for the treatment of chronic diseases.

- A change in attitude by regulators and industry from pre- and post-marketing safety assessment being viewed as separate activities to the assessment of product safety being a continuous process that starts early in product development and continues throughout the life of a marketed product.

- A shift from postmarketing safety assessment relying almost solely on individual case reports from practitioners and clinical trials to a modern system using large quantities of information collected by a number of different computerized systems (i.e., administrative claims data, electronic medical records) for both active surveillance and evaluation of safety signals.

- An increased use of retrospective pharmacoepidemiologic studies to evaluate safety signals.

- Increased prescription product litigation and the need to better manage the understanding of drug risks by practitioners and the public.

As a result of these changes and the possible paradigm shift, pre- and post-marketing safety surveillance, which were once viewed as separate activities, are now viewed as a continuum of "risk management" activities for pharmaceutical manufacturers, drug safety regulators, and health care providers. In the United States, assuring the safety of drug products is the responsibility of the Food and Drug Administration (FDA). According to the FDA Guidances for Industry,[1] risk management is an iterative process designed to optimize the benefit–risk balance for regulated prescription drug products. A brief history of drug regulation in the United States is provided later in this chapter that illustrates how the authority of the FDA has expanded over time and how current regulations have evolved to address the need to continuously assess drug safety throughout the life cycle of a drug product.

It is important to note that all drugs have some risks and that FDA approval of a new drug entering the market is based on an evaluation of the relative benefits of the drug compared to the risks of the condition and all currently available treatment options. Ideally, the FDA, manufacturers, and practitioners would find ways to treat medical conditions and diseases without the treatment posing any risk; however, this is seldom, if ever, the case. Therefore, the realistic goal in regulating pharmaceutical products is to approve only products that are believed to provide greater treatment benefit than risk and to monitor the safety of these products as new information is gathered continuously to assess this benefit–risk balance. Although pharmacoepidemiology studies can contribute to the assessment of premarket safety, their primary value is in postmarket evaluation of safety and the continuous monitoring and assessment of the benefit–risk balance of marketed products.

This chapter provides an overview of the terminology used in drug safety evaluation, the history of the FDA and U.S. drug regulation regarding safety and efficacy, and a discussion of how pharmacoepidemiology is used in the United States and other countries to monitor drug safety of marketed products.

THE TERMINOLOGY OF DRUG SAFETY

There have been a variety of terms and definitions used to describe, discuss, and regulate drug safety over the years. The similarity between many of the terms and the casual use of these terms, as if they are truly interchangeable, can result in confusion. Sometimes, the differences in terms simply has to do with the point of view being expressed. For example, the terms "adverse reaction" and "adverse effects" refer to the same phenomenon. *Adverse effect* is describing the phenomenon from the perspective of the drug—the drug causes an effect. The term *adverse reaction* is viewing the phenomenon from the point of view of the patient—the patient has a reaction to the drug.

The key terms that are important for practitioners to understand are described in this section. For a more comprehensive review of the terminology used in this area, the reader is referred to the article "Clarification of Terminology in Drug Safety," published by Aronson and Ferner in 2005.* The "official" and accepted definitions used in the United States and most developed countries for the key terms (adverse event and adverse reaction) are based on the International Conference on Harmonization (ICH) Guidelines.[2] The ICH definitions were developed with input from more than 30 Collaborating Centers of the World Health Organization (WHO)

---

*Aronson JK, Ferner RE. Clarification of terminology in drug safety. *Drug Saf.* 2005;28(10):861-870.

International Drug Monitoring Centre (Uppsala, Sweden).

Safety Signals

As mentioned in the introduction of this chapter, pharmacovigilance primarily involves the identification and evaluation of safety signals. An enormous effort is made to collect adverse event data by pharmaceutical manufacturers, government agencies, and others. However, the collection of these data is meaningless without a systematic method for organizing and analyzing the data in order to detect potential safety problems that were previously unknown.

The FDA defines a *safety signal* as "a concern about an excess of adverse events compared to what would be expected to be associated with a product's use."[1] Safety signals are reported information on a possible causal relationship between a drug and an adverse event when the relationship has previously been unknown or incompletely documented.

Safety signals are looked for in multiple ways. The oldest method is a passive approach that relies on the collection of spontaneous adverse event reports by pharmaceutical manufacturers, government health authorities (the FDA in the United States), or third-party organizations (academic centers, medical registries, etc.). These spontaneously generated reports are then reviewed to identify "striking," "unusual," or "unexpected" adverse events. Obviously this technique relies heavily on the good will and astuteness of the reporting physicians, nurses, pharmacists, and patients to send in notifications about adverse event reports and the competence of the data analysts reviewing the information. This technique is time consuming and labor intensive, but with good reporting by practitioners and patients and competent reviewers, the system has proven to be effective at identifying major problems and remains the cornerstone of signal generation and identification in the United States and in many countries around the world. Cobert[3] provides a detailed discussion of the generation and evaluation of safety signals in the book, *Manual of Drug Safety and Pharmacovigilance*. His list of the criteria that make spontaneous adverse event reports more sensitive or less sensitive when reviewed is provided in Table 9-1.

With the growth in available secondary data sources, especially large integrated administrative claims databases like those described in Chapter 4, active surveillance systems are being developed. Active surveillance systems use existing databases and various statistical techniques to identify safety signals that require further evaluation.

In pharmacovigilance, signals indicate the need for further investigation, which may or may not lead to the conclusion that the product caused the event. Safety signals that the FDA believes may warrant further investigation are listed in Table 9-2. Pharmacoepidemiology methods and statistical techniques play an important role in generating safety signals in active surveillance systems and in evaluating safety signals once they have been detected.

Adverse Events

Adverse events are unintended "bad things" that occur when taking a drug that may or may not be due to the drug itself. The ICH defines an *adverse event* as "any untoward medical occurrence in a patient or clinical investigation subject administered a pharmaceutical product and which does not necessarily have to have a causal relationship with this treatment."[1] As described in Chapter 1, practitioners and even patients are asked to spontaneously report adverse events through the FDA MedWatch program, and manufacturers are required to report serious adverse events to the FDA. It is important to note that adverse events are expected to be spontaneously reported to the FDA, even though they may not be caused by the drug product. The FDA then provides analysis of the adverse event reports received to determine whether a safety signal exists that warrants further investigation.

Adverse Drug Reactions

An adverse drug reaction (ADR) is an adverse event in which there is reasonable possibility of a causal relationship between the drug use and the event. The term ADR is slowly being replaced by the more precise term of *suspected adverse drug reaction* (SADR). The FDA and the ICH define a suspected adverse drug reaction as "a noxious and unintended response to any dose of a drug or biologic product for which there is a reasonable possibility that the product caused the response."[2] Further complicating the matter is the often interchangeable use of the terms ADR and SADR.

Table 9-1. Characteristics of adverse event reports that affect sensitiveness as safety signals*

Characteristics Making a Report More Sensitive:

1. The signal is very unusual and rarely seen in general (e.g., aplastic anemia).
2. The signal is rarely seen with that drug class (e.g., pulmonary fibrosis with beta-blockers—practolol).
3. The signal is rarely seen in that cohort of patients (e.g., cataracts in young nondiabetic patients).
4. The signal is fatal, particularly in patients groups who classically do not have high mortality rates (e.g., deaths in 20-year-olds).
5. The signal is expected to be seen because it has been reported in other drugs in the same class (e.g., rhabdomyolysis with a new statin).
6. The signal is expected because it is due to an exaggeration of the drug's pharmacologic effect (e.g., fainting in patients taking an antihypertensive).
7. The adverse event in question is seen almost exclusively with drugs (e.g., fixed drug reactions).
8. The causality is crystal clear (e.g., the tablet is large and sticky and gets stuck in the oral pharynx, producing obstruction, or immediate swelling and itching is seen at the site of a drug being injected).
9. No other drugs are being taken by the patient(s) in question.
10. The drug is being taken for a short time, and there are no or few confounders.
11. The patients are otherwise healthy and have no other medical problems beyond the one being treated with the drug in question.
12. There is a positive rechallenge (reaction reappears upon drug reintroduction after a positive dechallenge).

Characteristics Making a Report Less Sensitive:

1. The signal has a high background incidence in the general population (e.g., headaches, fatigue).
2. The signal has a high background incidence in the population being treated (e.g., myocardial infarction in elderly hypertensives).
3. The signal represents a worsening of the problem being treated (i.e., fialuridine producing worsening and fatal hepatitis in patients being treated for hepatitis).
4. The patients are taking multiple drugs (polypharmacy, intensive care unit).
5. The patients have major underlying medical problems producing disease, signs, and symptoms (e.g., oncology patients).
6. The drug is taken chronically, and many intercurrent illnesses and problems occur over time (confounders).
7. There is a negative dechallenge (reaction continues even after stopping drug), or the drug in question is not stopped in the patient and the adverse event disappears by itself anyway.

*Reprinted from: Cobert B. *Manual of Drug Safety and Pharmacovigilance.* Sudbury, MA: Jones & Bartlett Learning; 2007:46-47. www.jblearning.com. Reprinted with permission.

▶ The Classification of Adverse Drug Reactions

As with the terms used to describe different drug safety phenomenon, the terms used to classify SADRs have also evolved over time with only limited consensus at this point. Two systems that are used to classify SADRs are described below.

A/B Alphabetic Classification

In 1977, Rawlins and Thompson[4] suggested a division into two types of adverse drug reactions based on the relationship to dosing or cause. The initial types were labeled as type A, reactions that were predictable and dose related, and type B, reactions that were not predictable and not dose related. In order to

Table 9-2. Safety signals that may warrant further investigation by the FDA*

1. New unlabeled adverse events, especially if serious.
2. An apparent increase in the severity of a labeled event.
3. Occurrence of serious events thought to be extremely rare in the general population.
4. New product–product, product–device, product–food, or product–dietary supplement interactions.
5. Identification of a previously unrecognized at-risk population (e.g., populations with specific racial or genetic predispositions or comorbidities).
6. Confusion about a product's name, labeling, packaging, or use.
7. Concerns arising from the way a product is used (e.g., adverse events seen at higher than labeled doses or in populations not recommended for treatment).
8. Concerns arising from potential inadequacies of a currently implemented risk minimization action plan (e.g., reports of serious adverse events that appear to reflect failure of a RiskMAP goal).
9. Other concerns identified by the sponsor (*manufacturer*) or FDA.

*Source: *Guidance for Industry: Good Pharmacovigilance Practices and Pharmacoepidemiologic Assessment.* US Food and Drug Administration, 2005. www.fda.gov/downloads/Regulatory Information/Guidances/UCM126834.pdf. Accessed December 5, 2009.

make it easier to remember what each type was, Rawlins and Thompson invented a mnemonic in 1981—they called type A "augmented" and type B "bizarre."[5] In spite of the limitations of the A/B classification scheme, this classification system has persisted and has been expanded by several authors over the past few decades to address insufficiencies in the initial A/B categories. The current A/B classification system includes the following categories:

- Type A: augmented pharmacologic effects—dose dependent and predictable
- Type B: bizarre effects (or idiosyncratic)—dose independent and unpredictable
- Type C: chronic effects—long-term and continuous
- Type D: delayed effects
- Type E: end-of-treatment effects—includes withdrawal
- Type F: failure of therapy
- Type G: genetic/genomic

The Dose, Time, and Susceptibility (DoTS) Classification

The B portion of the A/B classification assumes that there are adverse events that are not dose related. However, as Aronson and Ferner[6] argue, "it is a basic pharmacological principle that effects of drugs involve interactions between chemical entities and are, therefore, subject to chemical laws, including the law of mass action. This implies that all drug effects, beneficial or adverse, including immunological reactions, are dose-related." For this reason, they proposed the dose, time, and susceptibility (DoTS) classification of adverse reactions.[7] This classification scheme considers the dose or concentration at which the adverse event occurs, the time in the course of therapy, and the susceptibility of the patient affected. A brief overview of the DoTS classification is provided below.

Relation to dose—In the A/B classification, type B reactions are defined as "totally aberrant effects that are not to be expected from the known pharmacological actions of a drug when given in the usual therapeutic doses,"[8] However, the concept of a usual therapeutic dose is flawed since (a) there is often wide variability in responsiveness to a given dose of a drug, (b) for some drugs the usual dose varies by indication, and (c) dose responsiveness can change from time to time, even in the same individual. Considering that all adverse drug events are related to the use of a specific drug, there is always some relationship to dose. The dose component of the DoTS classification is designed to take into account the fact that the active concentration of a drug may vary, even when the absolute dose is held constant, and that adverse events can occur even at subtherapeutic exposure to drugs. Aronson and Ferner proposed that the dose component of adverse event classification should be based on the therapeutic concentration in an individual at which the event occurs. The three proposed classification types are:

- Toxic effects: adverse effects that occur at supratherapeutic concentrations.
- Collateral effects: adverse effects that occur at standard therapeutic concentrations.
- Hypersusceptibility reactions: adverse reactions that occur at subtherapeutic doses in susceptible patients.

The term "side effects" is often used to refer to what Aronson and Ferner have labeled "collateral effects." The use of the term "side effects" can result in significant confusion, especially when discussing drug safety. The term "side effects" is most often used to reference all adverse effects associated with a drug. However, the WHO definition says that a side effect "is related to the pharmacological properties of the drug."[9] The ICH guidelines point out that the "term 'side effect' has been used in various ways in the past, usually to describe negative (unfavourable) effects, but also positive (favourable) effects."[2] The guidelines recommend that this term no longer be used and it specifically should not be considered to be synonymous with adverse event or adverse reaction.

Relation to time—In addition to their relationship with dose measure, adverse events can be classified on the basis of the relationship of the event to the time during a course of therapy. Aronson and Ferner have proposed the following classifications for time relatedness:

• Time-independent reactions occur at any time during a course of therapy (e.g., amount being administered changes due to a pharmaceutical formulation, concentration at site of action changes due to a pharmacokinetic mechanism such as digoxin toxicity with worsening renal function, pharmacological response is altered by a pharmacodynamic mechanism such as digoxin toxicity with potassium depletion).

• Time-dependent reactions are classified on the basis of the point at which they occur in the course of therapy. Six subtypes have been proposed:

  – Rapid reactions occur when a drug is administered too rapidly and are typically toxic reactions (e.g., red man syndrome with vancomycin[10]).

  – First-dose reactions occur after the first dose and not necessarily thereafter. They are typically hypersusceptibility reactions (e.g., hypotension after the first dose of an angiotensin converting enzyme inhibitor[11]).

  – Early reactions occur early in treatment and then abate with continuing treatment. These are typically collateral effects to which patients develop tolerance (e.g., nitrate-induced headache).

  – Intermediate reactions occur after some delay; however, during long-term therapy the risk of such a reaction falls over time. These can be collateral or hypersusceptibility reactions (e.g., thrombocytopenia due to quinine, ampicillin/amoxicillin pseudoallergic rash[12]).

  – Late reactions occur rarely or not at all initially with use of the drug, but the risk increases with continued or repeated exposure, such as late reactions like tardive dyskinesia with dopamine receptor antagonists. This classification includes withdrawal reactions (e.g., opiate and benzodiazepine withdrawal syndromes).

  – Delayed reactions are observed some time after exposure, even if use of the drug has ceased before the reaction appears. These are typically collateral reactions (e.g., vaginal adenocarcinoma in women whose mothers took diethylstilbestrol during pregnancy; phocomelia due to thalidomide).

Susceptibility factors—The final component of the DoTS classification system is susceptibility. The idea that adverse drug reaction classification should include susceptibility factors is because the risk of an adverse reaction can differ for different members of an exposed population. In this context, susceptibility refers to the proneness of an individual to have an adverse reaction. As described previously in this chapter, hypersusceptibility reactions are those that occur at subtherapeutic dosage levels in hypersusceptible patients.

The actual reasons for hypersusceptibility are not always known or understood, but there are several clear types of hypersusceptibility population subgroups that are known to exist for some drugs. These include the following:

• Genetic factors

• Age

• Sex

• Physiological factors (e.g., pregnancy)

• Endogenous factors (e.g., other drugs and foods)

• Diseases

The advantage of using the concept of susceptibility is that the term "hypersusceptibility" is a general term that can be used appropriately to describe an individual's increased susceptibility to an adverse reaction. Similar terms that have been used by other authors to describe these types of events are idiosyncrasy, hypersensitivity, and intolerance. Each of these terms has limitations and multiple meanings that restrict their ability to describe adequately the specific type of adverse event included in this category.

▶ Seriousness and Severity of Adverse Drug Reactions

Other criteria used to classify adverse drug reactions are the seriousness and severity of the reaction. In the United Kingdom, prescribers are asked to report all suspected adverse reactions to new and some intensely monitored drug products and all "serious" suspected reactions to established drugs. In the United States, the FDA requests that practitioners and patients voluntarily report serious suspected adverse events directly to the FDA or indirectly through the manufacturer. Since "serious" adverse events are supposed to be reported, it is important that we have clear definitions of seriousness. Although the terms "seriousness" and "severity" are similar, it is important to note that, in the context of drug safety, they refer to two distinctly different concepts.

Seriousness of an adverse drug event is the extent to which the reaction can or does cause harm. The FDA defines a serious adverse drug event to be any untoward medical occurrence where the patient outcome is one of the following,

- Death
- Life threatening
- Hospitalization (initial or prolonged)
- Disability
- Congenital anomaly
- Requires medical or surgical intervention to preclude permanent impairment or damage

Severity (or intensity) of an adverse drug event is a measure of the extent to which the adverse event develops in an individual. A severe reaction is not always serious. For example, discoloration of the urine by refampicin, even if very pronounced (severe) would not be considered serious.

MONITORING DRUG SAFETY

A primary mission of the Center for Drug Evaluation and Research (CDER) of the FDA is the review and approval for marketing of drug and biologic products. As previously stated in this chapter, current FDA approval of a new drug for marketing in the United States is based on an evaluation of the relative benefits compared to the risks of the condition and the currently available treatment options. The current level of regulatory authority granted to the FDA has evolved over the past century. Many of the major expansions of the FDA's regulatory authority and responsibility have come as the result of major safety problems that have occurred with pharmaceutical products. A brief history of the FDA is provided in the following section. A more detailed history is available at the FDA Web site.[13]

▶ Evolving Role of the FDA in Monitoring Drug Safety

The history of the FDA includes several major changes to their authorizing legislation that address the evolving view of their role in drug product regulation. In 1906, the Food and Drug Act was initially signed into law. The act prohibited, under penalty of seizure of goods, the interstate transport of "adulterated" drugs. Adulterated drugs were considered to be products for which the standard of strength, quality, or purity of the active ingredient was either not stated clearly on the label or listed in the U.S. Pharmacopoeia or the National Formulary. The initial act also banned the misbranding of drugs.

Initial responsibility for enforcing the act was given to the U.S. Department of Agriculture (USDA) Bureau of Chemistry. When the department tried to aggressively target drugs with false claims of therapeutic equivalency, a 1911 Supreme Court decision ruled that the 1906 Act did not grant the FDA this authority. In response, a 1912 amendment added "false and fraudulent" claims of "curative or therapeutic effect" to the act's definition of "misbranded." The major focus at this time was to assure basic levels of accuracy in labeling and product quality. During this period, drug safety and efficacy as we know them today were not regulated. This early incarnation of the FDA had the authority to regulate misbranding of drugs, but their powers were very limited by the court's interpretation that it was the burden of the FDA to prove that claims were fraudulent.

It was not until 1927 that the Bureau of Chemistry's regulatory powers were reorganized under a new USDA Food, Drug, and Insecticide organization. Three years later the name was shortened to the current name of Food and Drug Administration (FDA).

As more and more pharmaceutical products were being developed, there was increased public outcry for stronger regulatory authority. Even with considerable publicity about injurious products and worthless cures, initial attempts in the early 1930s to pass stronger FDA regulations failed. However, following the 1937 Elixir Sulfanilamide tragedy (see Case Study 9-2—Sulfanilamide Disaster), the 1938 amendments to the Food and Drug Act were quickly passed. The new legislation significantly increased the federal regulatory authority over drugs by granting a variety of new powers to the FDA. Under the 1938 amendments, the FDA could require a premarket review of the safety of all new drugs, ban false therapeutic claims in drug labeling, or inspect factories. A major shift was that now the FDA could ban false therapeutic claims without having to prove fraudulent intent. Soon after the 1938 amendments were passed, the FDA began to designate drugs as *safe for use* only under the supervision of a medical professional, and the category of "prescription-only" drugs was securely codified into law by the 1951 Durham–Humphrey Amendment.

The next major change in FDA legislation came as a result of hearings held by Senator Estes Kefauver in 1959. Senator Kefauver had concerns about pharmaceutical industry practices, such as the high cost and uncertain efficacy of drugs promoted by manufacturers. At that time, there was strong opposition to a new law expanding the FDA's authority. However, this rapidly changed after the thalidomide tragedy (see Case Study 9-3 Thalidomide Tragedy). The 1962 Kefauver–Harris Amendment to the Food, Drug and Cosmetic Act represented a major strengthening of the FDA regulatory authority. The most important changes in the amendments were as follows:

- The requirement that all new drug applications had to demonstrate "substantial evidence" of the drug's

efficacy for a marketed indication, in addition to the existing premarket requirement for demonstrating safety.
- The requirement that manufacturers use the "established" or "generic" name of a drug along with the trade name.
- The restriction of drug advertising to FDA-approved indications.
- The expansion of FDA powers to inspect drug manufacturing facilities.

Passage of the Kefauver–Harris amendments marked the beginning of the FDA approval process that is currently used in the United States. The next major change in U.S. drug product regulations was not driven by safety or efficacy concerns, but by economic concerns. In 1984, the Drug Price Competition and Patent Restoration Act was passed. This act extended the patent exclusivity terms of new drugs and tied the extensions, in part, to the length of the FDA approval process for each individual drug.

After the 1962 amendments, the FDA had full authority to require documentation of the risks (safety) and benefits (efficacy) of new drugs and to base approval of marketing for new drug products on their assessment of the relative risks and benefits of the products. However, until quite recently they did not have an explicit program for postmarket assessment of drug safety and had only limited responsibility or authority for assuring postmarket safety. The widely publicized recall of Fen-phen (fenfluramine and phentermine) in 1997 and of rofecoxib (Vioxx) in 2004 played a major role in driving a new wave of safety reforms at both the FDA regulatory and statutory levels (see Case Study 9-1 Vioxx Withdrawal). The FDA Amendments Act (FDA AA) of 2007 included a wide range of changes for the FDA. The amendments and the current FDA activities related to drug safety surveillance are described in detail in Chapter 10. Several major changes were included that are directly related to monitoring and managing the safety of marketed pharmaceutical products. Some of the changes that most directly involve pharmacoepidemiology have to do with the FDA's expanded authority for post-marketing safety.

CASE STUDY 9-1

Vioxx Withdrawal

Vioxx (rofecoxib) is a nonsteroidal antiinflammatory drug. Vioxx was approved by the FDA in 1999. The initial belief was that cyclooxygenase-2 (COX-2) inhibitors, like Vioxx, would be a safer antiinflammatory treatment than the dominant nonsteroidal antiinflammatory drugs (NSAIDs) that were linked to an increased risk of intestinal tract bleeding. However, a number of pre- and post-marketing studies suggested that Vioxx might increase the risk of myocardial infarction. The Vioxx Gastrointestinal Outcomes Research (VIGOR) study was designed to provide longer-term clinical outcome data to confirm the shorter-term findings about reductions in intestinal track bleeding and to evaluate overall safety. This was a large study conducted among rheumatoid arthritis patients who typically require higher doses of antiinflammatory medicines. Results of the VIGOR study were initially published in the New England Journal of Medicine in 2000. The publication did not include the findings from the study showing that Vioxx was associated with increased cardiovascular events. After

further review of the VIGOR results, the FDA approved extensive labeling changes for Vioxx and a new indication in the treatment of rheumatoid arthritis. The FDA continued to monitor the scientific literature, reviewing several retrospective epidemiologic studies. Some of these studies suggested an increased risk for cardiovascular events, especially with the higher 50 mg dose, but the study results were not consistent. In August 2004, results were released from the Adenomatous Polyp Prevention on Vioxx (APPROVe) Trial that included the first comparison to a placebo group and supported the previous signal seen in the VIGOR trial and some of the epidemiologic studies. The data demonstrated an increase in cardiovascular risk and stroke starting at the 18th-month time point compared to placebo. Merck voluntarily withdrew Vioxx from the market in September 2004. Lawsuits are still pending, but as of January 2010, Merck was already committed to paying claims for more than 3,100 deaths attributed to use of the product, with a settlement fund of $4.85 billion.

▶ FDA Premarket Assessment of Drug Safety

As mentioned in the introduction, all prescription drug products have some risks and FDA approval is based on a belief that the benefits of a drug outweigh the documented risks at the time of approval. The FDA continues to evaluate the benefits and risks of a drug as additional data become available. This reality was very clearly stated by Sandra Kweder, deputy director of the Office of New Drugs at the FDA, when she testified to Congress on drug safety and the withdrawal of Vioxx from the market.[14]

It is important to understand that all approved drugs pose some level of risk, such as the risks that are identified in clinical trials and listed on the labeling of the product. Unless a new drug's demonstrated benefit outweighs its known risk for an intended population, FDA will not approve the

drug. However, we cannot anticipate all possible effects of a drug during the clinical trials that precede approval. An adverse drug reaction can range from a minor, unpleasant response to a drug product, to a response that is sometimes life-threatening or deadly. Such adverse drug reactions may be expected (because clinical trial results indicate such possibilities) or unexpected (because the reaction was not evident in clinical trials). It may also result from errors in drug prescribing, dispensing or use. The issue of how to detect and limit adverse reactions can be challenging; how to weight the impact of these adverse reactions against the benefits of these products on individual patients and the public health is multifaceted and complex, involving scientific as well as public policy issues.

As pointed out by Dr. Kweder, clinical trials prior to product approval cannot be expected to detect all adverse reactions since some may occur too infrequently; however, they are designed to balance the cost of conducting trials against the likelihood of detecting all of the serious adverse events that may occur with a new product. As described in Chapter 1, Phase 3 clinical studies are conducted to rigorously evaluate a drug's efficacy and safety. At least one of the Phase 3 studies must be a randomized clinical trial designed to capture the required database for evaluating safety. The size of the premarketing trial used for safety evaluation depends on the following factors about the product:[15]

- Its novelty (i.e., whether it represents a new treatment or is similar to available treatments).
- The availability of alternative therapies and the relative safety of those alternatives as compared to the new product.
- The intended population and condition being treated.
- The intended duration of use.

Although the trial used for safety evaluation will also be used to further document efficacy, the sample size for this trial is driven by the need to adequately document safety. The required sample size for a new product will be set by the FDA on the basis of what is believed to be a sufficient sample to detect less common adverse events with a reasonable level of confidence. A more detailed explanation is provided in the *Textbook of Pharmacoepidemiology.***

Randomized clinical trials used to establish safety in the United States typically will include 500 to 3,000 patients who are exposed to the new drug even if the efficacy of the drug could be documented with fewer patients. If a study was conducted with 3,000 patients, the researchers would be 95% certain of detecting any adverse reactions that could occur in at least 1 patient out of 1,000 exposed patients. The smaller sample of 500 patients would be expected to have 95% confidence in detecting an adverse event occurring in 6 or more patients out of 1,000 exposed patients. As

demonstrated by these numbers, larger samples would be more likely to detect all of the significant adverse events that might occur with a new drug; however, costs of clinical trials are so high that it is imperative that the FDA and the manufacturer work with what is known about the new product, similar products, and the disease being treated to determine an appropriate sample size for the safety study that considers both cost and the need to be reasonably certain about the drug's safety.

▶ FDA Postmarketing Safety Surveillance

Even large clinical development programs for new products cannot reasonably be expected to identify all of the risks associated with a new pharmaceutical product. Therefore, it is expected that, even when a product is rigorously tested in preapproval studies, some risks will only become apparent when the product is used in thousands or even millions of patients in a real-world setting.

One of the 2007 FDA amendments addresses the need for rapid approval of new products and the limitation of approval trials to identify and evaluate all of the potential risks associated with a new product. Section 901 of the FDA AA (Postmarket Studies and Clinical Trials Regarding Human Drugs, Risk Evaluation, and Mitigation Strategies) gives the FDA authority to require postmarketing studies or clinical trials at the time of approval or afterwards if the FDA becomes aware of new safety information. FDA defines *postmarketing studies* as investigations with humans other than clinical trials and laboratory experiments. Postmarketing studies can be, but are not limited to, observational pharmacoepidemiological studies. These studies will often make use of administrative health claims data, electronic medical records, and patient/disease registries.

Section 905 of the FDA AA (Postmarket Risk Identification and Analysis System for Active Surveillance and Assessment) was another change that elevated the importance of pharmacoepidemiology in postmarketing safety surveillance. This section mandated that the FDA establish a postmarket risk identification and analysis system for monitoring drugs that

---

**Strom BL. Sample size considerations for pharmacoepidemiology studies. In: Strom BL, Kimmel SE, eds. *Textbook of Pharmacoepidemiology*. West Sussex, England: John Wiley & Sons Ltd., 2006:25-33.

CASE STUDY 9-2

Sulfanilamide Disaster[†]

In the 1930s, sulfanilamide, a drug used to treat streptococcal infections, had been shown to have dramatic curative effects and had been used safely for some time in tablet and powder form. In June 1937, a salesman for the S.E. Massengill Co., in Bristol, Tennessee, reported a demand in the Southern states for the drug in a liquid form. The company's chief chemist and pharmacist experimented and found that sulfanilamide would dissolve in diethylene glycol. The company's quality-control lab tested the mixture for flavor, appearance, and fragrance and found it satisfactory. Immediately, they compounded a quantity of the elixir and sent 633 shipments all over the country. The new formulation had not been tested for toxicity. At the time, the food and drug laws did not require that safety studies be conducted on new drugs. Because no pharmacological studies had been done on the new elixir, the company failed to note that diethylene glycol, a chemical normally used as antifreeze, is a deadly poison.

The first shipments of the elixir were shipped in early September. On October 11, the American Medical Association (AMA) received reports that an unfamiliar sulfanilamide compound was responsible for a number of deaths. The AMA obtained samples of the elixir, their laboratory isolated diethylene glycol as the toxic ingredient, and they immediately issued a warning. On October 14, the FDA was notified of this development by a New York physician. Inspectors immediately went to the Massengill headquarters and learned that the company already had been informed of the problem and had issued telegrams requesting the return of the product. The FDA got the company to issue a stronger recall notice and worked diligently with the company to recover all of the distributed product. Of the 240 gallons manufactured, 234 gallons and 1 pint were recovered. Even with this effort, more than 100 people died after using the drug.

would rely on electronic data from health care information holders. The FDA now had the responsibility, authority, and funding to collaborate with public, academic, and private entities to develop methods to obtain ready access to a variety of data sources and to develop methods to link and analyze safety data from multiple sources. The FDA Sentinel System is described in more detail in Chapter 10.

▶ A Shift to Relative Risk

Obviously, when large administrative claims databases are used for retrospective analyses, the samples can be many times larger than the samples used in randomized control trials. A larger sample makes it possible for researchers to study differences in the risk of adverse events, even for events that occur very infrequently. This has resulted in a shift from detection and analysis of drug safety based more on "visible harm" to one based on measures of "relative risk."

Visible harm refers to adverse events that are serious enough and are easy enough to be associated with the use of a specific drug that they result in spontaneous case reports. These reports serve as signals that then lead to additional studies to more precisely determine whether there is a cause and effect relationship between use of the drug and the adverse event. In the past, the follow-up evaluation would be a more systematic collection of case reports. The sulfanilamide disaster (Case Study 9-2) and the thalidomide tragedy (Case Study 9-3) are examples of visible harm resulting in safety signals, follow-up research, and regulatory safety actions. In both cases, the adverse events were severe, easily observed, and of high incidence among users. This made it fairly easy

---

[†]Summarized from: Ballentine C. Taste of Raspberries, Taste of Death: The 1937 Elixir Sulfanilamide Incident. *FDA Consumer Magazine*, June 1981. www.fda.gov/AboutFDA/WhatWeDo/History/ProductRegulation/SulfanilamideDisaster.

Thalidomide Disaster

Thalidomide has indications as a sedative-hypnotic and for the treatment of multiple myeloma. It was sold in a number of countries from 1957 until 1961 when it was withdrawn from the market after being found to be a cause of birth defects in what is considered to be one of the biggest medical tragedies of modern times. In 1957, thalidomide was first sold in Germany under the brand name of Contergan. By 1960, it was the top-selling sedative. In the late 1950s and early 1960s, more than 10,000 children in 46 countries were born with severe physical deformities, such as phocomelia, as a consequence of their mothers having taken thalidomide. The exact number of victims is not known, but estimates ranged from 10,000 to 20,000. The Australian obstetrician William McBride and the German pediatrician Widukind Lenz suspected a link between the birth defects in these children and use of thalidomide by their mothers. This relationship was proven by Lenz in 1961. The impact in the United States was minimized when Frances Oldham Kelsey, a pharmacologist and physician, refused FDA approval for an application to market the product in the United States. However, thousands of "trial samples" had been sent to U.S. physicians during the "clinical investigation" phase of the drug's development, which at the time was totally unregulated by the FDA. In spite of the product never being approved for sale in the United States as a sedative-hypnotic, 17 children were born in the United States with defects linked to thalidomide use. In July 1998, the FDA approved the use of thalidomide for the treatment of lesions associated with Erythema Nodosum Leprosum. In May 2006 they approved its use for the treatment of newly diagnosed multiple myeloma patients. In both cases, special risk management procedures were required to tightly control its use for the approved conditions and with appropriate patients.

to establish the relationship between the events and the use of the drugs.

The concept of relative risk refers to comparing the risks in two different groups of people. Relative risk is in essence a ratio measure of one group (the exposed group) to another group (the control group). Relative risk indicates how much more likely one group is to have an event than is the other group. With large databases and retrospective studies, a sufficient number of patient cases can be identified to measure differences in relative risks for outcomes that are fairly rare. When results from these studies are being interpreted, it is important to remember the difference between relative risk and absolute risk. As stated, relative risk is the comparison of risk for one group to another. Absolute risk is the risk of developing a disease or having an event over a specified time period. When the event being studied has a very low incidence rate, relative risk measures can be somewhat misleading.

The importance of distinguishing between the two terms can be seen when we look at the result of the APPROVe Trial that led to the withdrawal of Vioxx.[16] The risk of a confirmed thrombotic event among the rofecoxib patients was 1.50 events per 100 patient-years of follow-up compared to 0.78 events per 100 patient-years for the placebo patients. The increase in absolute risk when taking rofecoxib was 0.72 events per 100 patient-years and the relative risk was 1.92. This indicates that the rofecoxib patients were almost twice as likely to have a thrombotic event, even though the absolute risk of having such an event was still fairly small. Although this sounds like a very large risk difference, in absolute terms, it was not even an increase of 1% per year on treatment of having an event. Another heavily publicized study that demonstrates the need to consider the absolute risk as well as the relative risk is the meta-analysis conducted on the effect of rosiglitazone (Avandia) on the risk of myocardial infarction.[17] The relative risk of myocardial infarction when taking rosiglitazone was 1.43 compared to the control group. However, the increase in absolute risk was approximately 0.1%.

As pharmacoepidemiology techniques for designing and analyzing retrospective studies with large databases are further developed and improved, researchers will be even better equipped to examine the relative risk associated with infrequent events. This can be of significant benefit in terms of improving the quality of care provided. However, it also runs a risk if relatively rare safety issues are detected in postmarketing monitoring and we fail to remember that it is impractical, if not impossible, to detect all adverse events before approval. The large number of lawsuits related to the Vioxx withdrawal, the Avandia safety warnings, and other postmarketing safety events demonstrate the increasing product liability faced by manufacturers. During a presentation at the 2009 Harvard Medical School Postapproval Summit, Dr. Daemmrich even went so far as to question whether we were entering an era of "pharmacovigilantes."[18]

PHARMACOEPIDEMIOLOGY AND DRUG SAFETY EVALUATION

As previously stated, during the past two decades the evaluation, assessment and management of prescription drug safety has shifted to include risk management as an integral part of the development and life-cycle management of all drugs in the United States and most other countries. At the same time, large administrative claims databases have become more accessible and the number of researchers trained in how to use these databases to conduct analyses that integrate claims for prescription drug, inpatient care, and outpatient care using sound research methods has grown. With these changes, the fields of pharmacoepidemiology and drug safety have become more closely linked than ever before. The FDA and regulatory agencies in other countries increasingly require pharmaceutical manufacturers to conduct epidemiologic safety studies. As a result of the growing importance of pharmacoepidemiology, most pharmaceutical companies now have risk management/pharmacoepidemiology departments, and these companies more frequently support pharmacoepidemiology studies conducted by academics and others.

The number of publications from pharmacoepidemiology studies, especially those using large administrative claims databases, will certainly increase in the next decade. These studies will also become increasingly important in regulatory decisions as well as decisions about third-party coverage and clinical practice standards. As reports from retrospective studies using large claims databases become more prevalent and play an increasingly important role in drug product regulation and how pharmaceutical products are used, it will become even more important for practitioners to have a good working knowledge of pharmacoepidemiology and how to accurately interpret results from these studies.

SUMMARY

Health care professionals have a responsibility to assure the safe and appropriate use of drugs in their everyday work settings. In order to do this well, they must be knowledgeable about the known risks associated with marketed products and appropriately communicate this information to their patients. Postmarketing surveillance plays an important part in the continuous monitoring of drug product safety. Although practitioners are not typically involved in the analytical evaluation of potential drug safety signals, they do have an important role in drug safety monitoring. Drug safety signals most often are triggered by self-reports from practitioners of the serious adverse reactions observed in their practices. Once safety signals have been generated, various pharmacoepidemiology methods are typically used to evaluate the signal and determine if FDA action is required. It is important that public health professionals and practitioners understand the importance of reporting serious adverse events as well as the process by which safety signals are evaluated. Only by understanding the process used to monitor and assure drug safety and communicating appropriate safety information to patients can health care professionals be sure that the highest possible quality of health care is being provided.

DISCUSSION QUESTIONS

1. Describe "safety signal" and identify two methods used by the FDA to identify safety signals for further evaluation.

2. What are the major classifications of adverse drug events related to dose and time?

3. Discuss the implications to practitioners and regulators of different types of adverse drug events.

4. Do an on-line search to identify and describe four recent safety signals that have been identified as concern for further evaluation by the FDA.

5. Discuss the advantages and disadvantages of requiring larger premarket clinical studies that could better identify rare adverse drug events.

6. Provide your opinion regarding the accuracy of consumer's perceptions about the risks of prescription drug products.

   a. Describe what prescribers and pharmacists should do to be sure patients have an accurate understanding of the benefit–risk balance of the drugs they are taking.

7. Do an online search regarding litigation related to Vioxx, Avandia, or another recent product with postmarket identification of safety issues.

   a. Summarize the research findings (be sure to examine the relative risk and the absolute risk of the adverse event).

   b. Summarize the information and methods used by legal firms to solicit plaintiffs.

   c. Present your opinion about the appropriateness of the litigation within the context of drug product regulation and marketing.

REFERENCES

1. US Food and Drug Administration. Guidance for Industry: Good Pharmacovigilance Practices and Pharmacoepidemiologic Assessment. Available at: www.fda.gov/downloads/Regulatory Information/Guidances/UCM126834.pdf. Accessed December 5, 2009.

2. International Conference on Harmonisation of Technical Requirements for Registration of Pharmaceuticals for Human Use E2a. 1994. Clinical Safety Data Management: Definitions and Standards for Expedited Reporting. Available at: www.ich.org/cache/compo/475–272-1.html#E2A. Accessed November 15, 2009.

3. Cobert B. Manual of Drug Safety and Pharmacovigilance. Boston, MA: Jones & Barrlett Publishers, 2007.

4. Rawlins MD, Thompson JW. Pathogenesis of adverse drug reactions. In: Davies DM, ed. Textbook of Adverse Drug Reactions. Oxford: Oxford University Press, 1977:44.

5. Rawlins MD, Thompson JW. Pathogenesis of adverse drug reaction. In: Davies DM, ed. Textbook of Adverse Drug Reactions, 2nd ed. Oxford: Oxford University Press, 1981:11.

6. Aronson JK, Ferner RE. Clarification of terminology in drug safety. Drug Safety. 2005;28(10):861-870.

7. Aronson JK, Ferner RE. Joining the DoTS: Classifying adverse drug reactions by dose responsiveness, time course and susceptibility. BMJ. 2003;327:1222-1225.

8. Rawlins MD, Thomas SHL. Mechanisms of adverse drug reactions. In: Davies DM, Ferner RE, De Glanville H, eds. Davie's Textbook of Adverse Drug Reactions, 5th ed. London: Chapman & Hall Medical, 1998:40.

9. Stephens MBD, Talbot JCC, Routledge PA, eds. The Detection of New Adverse Drug Reactions, 4th ed. London: Macmillian, 1998:32-44.

10. Wallace MR, Mascola JR, Oldfield BC. Red man syndrome: Incidence, etiology and prophylaxis. J Infect Dis. 1991;164: 1180-1185.

11. Alderman CP. Adverse effects of the angiotensin-converting enzyme inhibitors. Ann Pharmacother. 1996;30:55-61.

12. Geyman JP, Erickson S. The ampicillin rash as a diagnostic and management problem: Case reports and literature review. J Fam Pract. 1978;7:493-496.

13. US Food and Drug Administration. FDA History. Available at: www.fda.gov/AboutFDA/WhatWeDo/History/default.htm. Accessed October 12, 2009.

14. US Food and Drug Administration. Kweder, S. Vioxx and Drug Safety. Testimony Before the Senate Committee on Finance. November 18, 2004. Available at: www.fda.gov/NewsEvents/ Testimony/ucm113235.htm. Accessed November 18, 2009.

15. US Food and Drug Administration. Guidance for Industry: Premarket Risk Assessment. Available at: www.fda.gov/downloads/Drugs/GuidanceComplianceRegulatoryInformation/Guidances/ucm072002.pdf. Accessed December 5, 2009.

16. Bresalier RS, Sandler RS, Quan H, et al. Cardiovascular events associated with rofecoxib in a colorectal adenoma chemoprevention trial. NJEM. 2005;352:1092-1102.

17. Nissen SE, Wolski K. Effect of rosiglitazone on the risk of myocardial infarction and death from cardiovascular causes. NEJM. 2007;356:2457-2471.

18. Daemmrich A. Drug Safety: Historical and Business perspectives. Presentation at Harvard Medical School Postapproval Summit, 2009. Agenda available at: www.postapproval.org/summit.htm. Accessed January 20, 2010.

The FDA Perspective on Postmarket Drug Safety

10

Heidi C. Marchand

▼ OBJECTIVES

At the end of the chapter, the reader will be able to:

1. Discuss the specific provisions of the Food and Drug Administration Amendments Act that address drug safety
2. Describe the scenarios under which the FDA requires postmarket studies and clinical trials to be conducted
3. Describe the various Risk Evaluation and Mitigation Strategies in place to minimize the occurrence of adverse events
4. Understand the FDA's efforts toward establishing a Postmarket Risk Identification and Analysis System
5. Discuss the potential role of health care providers in postmarket drug safety

INTRODUCTION

Today, millions of people depend on medications to sustain their health. However, the consequence of this success is that many Americans are exposed to multiple prescription drugs each year (on average, more than 10^1), and many individuals, particularly the elderly, take more than five separate medications on a chronic basis. Because of such widespread use, an unanticipated drug safety problem can evolve into a public health risk. Until recently, the Food and Drug Administration (FDA)'s authority in regulating drug safety was mostly restricted to the pre-marketing stage of drugs. However, several concerns with postmarketing drug safety have been highlighted throughout the book, with the recall of several FDA-

approved drugs. Alosetron was withdrawn and then returned to market with restrictions and a label warning. Troglitazone, propulsid, cerivastatin, rofecoxib, and valdecoxib have been withdrawn. Celecoxib and other nonselective, nonsteroidal, antiinflammatory drugs have had boxed warnings added to their labels. Additional warnings have been added to all antidepressant labels. The FDA identified the need to improve postmarket assessment of drug safety reporting and adverse drug reactions in a timely and efficient manner.

In 2005, the FDA asked the Institute of Medicine (IOM) to convene a committee to assess the U.S. drug safety system and to make recommendations to improve risk assessment, surveillance, and the safe use of drugs. As a result of the committee's work, in 2006, the IOM issued a report, *The Future of Drug Safety—Promoting and Protecting the Health of the Public*,[2] which offered 25 recommendations. Some of these recommendations were directed to the FDA, particularly its Center for Drug Evaluation and Research (CDER). The CDER-directed recommendations proposed ways the agency could improve programs related to drug safety. Recommendations directed to governmental organizations other than the FDA discussed the development of a more robust and comprehensive system for ensuring the safe use of medical products. The remaining recommendations were directed to Congress and called for the FDA to have adequate authority to require postmarketing risk assessment and risk management programs. The IOM also recommended that Congress enact legislation to ensure compliance by pharmaceutical manufacturers for drug safety commitments by increasing the FDA's enforcement authority and tools to include fines, injunctions, and withdrawal of drug approval.[3]

In September 2007, Congress passed the Food and Drug Administration Amendments Act (FDA AA)[4] to provide the FDA the authority and the resources to prevent, detect, and respond to safety problems in a timely way. Many of these new authorities addressed the recommendations from the 2006 IOM Report. Some of the key provisions of the act were

- The Prescription Drug User Fee Amendments of 2007 (PDUFA) (Title I),
- The Medical Device User Fee Amendments of 2007 (MDUFA) (Title II),
- The Pediatric Medical Device Safety and Improvement Act of 2007 (Title III),
- The Pediatric Research Equity Act of 2007 (PREA) (Title IV),
- The Best Pharmaceuticals for Children Act of 2007 (BPCA) (Title V),
- Clinical Trial Databases (Title VIII),
- Enhanced Authorities Regarding Postmarket Safety of Drugs (Title IX).

The FDA AA enacted Title IX, giving the FDA new authorities related to postmarket drug safety, effective March 25, 2008. The statute renders the FDA the authority to enforce postmarket studies and clinical trials, safety-labeling changes, and risk evaluation and mitigation strategies (REMS, Section 901). The FDA now has the authority to impose civil penalties for violations. Title IX, Section 905 of the FDA AA also mandated the FDA to establish a postmarket risk identification and analysis system (i.e., the Sentinel Initiative) for monitoring drugs that would rely on electronic data from health care information holders.

The FDA plans to apply new scientific and technological advancements and methods to build upon postmarketing drug safety evaluation. The emerging "science of safety" includes understanding the cause of adverse events based on a full characterization of the product, even to the molecular level. For example, the Sentinel Initiative, as discussed later in the chapter, is under development within the FDA and in collaboration with external stakeholders to create a national, integrated, electronic system for monitoring medical product safety. These new enhancements to the postmarketing safety system are expected to improve the exchange of information gathered across a drug product's development as part of clinical testing and throughout its lifecycle. The FDA will enhance postmarketing safety systems to better track and assess adverse events to help ensure safe use of medications. The FDA is already relying upon electronic health information to conduct robust surveillance to detect previously unrecognized adverse events. It is these new FDA initiatives that highlight the need for health care professionals to understand drug product safety and pharmacoepidemiology.

This chapter will elaborate on the provisions under Section 901 and Section 905 within the FDA AA that address the postmarket safety of drugs. A summary of the FDA's plans to address medication safety problems is provided. The chapter also includes a discussion of the role of health care providers in postmarket adverse event reporting via the MedWatch program.

POSTMARKET STUDIES AND CLINICAL TRIALS REGARDING HUMAN DRUGS

Drug manufacturers and/or researchers may conduct studies or clinical trials on drug products after they are marketed to the public. Research may be conducted on a product after its approval to identify new dosing regimens or to evaluate new indications. Results from these studies may support new information about the product meeting a regulatory threshold for inclusion into the product's labeling. For example, information from studies conducted after the product's approval may include dosing modifications in renal or hepatic impairment. Often such information is submitted to the FDA as a supplement to the New Drug Application, and upon the FDA's evaluation and review this information is included into the product's approved labeling. Alternatively, some studies are conducted for marketing or reimbursement purposes and not to meet the FDA's regulatory standards. A pharmaceutical manufacturer may conduct a study, comparing their drug with another treatment with the same approved indication. The comparison provides information on a range of health outcomes that could have marketing or reimbursement implications. However, because the study was not designed to meet well-defined regulatory standards that address endpoints, statistical significance, and so on, it is unlikely that the study's results will meet regulatory requirements for approval of a new marketing message or a new indication or statement within the drug's labeling. These studies are often conducted at the discretion of the pharmaceutical manufacturer and not as a requirement by the FDA.

Prior to the FDA AA, the FDA could enforce postmarketing studies only in certain situations. These studies were intended to further refine the safety, efficacy, or optimal use of a product or to ensure that the product's manufacturing processes met the required quality and reliability standards. Such studies were either agreed upon by the FDA and the pharmaceutical manufacturer or, under certain circumstances, required by the FDA. The FDA required postmarket studies for products because they were provided accelerated approvals, were approved with waiver of the required pediatric studies, or were approved on the basis of animal efficacy data. Since the time FDA AA came into force, the FDA retains its authority for these situations; however, the FDA now may require postmarketing studies or clinical trials at the time of approval or after approval if the FDA becomes aware of new safety information.

Postmarketing studies and clinical trials may be required for any or all three purposes:

- To assess a known serious risk related to the use of the drug,
- To assess signals of serious risk related to the use of the drug,
- To identify an unexpected serious risk when available data indicate the potential for a serious risk.

The primary goal of an FDA-required postmarketing study is to evaluate safety. Efficacy may also be included in any study conducted; however, the FDA's requirements are directed toward a safety-related outcome or endpoint. A postmarketing study required by the FDA under the FDA AA can be an observational pharmacoepidemiologic study or other type of study. These studies are designed to assess a serious risk attributed to a drug exposure, to quantify the risk associated with a drug exposure, or to evaluate factors that affect the risk of serious toxicity, such as drug dose, timing of exposure, or patient characteristics.[5] To facilitate interpretation of the findings, the studies should have a protocol (including prospectively defined objectives, methods, and an analysis plan) and a control group, unless there is a scientifically valid reason to exclude controls, and should test a prespecified hypothesis. Data sources for these studies can include administrative claims data, electronic medical records, disease registries, prospectively collected observational data, or other sources of observational data. A detailed explanation of the various study designs and data sources is provided in Chapters 3 and 4. Some examples of postmarket studies to evaluate product safety are listed in Table 10-1.

Additionally, the FDA may require further evaluation of safety (toxicity) in animal studies or other nonclinical studies that evaluate the safety of manufacturing controls. Safety studies in animals investigating specific end-organ toxicities include carcinogenicity and reproductive toxicity studies. Safety evaluation of the manufacturing process may include determining the risk of cross-contamination between products that could result from sharing product-contacting equipment and parts.

RISK EVALUATION AND MITIGATION STRATEGIES (REMS)

Because of the FDA's commitment to postmarketing surveillance, the number of drug products with risk evaluation and mitigation strategies (REMS) is

Table 10-1. Examples of postmarket studies with safety evaluations.

- Estimate the relative risk of a serious adverse event or toxicity associated with use of a drug.
- Provide estimates of risk (e.g., incidence rates) for a serious adverse event or toxicity. Obtain long-term clinical outcome data, including information about potentially rare serious adverse events in patients taking the drug compared to patients not exposed to the drug.
- Compare pregnancy outcomes and fetal/child outcomes after drug exposure during pregnancy to patients who did not receive the drug.
- Evaluate the occurrence of asthma exacerbations associated with the use of inhalation treatments for asthma in a controlled clinical trial.
- Determine the incidence of myocardial ischemia or infarction, malignancy, and mortality in patients treated with an approved drug on a chronic basis.
- Evaluate differences in safety between patients withdrawn from treatment after some period of treatment and patients who remain on the treatment.
- Determine growth and neurocognitive function in pediatric patients treated chronically with the drug.
- Evaluate safety in a particular racial or ethnic group or vulnerable population such as the immunocompromised.
- Evaluate the safety of the drug in pregnant women.
- Evaluate drug toxicity in patients with hepatic or renal impairment.
- Evaluate long-term safety of cell and gene therapy products depending on the type of vector used and the inherent risk of integration.
- Evaluate the safety of a drug in patients with HIV-1 coinfected with hepatitis C.
- Studies or clinical trials to evaluate the pharmacokinetics of the drug in the labeled population or in a subpopulation at potential risk for high drug exposures that could lead to toxicity.

increasing. The FDA can require REMS to manage known or potential serious risks from certain drug products. REMS are approaches established by the FDA and the pharmaceutical manufacturer to reduce risk from the use of a specific product. The strategies or approaches to reduce risk will vary by drug product; however, there is a common framework that may include the following components.

▶ Medication Guides and Patient Package Inserts

Medication guides and patient package inserts are printed information sheets written in nontechnical language that provide information to patients or their caregivers. These medication information sheets are often distributed by the pharmacist or other health care provider at the time the prescription is dispensed or prescribed. In the past, the FDA determined that the safe and effective use of some prescription drugs, such as oral contraceptives and estrogens, required patients to have additional information. Therefore, the FDA required that manufacturers make these information sheets available to patients. Medication information sheets are approved by the FDA and are regulated by the FDA as part of the product's labeling. For other medications, manufacturers may provide package inserts or information sheets to patients voluntarily.

More recently, the FDA has mandated patient labeling in the form of medication guides for prescription drugs that pose a serious and significant public health concern and for drugs for which FDA-approved patient information is necessary for safe and effective use of the product. Medications guides are required if the FDA determines that one or more of the following circumstances exists:

- Patient labeling could help prevent serious adverse effects.
- A drug product has serious risk(s) (relative to benefits) of which patients should be made aware because information concerning the risk(s) could affect a patient's decision to use or to continue to use the product.
- A drug product is important to a patient's health, and patient adherence to directions for use is crucial to the drug's effectiveness.

Medication guides are required to be distributed to the patient or the caregiver at the time the medication is dispensed. Medication guides are required to contain specific headings relevant to the drug product, an example of which is provided in Figure 10-1.

▶ Communication Plan

A communication plan is a plan prepared by the pharmaceutical manufacturer that provides information to health care providers directly or through professional societies to support implementation of the REMS. The

Medication Guide
Actiq® (AK-tik) CII
(oral transmucosal fentanyl citrate)
200 mcg, 400 mcg, 600 mcg, 800 mcg, 1200 mcg, 1600 mcg

▼ **WARNING:**

1. **Do not use** *Actiq* **unless you are regularly using other opioid pain medicines around-the-clock for your constant cancer pain and your body is used to these medicines.**
2. **You MUST keep** *Actiq* **in a safe place out of the reach of children.** Accidental ingestion by a child is a medical emergency and can result in death. **Death has been reported in children who have accidentally taken** *Actiq*. **If a child accidentally takes** *Actiq*, **get emergency help right away.**

Read the Medication Guide that comes with *Actiq* before you start taking it and each time you get a new prescription. There may be new information. This Medication Guide does not take the place of talking to your doctor about your medical condition or your treatment. Share this important information with members of your household.

What is the most important information I should know about *Actiq*?

1. *Actiq* can cause life threatening breathing problems which can lead to death:
   - if you are not regularly using other opioid pain medicines around-the-clock for your constant cancer pain and your body is not used to these medicines. This means that you are not opioid tolerant.
   - if you do not use it <u>exactly</u> as prescribed by your doctor.

2. Your doctor will prescribe a starting dose of *Actiq* that is different than other fentanyl containing medicines you may have been taking. Do not substitute *Actiq* for other fentanyl medicines without talking with your doctor.

3. Use no more than 2 units of *Actiq* per episode of breakthrough cancer pain. You must wait at least 4 hours before using *Actiq* again for another episode of breakthrough cancer pain.

▲ **Figure 10-1.** The heading highlighted on the medication guide, "What is the most important information I should know about (name of drug) Actiq?" is required to be followed by a statement describing the particular serious and significant public health concern that has created the need for the Medication Guide. The statement should describe specifically what the patient should do or consider because of that concern, such as weighing particular risks against the benefits of the drug, avoiding particular activities, observing certain symptoms, or engaging in particular behaviors.

plan often details activities that will be undertaken by the pharmaceutical manufacturer to accomplish implementation of REMS. A communication plan may include a "Dear Health Care Provider Letter" to inform the providers about a possible side effect, the signs and symptoms, and the need to reevaluate benefits and risks. The letter may also include additional information the providers could discuss with their patients. Other communication plans may include Web-based materials and safety-related kits (e.g., a link on the drug product's Web site that directs users to a separate Web site introducing the REMS program). An example of safety-related material includes a pharmaceutical manufacturer medical scientific liaison's presentation at a national professional society meeting that informs health care providers about issues related to the occurrence of a particular side effect.

▶ **Elements to Assure Safe Use**

The elements in the REMS to ensure safe use are established to diminish a specific serious risk listed in the labeling of the drug. The establishment of safe-use criteria may comprise multiple or limited elements. For example, depending on the risk, the elements might include specific requirements such as follows:

- Prescribers and dispensers may need to be certified.
- The drug may only be dispensed in certain health care settings, such as hospitals.
- Patients may be required to have specific laboratory tests, be subject to monitoring, or be enrolled in a registry.

Prescriber certification may require that the health care provider demonstrate that he understands the risks and benefits of the drug. The prescriber may also have to demonstrate that he has read the educational materials, can diagnose the condition for which the drug is indicated, can diagnose and treat potential adverse reactions associated with the drug, and will perform monitoring as outlined in the REMS. The program may require periodic recertification and reenrollment, and the manufacturer may maintain a database of all certified prescribers. For pharmacists and others who dispense the medication, the elements to assure safe use may require that these individuals do the following:

- Understand the risks and benefits of the product,
- Have read the educational materials before the drug is dispensed,
- Agree to fill a prescription and dispense the drug only after receiving prior authorization,
- Agree to check laboratory values,
- Check for the presence of stickers that prescribers affix to prescriptions for specified products to indicate that the patient has met all criteria for receiving the product ("qualification stickers") before dispensing a drug,
- Agree to fill a prescription and dispense the drug only within a specified period of time after the prescription is written,
- Agree to fill prescriptions only from enrolled prescribers.

Training is often an important component of several of the elements. For example, as part of the certification process, prescribers and dispensers may be required to undergo specific training. This training (through manufacturer-developed materials, approved as part of the REMS) may eliminate the need for specific communication plans if the training is included as elements to assure safe use. Training could also include REMS Program overview brochures, educational presentations, and other materials. These materials might be made available in printed form or as Web-based education materials.

Health care institutions may have to meet certain requirements in order to distribute the drug product. Examples of REMS requirements for hospitals to assure safe use may include the following:

- Hospital is certified by enrolling into a drug manufacturer's REMS program.
- Hospital personnel must attest that educational materials have been received and distributed to the appropriate staff.
- Systems are in place for ensuring the drug is dispensed only to patients with evidence of safe use conditions.

Patients may also be expected to comply with certain requirements before they can obtain the drug. Often the REMS include elements that are specific to patients. Examples of patient elements to assure safe use are listed as follows:

- Patients may be required to demonstrate an understanding of risks and benefits of the medication.
- Patients can only receive the drug after specified authorization is obtained and verified by the pharmacy (e.g., checking laboratory tests such as a pregnancy test or liver enzyme test).
- Patients may be required to receive specified periodic monitoring; for example, they may be required to have a follow-up visit to the physician every 6 months to ensure they are still appropriate candidates for treatment.
- Patients may be required to enroll into a patient registry.

The various elements of REMS that assure safe use are not mutually exclusive; in fact, there is considerable overlap. Each REMS element to ensure safe use will be unique to the particular drug or therapeutic class, as their purpose is to mitigate the individual risk related to the drug or therapeutic class.

▶ Implementation System

The elements to assure safe drug use need to be implemented, and, thus, there is often an implementation system as part of REMS. An implementation system requires the pharmaceutical manufacturer to take reasonable steps to monitor and evaluate those in the health care system responsible for adopting the elements to assure safe use into practice. Implementation systems have included databases of certified hospitals or other health care settings or compliance

THE FDA PERSPECTIVE ON POSTMARKET DRUG SAFETY

monitoring with data collection requirements and periodic safety monitoring.

▶ Assessment Timetable

The only required REMS element is a timetable for submission of assessments of the REMS. The assessment is to determine whether the elements to assure safe use have met the goals of the REMS. This assessment must occur after 18 months, 3 years, and in the 7th year after the REMS is approved. More frequent assessments, or even less frequent assessments, may be deemed appropriate by the FDA. Certain situations may require additional assessments. One reason for requiring additional assessments is modification of the REMS, such as changing or adding elements to assure safe use. For example, if the goal of an element to assure safe use is not met, the element may be changed in order to help meet the goal. This change could require a new assessment. Another example is if a supplemental application is submitted for a new indication of the drug then additional elements to assure safe use may be required for the new indication. After 3 years, if the FDA determines that serious risks of the drug have been adequately identified, assessed, and are adequately managed, then the FDA can eliminate assessments.

Information needed such as the number of adverse events associated with the drug, the number of nonenrolled or noncompliant prescribers (or health care settings), or the number of patients who were monitored for potential adverse events during the treatment can be obtained from a variety of sources. Drug use data provide information on patients receiving the drug with the REMS and the conditions of use. Patient registries, if in place, can also provide information. Surveys can be employed to learn more about health care professionals' knowledge of the drug and the REMS' effectiveness. For example, a survey might be used to measure health care providers' understanding about the safe use of the drug.

SENTINEL INITIATIVE

With the passage of the FDA AA, and specifically Section 905, the FDA was mandated to establish an active surveillance system for monitoring drugs, relying on electronic data from health care information holders.[6] The Sentinel Initiative is the FDA's response to that mandate. Its goal is to build and implement a new active surveillance system that will eventually be used to monitor all FDA-regulated products. The FDA AA also established goals for accessing the automated health care information of at least 25 million patients by July 1, 2010, and 100 million patients by July 1, 2012.[7]

Prior to this legislation, there were various calls for the FDA to expand its postmarket surveillance capabilities. During the past decade in particular, safety and quality have become a growing concern in the health care community. This increased focus on safety and quality is also a result of an emerging science of safety, which combines a growing understanding of disease and its origins with new methods of safety signal detection. The IOM focused on these concerns in a series of reports: *To Err is Human*, 1999; *Crossing the Quality Chasm*, 2001; *Patient Safety*, 2004; *The Future of Drug Safety—Promoting and Protecting the Health of the Public*, 2006;[2] *Safe Medical Devices for Children* and *Preventing Medication Errors*, 2007. The reports suggest the establishment of a modernized medical product safety system that enables exchange of information and feedback within the broad health care system.

In September 2005, the Secretary of Health and Human Services (HHS) asked the FDA to expand its current system for monitoring medical product performance. The Secretary recommended that the FDA explore the following:

- Augmenting their data-query capability by taking advantage of emerging technologies and building on existing systems and efforts, rather than creating new systems,

- Creating a public–private collaboration as a framework for such an effort,

- Leveraging increasingly available large, electronic databases.

In early 2007, in response to the Secretary's request in 2005, the FDA held a 2-day workshop with a diverse group of thought leaders from the Federal government, the pharmaceutical and medical device industries, academia, public and private health care facilities, health care professionals, bioinformatics institutions, and the public.[8] The workshop explored the concept of creating a national electronic system for monitoring medical product safety, based on multiple, broad-based partnerships (including public–private partnerships). The workshop concluded with broad support for developing such a process. There was a clear call to supplement the current, largely passive, system for monitoring postmarket adverse events and product problems with a proactive surveillance system. Such a system would enable the FDA to leverage existing large and growing health care databases so that the data could be electronically queried and analyzed within preestablished privacy and security safeguards.

In May 2008, the Secretary of HHS and the FDA Commissioner announced the Sentinel Initiative,[9] a long-term effort to create and implement a national electronic system for monitoring FDA-regulated product safety. The Sentinel System's goal is to transform the FDA's existing postmarket safety surveillance systems by enabling the agency to actively gather information about the postmarket safety and performance of its regulated products. The Sentinel System, once implemented, will fulfill many of the requirements of the FDA AA.

In the past, the FDA has used administrative and insurance claims data to investigate safety questions about FDA-regulated products, but generally it has only worked with one particular health care system at a time to evaluate a given safety issue. Its goal now is to create a linked, sustainable system—the Sentinel System—which will draw on existing automated health care data (e.g., electronic health record systems, administrative claims databases, registries) from multiple sources to actively monitor the safety of medical products continuously and in real time. The Sentinel System is intended to augment the FDA's existing surveillance capabilities, not replace them.

As currently envisioned, the Sentinel System will enable queries of disparate data sources quickly and securely for relevant product safety information. Data will continue to be managed by its owners, and only data of organizations who agree to participate in this system will be queried. Questions will be sent to appropriate, participating health care organizations with data sources, who in turn would, in accordance with existing privacy and security safeguards, evalu-

ate their data and send results for agency review (see Fig. 10-2).

This active electronic safety surveillance system would complement available methods for safety signal identification in the following ways:

- Improve capability to identify and evaluate safety issues in near real time,
- Expand capacity for evaluating safety issues,
- Improve access to subgroups and special populations (e.g., the elderly),
- Improve access to longer term data,
- Improve precision of risk estimates due to expanded number of drug product exposures available for study,
- Improve capability to identify increased risks of common adverse events (e.g., myocardial infarction, fracture) that health care providers may not suspect are related to drug products.

Before the Sentinel System is launched and is fully functional, substantial challenges need to be addressed. These include issues around data access and quality, data infrastructure, privacy and security of health care data, and statistical and epidemiological methodologies for active surveillance. To better understand these challenges and develop approaches to address them, a series of pilot programs are being conducted to inform how the Sentinel System should be organized and operated. These pilot programs along with active surveillance initiatives conducted outside the FDA (e.g., the foundation of the NIH's Observational Medical Outcomes Partnership, various active surveillance initiatives conducted in Europe, Canada, and Japan) will contribute substantial knowledge on how best to build the Sentinel System. Building this system will provide pharmacoepidemiologists with a significant resource to evaluate drug exposure and outcome associations as well as causality.

MEDWATCH: THE FDA SAFETY INFORMATION AND ADVERSE EVENTS REPORTING SYSTEM

The FDA's MedWatch program promotes, facilitates and supports the voluntary reporting of suspected serious adverse events to the FDA by clinicians who provide health care to patients in routine care

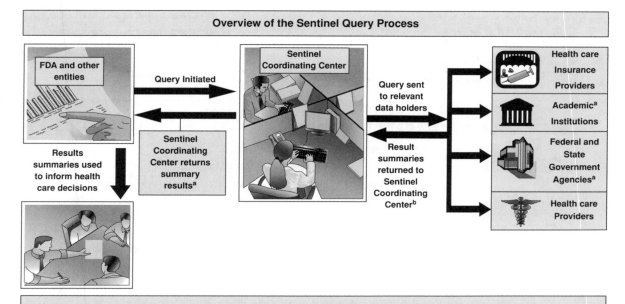

Figure 10-2. Overview of the Sentinel Query Process.

settings. The FDA relies upon the health care community's active support and collaboration. Continued monitoring of adverse events after the product is marketed is essential and depends on voluntary reporting of spontaneous adverse events, medication errors, and product problems by health professionals and consumers to the FDA.

A spontaneous report is an observation during direct patient care—not part of a clinical trial. The adverse event report is submitted voluntarily by a health care professional or patient either directly to the FDA or indirectly to the manufacturer and then to the FDA. Form FDA 3500 (MedWatch form), as shown in Figure 10-3, is used for all voluntary reporting for drugs, both prescription and over-the-counter, and biologics, medical devices, dietary supplements, infant formula, and cosmetics. An adverse event refers to any undesirable experience associated with the use of a medical product in a patient. The event is serious and should be reported

when the patient outcome is death, life threatening, hospitalization (initial or prolonged), disability, and congenital abnormality and requires intervention to prevent permanent impairment or damage. Examples of serious adverse events that should be reported to the FDA are presented in Table 10-2.

In 2008, the FDA received more than 30,000 adverse event reports directly from clinicians and their patients via the "MedWatch" process. The FDA also received some reports from clinicians indirectly through the manufacturers.

Health care professionals are encouraged to report any adverse event they judge to be clinically significant. Suspicion that a drug product may be related to a serious event is sufficient reason to submit a report. Pharmacists are often the primary source for reports of product quality problems, medication errors and near-misses, and reports of therapeutic inequivalence or failure that may be suspected with a switch

U.S. Department of Health and Human Services

Form Approved: OMB No. 0910-0291, Expires: 12/31/2011
See OMB statement on reverse.

MEDWATCH

For VOLUNTARY reporting of
adverse events, product problems and
product use errors

**The FDA Safety Information and
Adverse Event Reporting Program**

Page 1 of _____

FDA USE ONLY
Triage unit sequence #

A. PATIENT INFORMATION

1. Patient Identifier	2. Age at Time of Event or Date of Birth:	3. Sex	4. Weight
In confidence		☐ Female ☐ Male	_____ lb or _____ kg

B. ADVERSE EVENT, PRODUCT PROBLEM OR ERROR

Check all that apply:

1. ☐ Adverse Event ☐ Product Problem (e.g., defects/malfunctions)
☐ Product Use Error ☐ Problem with Different Manufacturer of Same Medicine

2. Outcomes Attributed to Adverse Event (Check all that apply)

☐ Death: _____ (mm/dd/yyyy)
☐ Life-threatening
☐ Hospitalization - initial or prolonged
☐ Required Intervention to Prevent Permanent Impairment/Damage (Devices)
☐ Disability or Permanent Damage
☐ Congenital Anomaly/Birth Defect
☐ Other Serious (Important Medical Events)

3. Date of Event (mm/dd/yyyy)	4. Date of this Report (mm/dd/yyyy)

5. Describe Event, Problem or Product Use Error

6. Relevant Tests/Laboratory Data, Including Dates

7. Other Relevant History, Including Preexisting Medical Conditions (e.g., allergies, race, pregnancy, smoking and alcohol use, and liver/kidney problems)

C. PRODUCT AVAILABILITY

Product Available for Evaluation? (Do not send product to FDA)

☐ Yes ☐ No ☐ Returned to Manufacturer on: _____ (mm/dd/yyyy)

D. SUSPECT PRODUCT(S)

1. Name, Strength, Manufacturer (from product label)
#1 Name:
    Strength:
    Manufacturer:
#2 Name:
    Strength:
    Manufacturer:

PLEASE TYPE OR USE BLACK INK

2. Dose or Amount	Frequency	Route
#1		
#2		

3. Dates of Use (If unknown, give duration) from/to (or best estimate)	5. Event Abated After Use Stopped or Dose Reduced?
#1	#1 ☐ Yes ☐ No ☐ Doesn't Apply
#2	#2 ☐ Yes ☐ No ☐ Doesn't Apply

4. Diagnosis or Reason for Use (Indication)	8. Event Reappeared After Reintroduction?
#1	#1 ☐ Yes ☐ No ☐ Doesn't Apply
#2	#2 ☐ Yes ☐ No ☐ Doesn't Apply

6. Lot #	7. Expiration Date	9. NDC # or Unique ID
#1	#1	
#2	#2	

E. SUSPECT MEDICAL DEVICE

1. Brand Name

2. Common Device Name

3. Manufacturer Name, City and State

4. Model #	Lot #	5. Operator of Device
		☐ Health Professional
Catalog #	Expiration Date (mm/dd/yyyy)	☐ Lay User/Patient
Serial #	Other #	☐ Other:

6. If Implanted, Give Date (mm/dd/yyyy)	7. If Explanted, Give Date (mm/dd/yyyy)

8. Is this a Single-use Device that was Reprocessed and Reused on a Patient?
☐ Yes ☐ No

9. If Yes to Item No. 8, Enter Name and Address of Reprocessor

F. OTHER (CONCOMITANT) MEDICAL PRODUCTS

Product names and therapy dates (exclude treatment of event)

G. REPORTER (See confidentiality section on back)

1. Name and Address
Name:
Address:

City: State: ZIP:

Phone #	E-mail

2. Health Professional?	3. Occupation	4. Also Reported to:
☐ Yes ☐ No		☐ Manufacturer
5. If you do NOT want your identity disclosed to the manufacturer, place an "X" in this box: ☐		☐ User Facility ☐ Distributor/Importer

FORM FDA 3500 (1/09)   Submission of a report does not constitute an admission that medical personnel or the product caused or contributed to the event.

▲ **Figure 10-3.** Form FDA 3500 (MedWatch Form).

U.S. Department of Health and Human Services

MEDWATCH

The FDA Safety Information and
Adverse Event Reporting Program

(CONTINUATION PAGE)
**For VOLUNTARY reporting of
adverse events and product problems**

Page 3 of ____

B.5. **Describe Event or Problem** *(continued)*

B.6. **Relevant Tests/Laboratory Data, Including Dates** *(continued)*

B.7. **Other Relevant History, Including Preexisting Medical Conditions** *(e.g., allergies, race, pregnancy, smoking and alcohol use, and hepatic/renal dysfunction)* *(continued)*

F. **Concomitant Medical Products and Therapy Dates** *(Exclude treatment of event)* *(continued)*

▲ **Figure 10-3.** *(Continued)*

Table 10-2. Examples of serious adverse events that should be reported to the FDA.

Serious adverse event category	Examples
Death	
Life-threatening event	Pacemaker failure Gastrointestinal hemorrhage Bone-marrow suppression Infusion-pump failure that permits uncontrolled free flow resulting in excessive drug dosing
Hospitalization (initial or prolonged)	Anaphylaxis Pseudomembranous colitis Bleeding causing or prolonging hospitalization
Disability	Cerebrovascular accident due to drug-induced hypercoagulability Toxicity Peripheral neuropathy
Congenital anomaly	Vaginal cancer in female offspring due to mother's use of diethylstilbestrol during pregnancy Malformation in the offspring due to mother's use of thalidomide during pregnancy
Event that requires intervention to prevent permanent impairment or damage	Acetaminophen overdose–induced hepatotoxicity requiring treatment with acetylcysteine to prevent permanent damage Burns from radiation equipment requiring drug therapy Breakage of a screw requiring replacement of hardware to prevent malunion of a fractured long bone

between brands of the same medication, generic or proprietary.

Submitting a voluntary report is quick and simple: A one-page paper form can be returned to the FDA by prepaid mail or fax. The four core elements of the report include a reporter's name, a suspect drug or device product, a narrative report of the adverse event or problem, and an identifiable patient. The FDA will hold the identity of patients in strict confidence, protected by Federal law and regulation. Since 1998, the MedWatch Web site, www.fda.gov/medwatch/report.htm, has offered an online reporting form as an alternative to reporting by mail or fax. Currently, more than 60% of voluntary MedWatch reports are submitted via the online form. In addition, a toll-free 800 number is available for inquires related to reporting and to submit a report.

When the FDA receives a report from a clinician about a suspected serious adverse event, the data in the report are entered immediately into the Adverse Event Reporting System (AERS) postmarketing sur-veillance database where it will be reviewed on a case-by-case basis by a safety evaluator. If the safety signal is determined to be potentially significant, the AERS database is examined further for similar reports to develop a case series. Each case report is evaluated for the adequacy of the information, the temporal association of the product and the event, potentially confounding factors such as patient disease or concomitant therapy, and dechallenge–rechallenge information. If the case series review by the CDER Office of Surveillance and Epidemiology staff suggests a new, unexpected safety signal for the product, the safety issue is evaluated further within the agency and by the manufacturer. Often, additional pharmacoepidemiologic investigations are performed to confirm the association between the product and the adverse outcome.

These investigations may lead to the development of a modified use or risk management program, thereby allowing the product to remain available for those whom it may benefit while mitigating the potential harm for those who are at risk of the adverse event. Changes to the labeling, also known as the prescribing information or package insert, are the most commonly used mitigation strategy. These labeling changes range from boxed warnings placed at the top of the prescribing information to additional statements in contraindications, precautions, or adverse reactions sections about new interactions, monitoring recommendations, or dosage adjustments. Certain drugs are required to have medication guides as part of a REMS. Medication guides are a "patient friendly" instruction sheet that is provided to the patient by the pharmacist each time a prescription is dispensed.

Cumulative MedWatch reports may result in valuable new safety information that may be addressed via a labeling change and may also need to be quickly disseminated to the practitioner. For example, adverse event reporting may demonstrate a new drug–drug interaction, requiring dose reductions in a certain patient subpopulation. Before the availability of the Internet, the FDA primarily communicated this new drug safety information "in the labeling" with the expectation that the end user would find the new information by accessing the label. However, with the current widespread use of the Internet and other electronic means for capture and display of information, the FDA is reaching "beyond the label." The Internet has greatly facilitated dissemination and retrieval of new safety information. The health care professionals are empowered with the easy ability to access timely, science-based, FDA-endorsed safety information at the point of care, whether at a desktop computer, handheld smartphone, or other portable device.

With e-mail, a daily tool in the practices of most clinicians, Medwatch provides a service that sends out timely, clinically useful safety alerts as e-mail notification bulletins at the same time the new safety information is posted on the FDA's MedWatch Web site. As of 2009, more than 150,000 subscribers of the MedWatch e-list receive a concise e-mail message about important labeling changes for drugs (e.g., boxed warnings or newly discovered drug–drug interactions), Class I recalls, announcements of product tampering or counterfeit products, and public health advisories.

The FDA is now providing practitioners and the public with earlier communications about emerging safety issues. These early communications about ongoing safety reviews offer the public access to interim scientific data known to the FDA for products of interest that remain under surveillance and monitoring. The FDA is using communication channels ranging from podcasts to text messaging and Really Simple Syndication (RSS) feeds to reach the widest audience possible. The FDA's goal is to deliver targeted, product-specific, and actionable information to both providers and their patients, ideally at the point of care, so that this information can be considered in the shared decision making about both diagnostic and therapeutic measures.

SUMMARY

The passage of the FDA AA in 2007 has provided the FDA with new authoritative powers to help better regulate postmarket studies and clinical trial regarding human drugs in order to reduce the incidents of adverse events and provide timely intervention. The chapter discusses various situations in which the FDA can mandate clinical trials and various REMS that could be implemented to avoid adverse events. The FDA is also working toward establishing an extensive surveillance system—the Sentinel System—which will link health care data from various sources and enhance the agency's safety surveillance capabilities. Apart from these, there are certain programs such as the MedWatch process that enable health care providers to report adverse events so that the FDA can take subsequent action.

DISCUSSION QUESTIONS

1. Under what scenarios does the FDA mandate the conduction of a postmarket clinical studies or trials?

2. List three elements that may be used to assure safe use in Risk Evaluation and Mitigation Strategies. Discuss how each element will help reduce the risk associated with the use of a drug product.

3. Describe the Sentinel System that is currently being developed by the FDA. What will be the benefits of such a system, when created?

4. Describe the role of clinicians in reducing the number of adverse drug reactions. Suggest strategies by which their role in risk management can be increased.

5. Apart from the strategies enlisted by the FDA AA, what other measures can be taken to better manage and mitigate potential adverse drug reactions?

ACKNOWLEDGMENT

The author wishes to thank the following individuals for their contribution to this chapter: Norman S. Marks, MD, MHA; Judith A. Racoosin, MD, MPH; Melissa Robb, R.N.; Theresa Toigo, RPh, MBA.

REFERENCES

1. Cox E, Mager D, Weisbart E. Express Scripts 2008. http://www.express-scripts.com/industryresearch/outcomes/onlinepublications/study/geoVariationTrends.pdf Accessed October 13, 2009.

2. Baciu A, Stratton K, Burke SP, eds. *The Future of Drug Safety: Promoting and Protecting the Health of the Public.* Washington, DC: The National Academies Press, 2007.

3. News and events. Food and Drug Administration Web site. http://www.fda.gov/NewsEvents/Newsroom/PressAnnouncements/2007/ucm108833.htm. Accessed February 18, 2010.

4. Food and Drug Administration Amendments Act of 2007. Food and Drug Administration Web site. http://www.fda.gov/RegulatoryInformation/Legislation/FederalFoodDrugandCosmeticActFDCAct/SignificantAmendmentstotheFDCAct/FoodandDrugAdministrationAmendmentsActof2007/default.htm. Accessed February 18, 2010.

5. Guidance for industry post-marketing studies and clinical trials—implementation of section 505(o) of the federal Food, Drug, and Cosmetic Act. http://www.fda.gov/downloads/Drugs/GuidanceComplianceRegulatoryInformation/Guidances/UCM172001.pdf. Accessed February 18, 2010.

6. Food and Drug Administration Amendments Act of 2007 Public Law 110–85 Section 905 (a.3.B). Food and Drug Administration Web site. http://frwebgate.access.gpo.gov/cgibin/getdoc.cgi?dbname=110_cong_public_laws&docid=f:publ085.110. Accessed February 18, 2010.

7. Food and Drug Administration Amendments Act of 2007 Public Law 110–85 Section 905 (1.3.B.ii). Food and Drug Administration Web site. http://frwebgate.access.gpo.gov/cgibin/getdoc.cgi?dbname=110_cong_public_laws&docid=f:publ085.110. Accessed February 18, 2010.

8. The FDA responded to the IOM report in 2007 and is implementing many of its recommendations. See *The Future of Drug Safety—Promoting and Protecting the Public Health, FDA's Response to the Institute of Medicine's 2006 Report,* January 2007. Food and Drug Administration Web site. http://www.fda.gov/oc/reports/iom013007.pdf.

9. The Sentinel Report, National Strategy for Monitoring Medical Product Safety. Food and Drug Administration Web site. http://www.fda.gov/downloads/Safety/FDAsSentinelInitiative/UCM124701.pdf. Accessed February 18, 2010.

Glossary

Absolute risk reduction   The absolute value of the arithmetic difference in the event rates of the treated and untreated groups.

Adherence   The extent that a patient follows the recommendations about day-to-day treatment by a provider with respect to timing, dosage, and frequency. The measure presumes that the provider received input from the patient. Typically measured as a proportion of the number of doses consumed, compared to the number of doses expected to be consumed. SYNONYM compliance.

Adjusted estimate   The measure of association estimated in the presence of the potential confounders; it can be thought of as the association between exposure and outcome while mathematically holding constant all of the observed confounding variables.

Adverse event   Any untoward medical occurrence in a patient or clinical investigation subject administered a pharmaceutical product and which does not necessarily have to have a causal relationship with the product.

Adverse drug reaction or adverse drug effect   An adverse outcome that is harmful or unpleasant that occurs while a patient is taking a drug product and has a causal relationship with the drug.

Age-adjusted mortality rate   The death rate that would occur if the observed age-specific death rates were present in a population with an age distribution equal to that of a standard population.

Age-specific mortality rate   The total number of deaths from all causes during a specified period of time in a specific age category divided by the total number of persons in that age category in the population during that period.

Alternative hypothesis   A statement of what one chooses to believe if the evidence provided in the sample data lead to a rejection of the null hypothesis.

Analysis of variance (ANOVA)   A procedure that can be used to compare the means from populations defined by three or more groups (can actually be used for two groups as well as the *t* test is actually a special case of ANOVA).

Association   When two events occur together repeatedly. This repeated occurrence takes place more often than a chance occurrence.

Atomistic fallacy   The fallacy associated with taking conclusions from a study looking at individual patients and applying them to entire groups; this fallacy occurs because relationships and characteristics at the individual patient level may not apply categorically to an overall group of patients; compare with the ecologic fallacy.

Automated health care database   A database that consists of data automatically captured as the result of the provision of care; contents of these databases may include administrative claims or transactional or operational data, such as drug dispensing data.

Bias   It occurs when the groups under study are treated in a consistently different manner. The existence of a bias causes a study to produce incorrect results.

Biostatistics   The application of statistical methods to the medical and health sciences, including epidemiology.

Black box warning   A type of warning about serious adverse events associated with the drug that appears on the package insert.

Case–control study   An observational study design that begins by identifying a group of individuals with the outcome of interest and a group without the outcome of interest, then compares the exposure status of individuals between those groups.

Case-crossover study   An observational study design where participants are observed at more than one point in time, to compare the exposure status within each individual across various periods where the outcome occurred in at least one period and did not occur in at least one. These are particularly useful for transient exposures and are analogous to the experimental crossover design.

Case fatality   The propensity of a disease to cause the death of affected persons. Case fatality is calculated as the total number of deaths from a disease during a specified period of time divided by the total number of persons diagnosed with the disease during that period.

Case report　A study design that describes the clinical experience of one patient with a particular drug; these frequently describe unexpected or previously undescribed events, both adverse and beneficial.

Case series　A study design that is similar to a case report, except it describes the experience of multiple patients.

Cause-specific mortality rate　Measures the total number of deaths from a specific cause. Cause-specific mortality rate is calculated using the total number of deaths for a specific cause during a specified period of time divided by the total number of persons in the population during that period.

Causation　When an event triggers another event. In order for this to happen, the first event must precede the second event.

Closed cohort　A type of cohort in which all participants begin the study at the same time and no additional participants are allowed to be included once the study begins; exposure is defined at the beginning of the study, and no one switches from the exposed to unexposed group, or vice versa; there is no loss to follow-up in a closed cohort.

Coefficient of determination　Provides information about the percentage of variation in one variable that is explained by, or is accounted for, by knowing the value of another variable. It is the square of the correlation coefficient.

Coefficient of variation　A distribution's standard deviation divided by its mean; it provides a measure of dispersion that is independent of the unit of measurement.

Cohort study　An observational study design that begins by identifying an outcome-free group (i.e., a cohort) and then determines the exposure status of the individuals within that group; the occurrence of outcomes in the exposed group is compared to that in the unexposed group.

Comorbidity index　A composite score based on assignment of weights to each of the comorbidities present. The weights are added to arrive at a comorbidity score, referred to as index.

Compliance　The extent of conformity to the recommendations about day-to-day treatment by a provider with respect to timing, dosage, and frequency. It is typically measured as a proportion of the number of doses consumed compared to the number of doses expected to be consumed. SYNONYM adherence.

Concordance　Involvement of patients in decision making to improve patient compliance with medical advice. Concordance is measured typically as a proportion of the number of doses consumed compared to the number of doses expected to be consumed.

Confounder　A confounder is a third variable that is independently correlated with both the treatment and outcome variables. This correlation may create a spurious association or mask a true association.

Confounding by indication　Occurs when the underlying condition, disease severity, or any other characteristics leads to prescribing or use of a certain drug and that condition, severity, or characteristic is also related to the patient outcome.

Confounding　A type of bias that is said to exist if meaningfully different interpretations of the relationship between the independent variable and the dependent variable result when the confounder is ignored or when it is included in the analysis.

Contingency table　A method to display data on nominal variables in which observations are cross-classified according to their membership in the categories of the variables.

Continuous variables　Variables that can take on any value within a defined range, sometimes referred to as a "quantitative" variable.

Correlation coefficient (r)　A measure of how two numerical variables are linearly associated in a sample.

Cox regression (proportional hazards model)　A regression technique used when the dependent variable of interest is a time-to-event variable.

Cronbach's alpha　A measure of internal consistency or reliability of a scale. Higher numbers (>0.70) indicate that the items of the scale are measuring the same thing.

Cross-sectional study　An observational study design that examines the relationship between an exposure and outcome at one point in time in a sample of participants (i.e., a cross section); also called prevalence studies.

Crude (or unadjusted) estimate　The measure of association estimated without the potential confounders (or control variables).

Crude mortality rate　The total number of deaths from all causes during a specified period of time divided by the total number of persons in the population during that period.

Cumulative incidence Measures the proportion of the population at risk that becomes cases over a specified period of time. SYNONYM risk or incidence proportion.

Daily dose The amount of drug that a patient receives over the period of 1 day.

Data dictionary A document that accompanies databases and describes the names of the variables included, the meaning of codes used in coded variables, the type of data in a given variable (e.g., character or numeric).

Data linkage The process of identifying unique individuals across separate data sources and matching data so that it can be brought together into one common data source.

Data use agreement (DUA) A business agreement entered into between a data provider and a data user that describes the conditions under which data are provided and acceptable uses of the data; these agreements are required under HIPAA for some data disclosures but are common in many situations where proprietary data are provided.

Days of therapy (DOT) The count of the number of days on which at least one dose of a drug being studied was given.

Defined daily dose (DDD) The assumed average maintenance dose per day for a drug used for its main indication in adults as determined by the World Health Organization; this is a standardized unit of measure and allows comparisons across countries or even drugs, but may not reflect actual prescribing practices.

De-identified datasets Datasets that have been stripped of elements specified by HIPAA that could reveal the identity of individuals contained within the dataset.

Dependent variable The response variable or the outcome of interest. It is what the investigator is attempting to describe in terms of other variables.

Descriptive statistics Methods and procedures for summarizing and describing data.

Detection bias An error that can occur when cases are given more importance than controls in collection of information, or when the exposed participants are followed more closely than the unexposed participants.

Dichotomous measure A variable that distinguishes participants by placing them into a two categories.

Differential misclassification When the information collected depends on whether the participant is exposed or unexposed or whether the participant is in the diseased or healthy group.

Directly observed therapy (DOT) Involves observing a patient consuming his or her medication to ensure that medications are taken at the correct time and for correct duration.

Discrete variables Variables comprised of distinct categories. The terms "qualitative" or "categorical" are sometimes applied to discrete variables.

Drug classification scheme A coding system that facilitates the grouping of drugs into meaningful pharmacologic and/or therapeutic classes (e.g., Anatomic Therapeutic Classification system).

Drug identification scheme A coding system that allows the user to identify a unique drug or drug product (e.g., National Drug Codes).

Ecologic fallacy The fallacy associated with taking conclusions from a study looking at groups and applying them to individual patients; this fallacy occurs because relationships and characteristics of the group may not apply to each member of that group; compare with atomistic fallacy.

Ecologic study An observational study design where relationships between exposures and outcomes are examined using higher-level units or groups, such as hospitals or states or medical practices.

Effectiveness The ability of an intervention (e.g., a drug) to produce the desired effect as implemented in actual clinical practice (i.e., in a "real-world" setting).

Efficacy The ability of an intervention (e.g., a drug) to produce the desired effect in a highly controlled experimental environment (i.e., in "ideal" conditions).

Electronic medical record An electronic version of the medical record used to document activities associated with providing health care to patients; these may be implemented within institutional settings like hospitals or at the individual physician practice level.

Epidemiology The study of the factors that determine the occurrence and distribution of diseases in populations.

Exclusion criteria   A set of factors that are used to determine whether a person will be excluded from participation in a study. These factors are determined before a study is conducted and may be helpful in removing confounding and producing unbiased and reliable results. Some of the examples of these criteria include age, gender, previous treatment history, comorbid conditions, and enrollment time period. These criteria may vary from one study to another.

Experimental study   A general type of research design where the researcher is actively involved in manipulating an experimental variable (e.g., drug vs placebo) and participants are assigned at random to either a comparison group or one or more treatment groups.

External validity   The degree to which the results of a study can be generalized or extended to the general population or another setting.

Factor   In the context of analysis of variance, it refers to a nominal variable that comprises group membership.

Fixed cohort   A type of cohort in which all participants begin the study at the same time, and no additional participants are allowed to be included once the study begins; exposure is defined at the beginning of the study, and no one switches from the exposed to unexposed group, or vice versa; loss to follow-up is possible in a fixed cohort.

Group-level data   Data collected that have been aggregated at some higher level unit, such as a hospital or a state or a medical practice; also known as aggregate data; compare with patient-level data.

Incidence   The number of new cases of a disease that occurs in a population at risk for developing the disease during a specified time period.

Incidence rate   The number of new cases of a disease divided by person-time of observation in the population at risk. SYNONYM: incidence density.

Inclusion criteria   A set of factors that are used to determine whether a participant will be included to participate in a study. These factors are determined before a study is conducted and may be helpful in removing confounding and producing unbiased and reliable results. Some of the examples of these criteria include age, gender, previous treatment history, comorbid conditions, and enrollment time period. These criteria may vary from one study to another.

Independent variable   Predictor variable or a variable used to describe or explain a dependent variable. Can be manipulated by the investigator (i.e., a treatment in an experimental design) or observed.

Index date   Represents the beginning of the time-window of observation for a cohort study. In case–control studies, this represents the date the outcome occurred; the period of time before this date is when exposure is determined. In studies of compliance/persistence this represents the date of first prescription for the medication of interest.

Induction period   The period of time between the exposure and occurrence of an outcome.

Inferential statistics   Statistical methods that are used to make statements about populations based on the information gathered from samples drawn from that population. Includes the functions of estimation and hypothesis testing.

Information bias   An error in the results of a study due to errors in measurement of information on the study participants.

Instrumental variable   A variable that is correlated with the treatment variable but not with the outcome. This variable is used in the instrumental variable analysis to correct for selection bias.

Internal validity   The degree to which any statements of effects under study are actually the result of the exposure or variable of interest, and not some other interfering variable.

Interquartiles range   The distance between the first and the third quartiles of a set of scores and thus describe the middle 50% of the data.

Interrupted time series design   A type of quasi-experimental design where repeated measurements over time are taken before and after a distinct change occurred; this is frequently used to examine effects associated with the initiation of some program or changes in policy.

Interval estimation   The process of associating with the point estimate a measure of statistical variation or random error.

Level   The different categories of a factor.

Linear regression   A regression technique used when the dependent variable of interest is continuous (i.e., numerical).

Logistic regression   A regression technique used when the dependent variable of interest is a binary (two-group, dichotomous) categorical variable rather than a numerical (or continuous) measure; can be generalized to the cases of a response variable with three or more categories or when the response variable is ordered categories.

Matching The process of taking one participant in a study and pairing them with another participant based on some common characteristic, such as age or disease; this is frequently used to eliminate the effects of potential confounders; participants may be matched in pairs or in larger groups (e.g., one case to two controls).

Mean Generally refers to the arithmetic mean or simply the average. Other means include the geometric mean and the harmonic mean.

Median The middle number or the value of a set of scores such that half of the data points are above it and half are below it.

Mediation An intervening variable effect, which suggests that one variable causes the mediator that in turn causes another variable.

Medication error Any preventable event that may lead to inappropriate use or patient harm.

MedWatch Safety Information and Adverse Event Reporting Program The FDA's adverse event reporting program that consists of a computer database that contains reports of adverse events that are used to identify potential problems with specific drug products. The MedWatch program accepts adverse event reports from health care professionals and patients as well as disseminates drug information to health care professionals and the public about safety issues with specific drug products.

Meta-analysis A systematic method of using statistical techniques to combine the results of various studies to arrive at an overall estimate of effect that has increased power and/or precision.

Misclassification bias The error resulting from misclassifying exposed as unexposed (and vice versa) or a misclassifying a diseased person as nondiseased (and vice versa).

Mode The most frequently occurring value in a set of scores.

Moderation A condition in which the strength or direction of the relationship between an independent variable and a dependent variable is different at different levels of a third variable, called a moderator.

Moderation involves the presence of a statistical interaction, often called effect modification.

Mortality Refers to the occurrence of death in a specified population during a specified period of time.

Multiple regression models In regression modeling, the inclusion of more than one predictor (the addition of predictors to a simple regression model).

Multivariable analysis Methods for exploring the relationship between a number of factors, or independent variables, and a single outcome or dependent variable.

Multivariate statistics Methods in which several dependent variables are considered simultaneously.

Nested case-control study A case–control study that is conducted within a fully defined cohort of individuals.

Nil hypothesis The null hypothesis of no difference (or no association).

Nondifferential misclassification When misclassification occurs independently of the exposure and outcome relationship. The degree of misclassification is similar for all patients regardless of exposure or outcome. Nondifferential misclassification may result in bias toward the null.

Nonparametric statistical methods Techniques that test hypotheses that are not statements about population parameters (i.e., truly nonparametric procedures) or those that make little or no assumptions about the sampled population (i.e., distribution-free procedures).

Null hypothesis The hypothesis to be tested in a hypothesis testing procedure; based on sample data, one will either reject or fail to reject the null hypothesis.

Number needed to harm A measure of the number of persons who would have to be treated for one person to experience an adverse event.

Number needed to treat The number of individuals who would have to receive the treatment for one of them to benefit from the treatment over a specified period of time.

Odds ratio The ratio of events over nonevents in the intervention (case) group over the ratio of events over nonevents in the control group.

Open cohort A type of cohort in which participants are free to enter (and leave) at various times after the study begins; also called a dynamic cohort.

Operationalization Defining a measure in a manner that makes it measurable or identifiable.

Parameters Measures computed from the data of a population (or assumed to represent a population).

Paternalistic A relationship where the authority (physician) provides for the needs of another person (patient) without giving them rights or responsibilities.

Patient-level data Data collected for each individual patient within a group; compare with group-level data.

Pearson chi-square test of independence (association) A procedure that can be used to assess whether two categorical variables are associated.

Percentage A proportion multiplied by 100.

Period prevalence The number of persons who have the disease at any point during a period of time, divided by the number of persons in the population during that period of time.

Persistence The length of time of taking a medication.

Pharmacoepidemiology The study of the use and effects of drugs in large numbers of people.

Pharmacology The study of the effects of medications in humans.

Pharmacovigilance The science relating to the detection, assessment, understanding, and prevention of adverse effects of medicines.

Point estimation The process of finding a single value, the point estimate, which is the best guess of a population parameter.

Point prevalence The number of people who have the disease of interest at a single point in time, divided by the number of people in the population at that specific time.

Post-marketing surveillance Any means of gathering information about a product after it has been approved for public use.

Power The probability of correctly rejecting the null hypothesis when it is false (it equals $1-\beta$).

Power analysis A sample size estimation technique where a researcher uses a predetermined α and attempts to achieve a desired level of β (or conversely power) by choosing an appropriate sample size to detect a clinically or scientifically meaningful effect.

Precision analysis A technique used to determine a sample size necessary to achieve confidence intervals of a sufficiently narrow width.

Predictive validity The extent to which a measure can predict subsequent behavior.

Prescribed daily dose (PDD) The average daily dose of a drug that is actually prescribed by providers in a given area or setting (e.g., a country or hospital); location-specific dispensing or prescribing data are required to calculate this measure.

Prevalence The number of existing cases (old and new) in the population (sick, healthy, at risk, and not at risk).

Primary data Data that were collected specifically for a given research project and were not previously available.

Primary diagnosis (principal diagnosis) According to the Uniform Hospital Discharge Data Set, the condition or disease determined to be responsible for requiring the admission of the patient to the hospital; the Veterans Administration defines this as the condition or disease that was primarily responsible for the length of hospitalization.

Propensity Score An approach to controlling for confounding that uses regression modeling to predict the probability of being in a particular treatment group. These probabilities are used to correct for selection bias.

Proportion A division of two numbers; the numerator and the denominator are related. The numerator is always a subset of the denominator.

Proportionate mortality The proportion of deaths that are attributable to a specific disease. It is calculated as the total number of deaths from a specific disease during a specified period divided by the total number of deaths during that period.

Protected health information (PHI) Individually identifiable information, such as demographics and other information related to the physical or mental condition of an individual or the provision of or payment for health care, which is created or received by health care providers, health plans, employers, and other covered entities.

P value (also called the observed significance level) The probability of obtaining, when the null is true, a value of a test statistic as extreme or more extreme (in the direction supporting the alternative) than the one actually computed; it quantifies how unusual the observed results would be if H_0 were true.

Quasi-experimental study A general type of research design where the researcher is actively manipulating an experimental variable, but participants are not assigned at random to study groups by the researcher; study groups are formed by self-selection of the participants or by some other process out of the control of the researchers (e.g., patients within a medical practice).

Random assignment The process of assigning individuals to one or more groups based on an accepted method that gives each participant the same probability of being in any given treatment group (e.g., active drug vs. placebo); some methods include tables of random numbers, flipping a fair coin, or using computer programs; the result is groups of participants that are statistically equivalent with respect to participant characteristics because any differences are the result of random variation.

Random error Processes that lead to estimates that depart from the true values due to chance alone. Error that is due to pure chance.

Range The difference between the smallest and largest observed values on a single variable.

Rate A type of ratio that includes a time component or some other physical unit; rates provide information about the frequency of occurrence of a phenomenon.

Ratio The value obtained by dividing one quantity by another. The numerator and the denominator are not necessarily related.

Recall bias When one study group is systematically different from the other group in the accuracy or completeness of the group participants' memory of past exposures or health events.

Recency effect Bias that results from the likelihood that patients will recall their most recent medication-taking behaviors rather than their behaviors at the beginning or middle of the period under interest.

Referral bias Error in the results of a study that occurs when the reasons for referring a patient for medical care are related to the exposure status.

Relative risk reduction The difference in the two event rates expressed as a proportion of the event rate in the unexposed group.

Reliability The consistency of a measure. Measures that are reliable are thought to be free from random error.

Risk A probability that an event will happen.

Risk adjustment Refers to evaluating the outcomes by statistically controlling for group differences when comparing dissimilar treatment groups. Risk adjustment is used to calculate an expected outcome measure based on risk factors considered and their relationship with outcomes.

Risk ratio The ratio of the risk of event (developing the disease or death) in exposed individuals to that in unexposed individuals.

Safety signal A concern about an excess of adverse events compared to what would be expected to be associated with a product's use.

Secondary data Data that were previously collected for purposes other than those of a particular pharmacoepidemiology research study such as health care billing or a clinical trial.

Secondary diagnosis Any disease or condition other than the primary diagnosis that was existing at the time of hospitalization or developed during the course of the hospitalization and affect the treatment received and/or the length of the hospitalization.

Selection bias Error in a study that is due to systematic differences in characteristics between those who are selected for the study and those who are not.

Self-selection The process by which participants determine their own study group; this can introduce bias because the groups formed are not random and there can be systematic differences between individuals in each group.

Sensitivity analysis Conducted by systematically repeating the analysis by varying assumptions each time to assess how sensitive the results obtained are to the variations in model assumptions and whether the results are consistent across the variations in assumptions.

Sentinel Initiative The creation of a national electronic system that will allow the FDA to track the safety of drugs, biologics, and medical devices.

Serious adverse drug reactions Any untoward medical occurrence that at any dose results in death, is life threatening, requires or prolongs hospital admission, results in significant disability/incapacity, requires medical or surgical intervention to preclude permanent impairment of a body function or permanent damage to a body structure, is a cancer or a congenital anomaly, or would be considered a serious medical event if it did not respond to acute treatment.

Seriousness The extent to which an adverse drug reaction can or does cause harm.

Severity A measure of the extent to which an adverse drug event develops in an individual.

Side effect A dose-dependent effect of a drug that is predictable and may be desirable, undesirable, or inconsequential.

Social desirability bias Bias in the data collected from interviews or a survey that is the result of respondents answering questions in the direction of socially desirable attitudes or traits. Answering questions as someone "should" rather than based on true beliefs or attitudes.

Spearman rank correlation (Spearman's rho) A measure used to describe the relationship between two ordinal (or one ordinal and one numeric) variables. It can also be used with numeric variables that are skewed with extreme observations (it is less sensitive to outliers when compared to Pearson's r).

Standard deviation The positive square root of the variance; it is an index of variability in the original measurement units.

Statistics The study of how information should be employed to reflect on, and give guidance for action in, a practical situation involving uncertainty; can also be used to describe measures computed from the data of a sample.

Stratification A technique in which analysis is performed for each stratum defined by the levels of the confounder. It is used to control for variation driven by the confounder.

Suboptimal medical consumption The number of doses not taken or taken incorrectly that places the expected therapeutic outcome in doubt.

Suspected adverse drug reaction A noxious and unintended response to any dose of a drug or biologic product for which there is a reasonable possibility that the product caused the response.

Systematic error When the study groups under investigation are selected in a manner that consistently treats one study group differently from the other groups. It leads to bias in results.

Systematic review A method to produce a review of the literature in a particular area; this method is characterized by transparent and rigorous methods in the identification and analysis of various study reports.

t **Test** A procedure used to test the null hypothesis that two different populations have the same mean.

Tests for equivalence A type of hypothesis testing procedure that can be used to provide evidence that treatments are not different by more than some prespecified amount (usually some clinically insignificant amount); in other words, suggesting that the effects of the interventions are very similar.

Tests for noninferiority A type of hypothesis-testing procedure that can be used to provide evidence that one treatment is not worse, or is as effective, than other treatment (and may even be better).

Type I error Rejecting a null hypothesis when it is true; the probability of a type I error is referred to as alpha (α).

Type II error Failing to reject a false null hypothesis; the probability of a type II error is referred to as beta (β).

Unit of analysis The things on which data are collected in a study; this could be a patient or some larger group, such as a hospital, state, pharmacy, or health plan; also referred to as level of analysis.

Univariate statistics Refers to the analysis of a single dependent variable, even though there may be multiple independent variables.

Validity The ability of measure to measure what it is intended to measure. The extent that a measure is free from systematic error.

Variance From a sample of observations, it is defined as the sum of the squared deviations of the values from the mean score divided by the sample size (n) minus 1.

Washout period A set period of time that the participant should be without treatment with the drug under investigation prior to the index date.

Index

Note: Page locators followed by f and t indicates figure and table respectively.